NATO Advanced Study Institute on "Motor Skill Acquisition in Children" (1985 : Maastricht, Netherlands)

Themes i

DATE			

Themes in Motor Development

NATO ASI Series

Advanced Science Institutes Series

A Series presenting the results of activities sponsored by the NATO Science Committee, which aims at the dissemination of advanced scientific and technological knowledge, with a view to strengthening links between scientific communities.

The Series is published by an international board of publishers in conjunction with the NATO Scientific Affairs Division

A	**Life Sciences**	Plenum Publishing Corporation
B	**Physics**	London and New York
C	**Mathematical and Physical Sciences**	D. Reidel Publishing Company Dordrecht and Boston
D	**Behavioural and Social Sciences**	Martinus Nijhoff Publishers Dordrecht/Boston/Lancaster
E	**Applied Sciences**	
F	**Computer and Systems Sciences**	Springer-Verlag Berlin/Heidelberg/New York
G	**Ecological Sciences**	

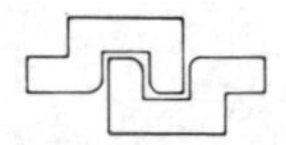

Series D: Behavioural and Social Sciences – No. 35

Themes in Motor Development

edited by

H.T.A. Whiting

Department of Psychology
Interfaculty of Human Movement Sciences
The Free University
Amsterdam
The Netherlands

M.G. Wade

Department of Physical Education
Southern Illinois University
Carbondale, Illinois
U.S.A.

1986 **Martinus Nijhoff Publishers**
Dordrecht / Boston / Lancaster
Published in cooperation with NATO Scientific Affairs Division

Proceedings of the NATO Advanced Study Institute on ''Motor Skill Acquisition in Children'', Maastricht, The Netherlands, July, 1985

Library of Congress Cataloging in Publication Data

NATO Advanced Study Institute on "Motor Skill
Acquisition in Children" (1985 : Maastricht,
Netherlands)
Themes in motor development.

(NATO ASI series. Series D, Behavioural and social
sciences ; no. 35)
"Proceedings of the NATO Advanced Study Institute
on "Motor Skill Acquisition in Children," Maastricht,
the Netherlands, July, 1985"--T.p. verso.
Companion Volume to: Motor development in children.
Includes bibliographies and indexes.
1. Motor ability in children--Congresses. 2. Learning
disabled children--Physiology--Congresses. 3. Movement
disorders in children--Congresses. 4. Cognition in
children--Congresses. I. Whiting, H. T. A. (Harold
Thomas Anthony), 1929- . II. Wade, Michael G.
III. North Atlantic Treaty Organization. Scientific
Affaris Division. IV. NATO Advanced Study Institute on
"Motor Skill Acquisition in Children" (1985 : Maastricht,
Netherlands) Motor development in children. V. Title.
VI. Series. [DNLM: 1. Child Development--congresses.
2. Child Development Disorders--congresses. 3. Motor
Skills--in infancy & childhood--congresses. 4. Movement
Disorders--in infancy & childhood--congresses.
WE 103 N2786 1985t]
BF723.M6N37 1985a 155.4'12 86-16423
ISBN 90-247-3390-1

ISBN 90-247-3390-1 (this volume)
ISBN 90-247-2688-3 (series)

Distributors for the United States and Canada: Kluwer Academic Publishers, 101 Philip Drive, Assinippi Park, Norwell, MA 02061, U.S.A.

Distributors for the UK and Ireland: Kluwer Academic Publishers, MTP Press Ltd, Falcon House, Queen Square, Lancaster LA1 1RN, UK

Distributors for all other countries: Kluwer Academic Publishers Group, Distribution Center, P.O. Box 322, 3300 AH Dordrecht, The Netherlands

Printed in The Netherlands

CONTENTS

Foreword

This book is divided into Sections. Each Section is devoted to a particular theme in Motor Development and comprises two or more contributions. The order of presentation is largely fortuitous and does not reflect any value judgement on the part of the editors as to the importance of any one theme in comparison to others addressed in the book.

This volume is to be seen as a companion volume to *'Motor Development in Children: Aspects of coordination and control'* in which the more general issues in motor development presented during the Institute are published. Together, the two volumes provide both a general and a theme specific approach to this expanding field of knowledge.

PREFACE

Books and conferences, on what in North America is euphemistically termed motor development, have been few and far between in the past 25 years. This is not to say that the study of how children acquire and develop motor skills has not been a subject on which scientists have focused their attention. In the United States in the 1930's and 1940's, Bayley (1935) and Gesell and Amatruda (1947) described and scaled the rates at which young children acquired motor skills. In Europe, the development of childrens' motor behaviour was of theoretical interest to Piaget (1952). Nevertheless, we feel that it is true to say that the study of motor skill acquisition in children has been overshadowed, certainly in the past 25 years, by the attempts of human movement scientists to establish the basic theory of action as it relates to the broad aspects of motor learning, control and coordination. As Wade (1976) noted, there has been no real theorising in motor development. This deficiency could be attributed to the fact that the field of motor learning was, at that time, trying to establish its own theoretical position - only since the late 1960's and early 1970's have theoretical models to predict and describe how motor skills are acquired become apparent (e.g. Adams, 1971; Schmidt, 1975).

Although considerable developmental research on motor skill acquisition exists (see for example reviews by Wade, 1976), publications specifically focusing on the topic have been meagre. A landmark conference organised by Connolly - funded by the CIBA organisation - produced a publication in 1970 called 'Mechanisms of Motor Skill Development' and a conference held at the University of Iowa in 1980 - sponsored by the Big Ten Committee on Institutional Cooperation - produced a publication in 1982 edited by Kelso and Clark (1982) entitled "The Development of Movement Control and Coordination". Both of these books cast the study of motor skills in a more theoretical light by asking questions as to *how* children acquire motor skills rather than describing what it is they acquire.

With respect to the study and focus of motor skills research within the framework of NATO Advanced Study Institute programmes, only the Institute on Motor Behaviour held in France in 1979 and co-directed by Stelmach (USA) and Requin (France) is of central concern. Nevertheless, given the considerable interest, both in Europe and North America, in theorising and active experimentation over the past 15 years, it seemed to the Co-directors of the ASI that it was high time that another conference, focusing on developmental issues, was held. Subsequently, a successful application was made to the NATO Scientific Committee. This led directly to the conference in Maastricht held in July 1985.

It was decided to develop the ASI along the lines of central issues in motor development with invitations being sent to senior scientists to provide keynote lectures each day on a specific topic and to have other participants react or present research material addressing related themes. The response to invitations was overwhelming to the point that it became necessary to publish two companion volumes in order to accommodate the wealth of original material presented. A decision as to which material to publish in which volume was not difficult since there was a natural division into those papers which presented material of a more general nature - the keynote addresses and reactions - and those which addressed more specific themes in motor development. The present text comprises the latter material. It is wished to emphasise that the two volumes are companion volumes and no value judgement is made as to the likely contribution of the one as against the other to an understanding of motor development. Undoubtedly, different readers will have different needs and this will determine the amount of attention paid to either volume.

Editors are always faced with the difficult task of classifying contributions under a particular heading. The task was no less easy for the present volume. However, a choice had to be made and while it was not arbitrary arguments could be provided for a completely different classification system. Nevertheless, the themes isolated: Postural control, Skill development and learning disabilities, The development of fine motor skills, Perceptual and cognitive control of motor behaviour, Posture and locomotion, Cultural influences, Speech and language, will be familiar to most workers in this area.

To a large extent, the number of papers included under any one theme reflects the amount of interest being shown in the literature. Thus, a rather large section on 'Skill development and learning disabilities' is to be expected. Even then, only a limited number of topics could be addressed in the time available. At the other extreme, the limited number of contributions to the theme 'Cultural influences' reflects this emerging field. It is interesting to note how salient issues in motor development - such as the development of coordinative structures - are addressed in a cultural context.

It would have been possible to have made considerable cross-referencing in terms of the sub-themes discussed in the different contributions. Thus, in many of the themes the 'motor systems/action systems controversy, which dominated to a large extent the companion volume, is also to be detected here under the various guises of movement and cognition and the development of coordination. The decision not to do so was made on the grounds that this might pre-set the reader in ways which were undesirable given the variety of other ideas which are also presented. Instead recourse is made to an elaborate subject index which will enable the reader to easily trace such sub-themes if wished.

The director and co-director wish to thank all of the participants, for their thoughtful presentations and comments and for the endurance that they showed over the ten-day working conference. Many of the participants had not met each other prior to convening in Maastricht, and it was gratifying to both the director and co-director that in a very short while, individuals from all over the participating NATO countries quickly became friends and participated in intense discussion and exchange of ideas which is the very essence of the NATO Advanced Study Institute programme.

The environment in which the Institute prospered was in large part due to the hard work of the staff of the Hotel Maastricht and of the conference secretariat provided by Mrs. Irma Reijnhout of the Free University of Amsterdam. In addition, to thanking Mrs. Reijnhout for her hard work the directors would also like to recognise the work of Ms. Pat Terneus of Southern Illinois University for the organising effort that she put in regarding the North American participants. In addition to the funding received from the NATO Scientific Committee, the directors would also like to recognise the funding provided by the *National Science Foundation* (Grant nr. 8505988) that provided travel support for the United States participants.

Mrs. Irma Reijnhout took on the thankless task of typing all the manuscripts and preparing the book for publication. The fact that it is in press so quickly is largely due to her efforts. We express our sincere appreciation as well as that of the publishers.

The present volume provides an up-to-date perspective on the current status of motor skills research as it relates to children and in that sense builds on the earlier volumes published by Connolly (1970) and Kelso and Clark (1982). It remains to be seen what the level and impact of the theorising presented in this volume will have on the theorising and research activities of those interested in motor skill acquisition in children in the ensuing decade. The effects of this will perhaps be assessed by another Advanced Study Institute towards the end of the present century!

H.T.A. Whiting
Amsterdam, Netherlands

M.G. Wade
Carbondale, IL

References

Adams, J.A. (1971). A closed-loop theory of motor learning. *Journal of Motor Behavior, 3,* 111-150.
Bayley, N. (1935). The development of motor abilities during the first three years. *Monographs of the Society for Research in Child Development, 1,* 1-26.
Connolly, K.J. (1970). *Mechanisms of motor skill development.* New York: Academic Press.
Piaget, J. (1952). *The origins of intelligence in children.* New York: International University Press.
Wade, M.G. (1976). Developmental motor learning. In J. Keogh and R.S. Hulton (Eds.), *Exercises and sport sciences reviews, 4,* 375-394.
Gesell, A. & Amatruda, C.S. (1947). *Developmental diagnosis.* (2nd. Ed.) New York: Harper and Row.
Kelso, J.A.S. & Clark, J.E. (1982). *The development of movement control and coordination.* New York: Wiley and Sons.
Schmidt, R.A. (1975). A schema theory of discrete motor skill learning. *Psychological Review, 82,* 225-260.

INVITED DELEGATES
(who contributed to this Volume)

Bairstow, P.J.	Wolfson Centre Mecklenburgh Square London WC 1N 2AP England
Berkson, G.	Department of Psychology University of Illinois-Chicago Box 4348 Chicago, Ill. 60680 U.S.A.
Bril, B.	Laboratoire de Psychologie Centre d'étude des processes cognitifs et du language 54, Boulevard Raspail F-75270 Paris Cedex 06 France
Das, J.P.	Department of Educational Psychology University of Alberta-Edmonton Alberta Canada T6G 2E1
Davis, W.E.	Department of Physical Education Kent State University Kent OH 44242 U.S.A.
Ferrandez, A.M.	Centre National de la Recherche Scientifique Laboratoire de Psychologie de l'apprentissage J.E. 16 IBHOP, Rue des Géraniums 13014 Marseille France
Henderson, S.E.	University of London Institute of Education 20 Bedford Way London WC1H 0AL England
Hulstijn, W.	Psychologisch Laboratorium Katholieke Universiteit Postbus 9104 6500 HE Nijmegen The Netherlands

Jeannerod, M.	Laboratoire de Neuropsychologie Experimentale 16, Avenue du Doyen Lépine 69500 Bron France
Konstantareas, M.M.	Clarke Institute of Psychiatry 250 College Street Toronto Ontario M5T 1R8 Canada
Molfese, D.L.	Department of Psychology Southern Illinois University Carbondale, Ill. 62901 U.S.A.
Molfese, V.J.	Department of Psychology Southern Illinois University Carbondale, Ill. 62901 U.S.A.
Reid, R.	Department of Physical Education University of Illinois 906 Goodwin Avenue Urbana, Ill. 61801 U.S.A.
Roberton, M.A.	Department of Physical Education University of Wisconsin Madison, WI 53706 U.S.A.
Sugden, D.A.	Department of Education University of Leeds Leeds England
Todor, J.I.	Department of Physical Education University of Michigan Ann Arbor, MI 48109 U.S.A.
Wann, J.P.	MRC Applied Psychology Unit 15 Chaucer Road Cambridge CB2 2EF England

Williams, H.

Department of Physical Education
University of South Carolina
Columbia, SC 29208
U.S.A.

Woollacott, M.H.

Department of Physical Education
University of Oregon
Eugene, OR 97403
U.S.A.

SECTION 1

POSTURAL CONTROL

POSTURAL CONTROL AND DEVELOPMENT

M.H. Woollacott

1. INTRODUCTION

Historically, the development of motor coordination in children has been viewed from the perspective of the acquisition and refinement of voluntary motor skills. Though the development of postural skills is mentioned briefly in many motor development texts, its description is largely confined to the first year of life in which the child learns to control the head, sit independently, and finally stand (Keogh & Sugden, 1985; Thomas, 1984). The role of postural control as a foundation for the accurate execution of voluntary tasks is ignored.

However, recent research on voluntary motor coordination in adults (Belinkii et al, 1967; Cordo & Nashner, 1982) has shown that postural muscles are automatically activated prior to the prime mover muscle in voluntary tasks, since they are required as a stabilising foundation upon which the voluntary movement takes place. Studies on the control of voluntary movement in animals have also shown that the nervous system pre-programs postural adjustments when a voluntary movement is made, and that the areas of the brain which control voluntary movement execution also activate postural adjustments (Gahery & Massion, 1981). It is thus possible that the postural and voluntary control systems develop as a unit and that the development of the postural control system is much more important to the development of voluntary movement control than was previously realised.

In the following pages we will explore recent research on both the development of the postural control system, and on the coordination of the postural and voluntary control systems in children. We will review evidence that the postural control system, like the voluntary movement control system shows a developmental progression from head to foot, with postural muscle responses first appearing in the neck, followed by the trunk, and legs. In addition, we will examine the changing roles of the visual, somatosensory and vestibular systems in postural control and the development of intersensory integration abilities.

Do newborn infants show any sign of postural control? And if so, what sensory inputs trigger postural responses? Previous studies by Yonas (1981) and others (Bower, 1972, 1974), though not directly exploring the development of postural control mechanisms in the infant, may give us evidence for the presence of visually elicited postural responses in the neonate. These authors describe stereotyped responses to "looming" objects (objects on a collision course with the infant). The behavioural response includes a backward movement of the head and raising of the arms, and has been observed in newborns (six to nine days of age) and in infants of two weeks of age (Bower, 1974; Bower, Broughton & Moore, 1970). Yonas (1981) has shown that infants have a strong tendency to track upward moving contours and concludes that the visual tracking of the upward moving contour of the "looming" object causes *backward head movement*, a *loss of balance* and a compensatory raising of the arms.

These head movements are interesting because they are similar to body sway movements seen in sitting and standing infants when they are presented with similar visual flow patterns created to simulate body sway (Lee & Aronson, 1974; Butterworth & Hicks, 1977). In experiments designed to test the effect of visual stimuli on postural control in children, both Lee and Aronson (1974) and Butterworth and Hicks (1977) placed infants on a stable floor inside a room whose walls and ceiling moved forward or backward as a unit. Lee and Aronson performed experiments on standing children 13-16 months of age. When the walls moved, the infants experienced optic flow patterns simulating body sway, compensated for this nonexistent sway, and as a result, fell, staggered or swayed in the direction of optical movement. In the experiments of Butterworth and Hicks, younger infants, who were capable of sitting, but not standing showed similar responses to these optic flow patterns, swaying forward or backward at the trunk. Because infants developed these sway responses before learning to stand, Butterworth and Hicks concluded that experience standing is not required for the development of postural responses to visual stimulation (Butterworth & Hicks, 1977; Butterworth, 1982).

The results of the above experiments have led Lee and Aronson to state that it is primarily visual cues which are used in posture control by infants who are first learning to stand. These cues are believed to be more potent than mechanical proprioceptive information, since visual cues dominated over mechanical cues under the above conflicting conditions. However, these conclusions have been based on experiments in which children were given only *dynamic* visual stimuli. Children were not tested under conditions in which only proprioceptive cues were presented, or under conditions in which proprioceptive cues indicated body sway while visual cues did not. These additional experiments need to be performed in order to determine conclusively the relative dominance of visual versus mechanical proprioceptive cues in the control of posture in the young child.

Recent experiments on the development of postural control in infants, both in our own laboratory and in the laboratory of Lew Nashner, have explored these specific questions. In order to examine the relative weighting given to visual, proprioceptive and vestibular cues during different periods in the development of balance control in children, we performed experiments in which the balance of a child was momentarily disturbed while sitting or standing on a platform capable of movements in the anterior or posterior direction (Forssberg & Nashner, 1972; Shumway-Cook & Woollacott, 1985; Woollacott et al, 1985). This could be considered to simulate momentary loss of balance on a slippery surface. During certain trials visual cues were removed (children wore opaque goggles) and in some cases the platform was made to rotate in exact proportion to body sway in the anterior or posterior direction. This allowed us to essentially eliminate sway-related ankle joint proprioception by keeping the ankle joint at a constant 90° angle. When eyes were closed and the platform was rotated in exact proportion to body sway, eliminating ankle proprioceptive cues, vestibular cues became the most relevant sensory stimuli. Children of a variety of age groups were tested in two separate studies in our laboratory. The first study (Shumway-Cook & Woollacott, 1985) included three age groups (15-31 months, four-six years and seven-ten years), while the second study (Woollacott et al, 1985;

Woollacott et al, in press) included five age groups (four-five months, eight-14 months, two-three years, four-six years, and seven-ten years). In both studies the responses of the children were compared to those of adults. The youngest children were tested in an infant seat, or when possible, sitting independently, whereas older children, capable of standing independently, were tested during quiet stance.

In order to more carefully analyse the nervous system changes correlated with the children's changing postural control abilities we made surface electromyographic (EMG) recordings from the muscles of the leg, trunk and neck during the platform movements. We compared onset latencies and temporal organisation of the muscle responses under the different sensory conditions, in order to determine if muscle responses elicited by visual vs. proprioceptive cues had different temporal characteristics for each of the age groups tested. Body sway was measured by a belt at the hips which was attached to a potentiometer at the base of the platform via a rod.

2. POSTURAL RESPONSES IN ADULTS

In order to have a baseline for comparing the developmental changes in the postural responses of the different age groups of children, we will first briefly review the muscle response organisation used by adults when compensating for platform-induced sway under different sensory conditions. Research on the responses of young adults to platform-induced sway under normal sensory conditions (visual and ankle proprioceptive cues present) (Nashner, 1977; Nashner & Woollacott, 1979; Woollacott & Keshner, 1984) has shown that adults compensate for sway by using a relatively stereotyped activation pattern of postural muscles, with responses beginning first in the muscles closest to the base of support (at about 70-100 ms after platform movement onset) and ascending upward to the trunk musculature. Thus, if the platform is moved backwards, causing forward (anterior) sway, muscle responses are activated first in the gastrocnemius (G) muscle, followed sequentially by the hamstrings (H) and trunk extensor (TE) muscles (Figure 1). If the platform is moved forward, simulating slipping forward and swaying backwards, muscles on the opposite side of the leg are activated in the same manner. These responses are believed to be elicited primarily by ankle joint proprioceptive inputs, since altering visual inputs and hip proprioceptive inputs does not affect their onset latencies (Nashner, 1976). In a recent theoretical paper, Nashner and McCollum (in press) have shown that this distal to proximal temporal organisation of contraction is the most efficient one which can be used for returning the body's centre of gravity to its initial position.

More recent research (Woollacott & Keshner, 1984) has shown that, in addition to these responses radiating upward from the ankle joint, very early responses are activated in the neck muscles and the trunk muscles on the *opposite* surface of the body from the leg muscles (when ankle extensors are activated, neck flexors are activated) (Figure 1). These responses are very interesting because they appear to be activated by different sensory stimuli from the leg responses. In adults, the neck and trunk muscle responses showed no significant changes in onset latency with eyes closed versus open, and has thus been concluded that visual inputs are not primarily responsible for the activation of these responses. However, the neck muscle responses occur significantly less often under conditions in which ankle joint inputs are strong, but head movements are minimal (during dorsi- or plantarflexing

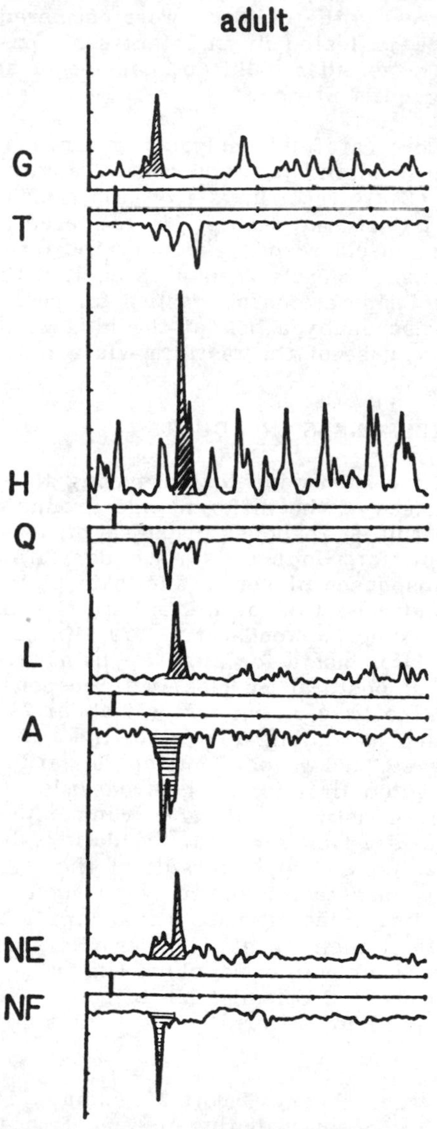

Fig. 1. Surface EMG recordings (rectified and filtered) of muscle responses of a single standing adult to a posterior platform translation causing forward sway. The two muscles recorded from each body segment are grouped together with the flexor muscle inverted. The line indicates the onset of platform movement. Time marks are at 100 ms intervals. G = gastrocnemius; T = tibialis anterior; H = hamstrings; Q = quadriceps; L = lumbar paraspinals; A = abdominals; NE = neck extensors; NF = neck flexors.

rotations of the ankle joint). Since conditions of minimal head movement reduce vestibular and neck proprioceptive inputs, we conclude that these neck responses may be activated via the vestibular or neck proprioceptive systems rather than ankle joint proprioceptors.

We have also tested adults in the seated condition (on a stool) and compared their muscle responses during platform-induced sway to those of the youngest children tested, who could not stand independently. When seated, adults show responses in the muscles of the neck and trunk which are

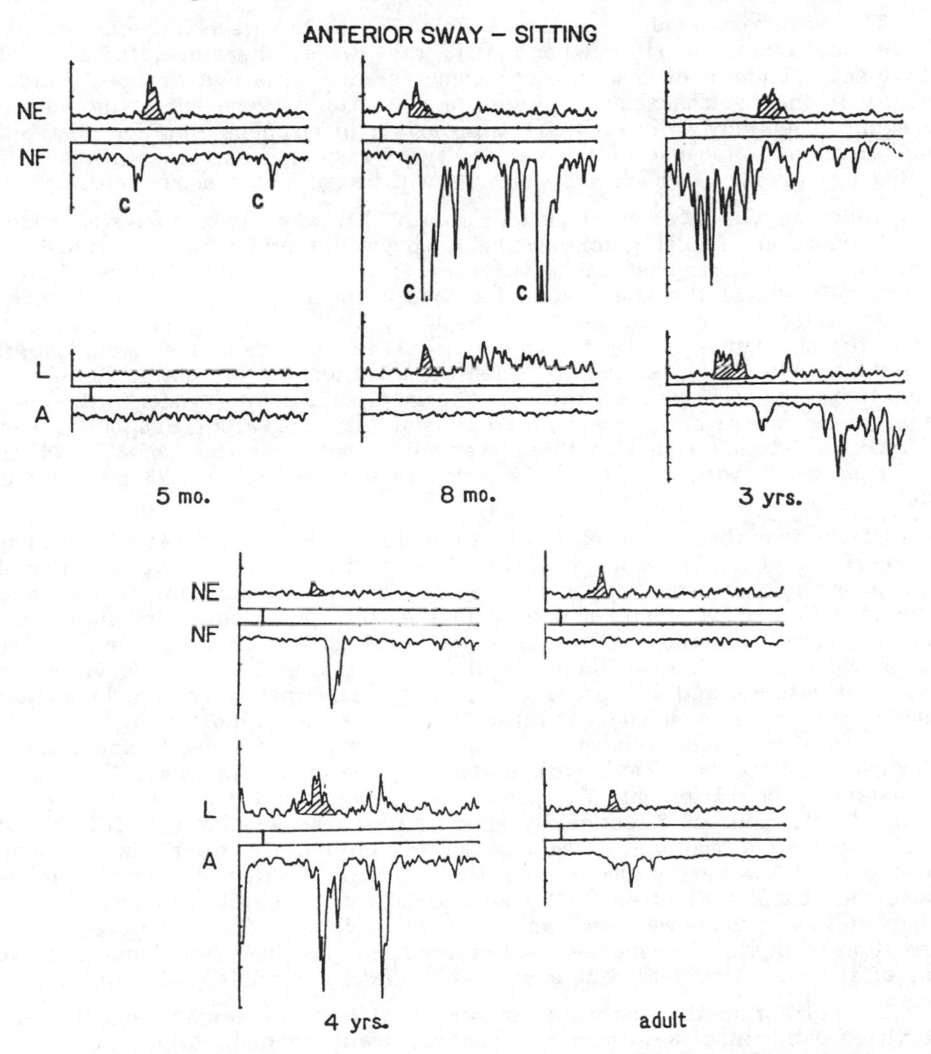

Fig. 2. Surface EMG recordings of muscle responses of individuals in each age group to posterior platform translations (anterior sway) while seated. Responses are represented as indicated in Figure 1. C = cardiovascular artifact (heartbeat) recorded by the electrodes over the neck flexor muscles in the youngest children.

directionally appropriate, and counteract the platform-induced sway. Thus, for platform movements causing forward sway, the trunk extensor and neck extensor muscles are activated before flexors, bringing the centre of mass back to its initial position. However, the temporal organisation of these responses is more variable than that seen during stance: either the neck or the trunk muscles may be activated first (see Figure 2).

3. POSTURAL RESPONSES IN CHILDREN-SITTING

The youngest group of children which we tested were four-five months of age, and unable to sit independently; they were, therefore, tested in an infant seat. Though each of the children tested in this age group showed activity in the neck muscles in response to platform movements, the responses were not consistently directionally appropriate in compensating for destabilising head movement. Because of the variability of response patterns within children of this age group, each child's patterns will be examined separately.

When the youngest child, a four month old, was given posterior platform translations (causing forward head movement) under *normal* visual conditions, the appropriate neck extensor (NE) muscles were activated first during only 60% of the trials while the inappropriate neck flexor (NF) muscles were activated the remaining 40% of the time. There were no responses in either the abdominal (A) or trunk extensor (TE) muscles. This would appear to indicate a lack of postural response organisation in this child. However, when the eyes were covered with opaque goggles blocking vision, NE muscles were, to our surprise, correctly and consistently activated. Responses were in the same latency range as those seen in the adult (a mean of 87 ± 24 ms for NE muscles, with no vision, compared to a mean of 110 ± 23 ms for the adults).

Of the two five month old children tested, the first repeatedly used an incorrect activation pattern, while the second showed consistent directionally appropriate neck muscle responses (see Figure 2). In addition, trunk muscle responses were occasionally activated in the first five month old child: for platform movements causing backward sway, abdominal muscles were activated 40% of the time, with mean latencies of 98 ± 11 ms. Both the wide variety of response patterns and the presence of many trials with no response in trunk muscles with eyes open, do not initially lend strong support to the concept that postural response synergies are genetically predetermined, and thus prewired prior to experience with stabilising the centre of mass. This initial inconsistency could indicate the presence of a trial and error learning period in the development of directionally specific postural responses in infants, in which the precise mapping of sensory inputs onto the postural musculature takes place. However, as mentioned earlier, it is of interest that in the four month old, consistent directionally appropriate neck muscle responses became apparent when vision was *removed*. It is possible that the proprioceptive activation of postural responses is prewired and becomes functional prior to that of the visual system, but is inhibited under normal visual conditions.

In contrast to the youngest age group of children tested while seated, the three children of 8-14 months, who could sit independently, showed clear directionally specific neck and trunk muscle responses which showed low variability in onset latency (see Figure 2 and Table 1). This was also true for the group of two-three year olds (Figure 2 and Table 1). As previously noted for responses in adults, there was no clear pattern of temporal sequencing of muscles beginning from the base of support and moving upward.

It thus appears that the temporal coupling of neck and trunk muscles is not as critical to balance control while sitting, as is the temporal coupling of the leg, trunk and neck muscles during stance.

Table 1. Muscle Response Latencies for Platform Translations - Seated (in ms)

	Neck Extensor	Trunk Extensor	Neck Flexor	Abdominal
Translations Causing Anterior Sway				
4 - 5 months	106 ± 24	NR	77 ± 21	NR
8 - 14 months	86 ± 28	94 ± 9	NR	NR
2 - 3 years	132 ± 47	90 ± 3	NR	NR
Adults	108 ± 20	107 ± 25	117 ± 27	107 ± 16
Translations Causing Posterior Sway				
4 - 5 months	94 ± 4	275 ± 14 N=1 NR N=2	138 ± 86	98 ± 11 N=1
8 - 14 months	125 ± 61	229 ± 38 N=1 NR N=2	106 ± 17	113 ± 20
2 - 3 years	200 ± 55 N=1	180 ± 6	98 ± 7	97 ± 2
Adults	113 ± 12	151 ± 91	98 ± 18	94 ± 30

NR= No response.

As in the younger age group, postural responses were also activated by platform movements when the childrens' eyes were covered with opaque goggles. Figure 3 shows an example of responses of a five month old and an eight month old to platform translations causing anterior sway with eyes covered. Note that the responses are still present when vision is removed.

4. POSTURAL RESPONSES IN CHILDREN- STANDING

Three children were tested in the eight-14 month old age range and represented the full range of stages seen in learning to stand (from no experience in independent stance (eight months) through minimal experience (10 months) and finally, to one and one-half months experience in stance and walking (14 months)). As we observed in the children of the youngest age group which were tested while sitting, these children showed an increase in response organisation with age and experience standing. The eight month old (lightly supported at the waist by the mother as an aid in standing) showed no responses to platform movements. Leg, trunk, and neck muscles were either tonically active or did not respond. Neither postural reflexes nor voluntary control of leg muscles in stance were apparent.

In contrast, the 10 month old showed appropriate responses in the G muscle during 40% of the platform movements causing anterior sway, but

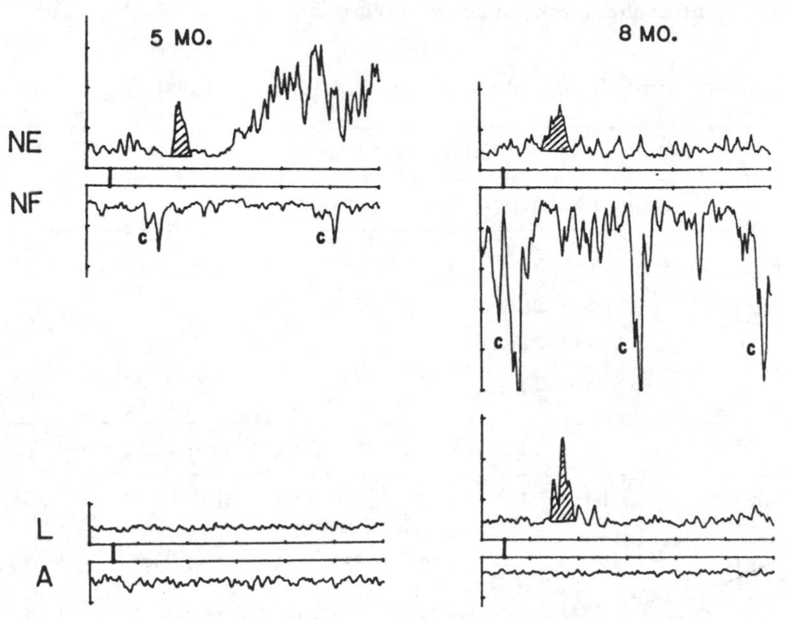

Fig. 3. Muscle responses of a seated 5 and an 8 month old child to a posterior platform translation (anterior sway) with vision removed. Note that responses are still present. Time marks are at 100 ms intervals. Abbreviations are noted in Figure 1.

responses were activated at very early, *monosynaptic latencies* (39 ± 8 ms) rather than the longer (85 ± 20 ms) latencies seen in the 14 month old and typical of adults. Upper leg muscles were activated in only one trial. Though trunk and neck muscles were activated in the majority of trials, they were not consistently directionally appropriate. Finally, the oldest child (the 14 month old), showed correctly organised responses in the leg muscles during all of the platform movements. (G latencies for anterior sway were 85 ± 20 ms; TA mean latencies for posterior sway were 119 ± 17 ms (see Table 2)). Neck and trunk responses, though often present, were not consistently organised in the temporal sequence seen in the adult.

We thus see a clear increase in both the level of activation and consistency of organisation of response patterns during the development of postural responses while standing. This is coincident with onset of voluntary use of the muscles in stance. Thus, the youngest child showed no responses, the middle child showed proprioceptive reflexes, and the oldest child, with experience standing, showed consistently correct responses in muscles of the leg, but less consistently organised responses in muscles of the trunk and neck (see Table 2).

Children in the next age group (one and one-half to three year olds) showed clearly organised leg muscle responses to platform movements given

Table 2. Muscle Response Latencies for Platform Translations - Standing (in ms)

	NE	NF	TE	A	H	Q	G	TA
Translations Causing Anterior Sway								
14 months	145±65	NR	115±76	NR	*	NR	85±20	94±10
2-3 years	109± 8	90±15	132±12	107±30	131±34	146±20	87± 8	125±25
4-6 years	135±23	106±36	149±18	95±33	113±23	NR	79± 5	157±26
7-10 years (gymnasts)	127±10	72± 7	104± 7	69±11	85±14	91±12	61± 9	106±23
Adults	104±21	84± 8	96±17	84±16	90± 6	108±12	75±12	94±23
Translations Causing Posterior sway								
14 months	NR	157±34	NR	NR	*	134±13	NR	119±17
2-3 years	105±27	111±13	86±19	168±62	145±10	137± 8	112±42	72± 5
4-6 years	109±22	174±19	159±34	97±23	122±10	116±29	101±49	78± 5
7-10 years (gymnasts)	83±16	88±21	59± 3 123±26	106± 6	89±73	77± 9	96±17	68± 5
Adults	77±11	90± 9	112±23	104±18	75±10	93±15	114±34	77±19

* Not recorded NR= No response

while standing. Previous studies (Forssburg & Nashner, 1982) and our first experiment (Shumway-Cook & Woollacott, 1985) on children in this age group, showed that distal muscles of the leg were activated before proximal muscles in children, as seen in adults. These postural responses were consistently large in amplitude and longer in duration than those seen in the adult. In fact, the postural responses often overcompensated for platform induced sway and thus produced greater body oscillation than in the older children tested. In addition to the activation of the appropriate agonist muscles, the children showed a large degree of activation of the antagonist leg muscles, at a slightly longer latency. This strategy may have been used to compensate for the unnecessarily large initial agonist muscle responses, or actually may have been due to a simple lack of refinement of the children's muscle response pattern.

Our more recent studies (Woollacott et al, 1985) have also analysed the responses of children's trunk and neck muscles to platform movements. The developmental emergence of the secondary response synergy in the upper body musculature, which was described above for adults, appears to occur later in childhood than the leg muscle response synergy. For example, the two and one half year old showed responses in the trunk musculature during only 20% of the trials. Early responses were apparent in neck flexor muscles during perturbations causing anterior sway, but never present in neck extensors in response to posterior sway. Neck flexor muscle responses were elicited in the two-three year old age group in response to anterior sway

42% of the time, while they occurred in *76%* of the trials in the adult age group. When the responses did appear in the two-three year olds, they occurred at approximately the same latency as in the adults (two-three year olds: 90 ± 15 ms; adults: 84 ± 8 ms) (see Table 2).

The results of our experiments analysing the onset latency and variability of the leg muscle responses of four-six year olds (Shumway-Cook & Woollacott, 1985) were unexpected. We found that four-six year olds appeared to regress in their postural response organisation: postural response synergies were more variable in this age group than in the 15-31 month olds, seven-ten year olds, or adults. In the four-six year olds, leg muscle postural synergies were more variable in both onset latencies and timing relationships (between distal and proximal leg muscle synergists) than in any other age group. The 15-31 month old children exhibited latencies comparable to seven-ten year olds and adults, while the four-six year old children were both significantly slower and more variable in the timing of their responses ($p < .01$). The four-six year olds also showed a longer temporal delay between the onset of responses in distal and proximal leg synergists. When we filmed the children during the platform movements and made a biomechanical analysis of joint angle changes associated with platform movements, we found that this diminished temporal coupling resulted in a buckling of the knee joint when the four-six year olds attempted to compensate for the platform induced body sway. We did not find this in the adult group, where compensation for platform induced sway occurred primarily at the ankle. We conclude that the activation of the proximal leg muscles of the four-six year olds was not sufficiently rapid to minimise the inertial lag associated with the mass of the thigh and trunk (Shumway-Cook & Woollacott, 1985).

Our recent studies (Woollacott et al, 1985) analysing the response of trunk and neck muscles in four-six year olds, support the earlier indication of high variability in response patterns. Under normal visual conditions, neck muscle responses occurred less often in the four-six year olds (22% of the trials) than in the two-three year olds (42% of the trials) or the adults (76% of the trials). When present they were both longer in latency and more variable (106 ± 36 ms) than the other age groups tested (2-3 years: 90 ± 15 ms; adults: 84 ± 8 ms) (see Table 2).

The seven-ten year olds analysed in our first study showed postural responses which were similar to those seen in the adults in that there were no significant differences between the two groups in onset latency, variability, or temporal coordination between muscles within the synergy. The seven-ten year olds used in our second study were a select group trained in gymnastics, and also showed responses in neck and trunk muscles similar to those seen in the adults, though somewhat shorter in latency. Thus we can conclude that postural responses are mature by seven-ten years of age (see Table 2).

5. POSTURAL RESPONSES - EYES CLOSED

The removal of visual inputs (the children wore opaque goggles) during platform movements had different effects on the various age groups tested. In all age groups (including the youngest children, tested in an infant seat) postural responses remained when visual cues were removed. In fact, the youngest child tested (four months) showed consistent, directionally appropriate neck muscle responses only when vision was removed. It is thus possible that removal of vision heightens the sensitivity of the system to proprioceptive and/or vestibular cues.

Figure 4 shows the differences in latency between eyes open and closed conditions for NF and G muscles for the two-three year olds, four-six year olds and adults for platform movements causing anterior sway. The adults showed no significant differences in the latency of these responses for the two conditions (Keshner & Woollacott, 1984). However, both groups of children showed changes in postural responses with visual cues removed. The two-three year olds showed a reduction in the mean latency of neck muscle responses from 90 ± 15 ms to 81 ± 8 ms with an additional increase in the frequency of occurrence of neck muscle monosynaptic reflexes. However, no changes were observed in the frequency with which the longer latency responses were observed in neck muscles (42% of the trials both with eyes open and closed). G response latencies were reduced from a mean of 87 ± 8 ms to 83 ± 9 ms (nonsignificant) and also showed an increase in monosynaptic reflex occurrence.

The four-six year old age group showed greater variability in neck and leg muscle latencies, and no reduction in response latency was apparent. However, with vision removed they showed an increase in the frequency of occurrence of postural responses in neck muscles from response activation in 22% of the trials to activation in 58% of the trials. In addition they showed an increase in the occurrence of monosynaptic reflexes in the G muscle of the leg.

What is the meaning of either a reduction in postural response onset latency or an increase in the frequency of occurrence of monosynaptic and longer latency responses when vision is removed? It is possible that visual cues are not required to activate postural responses in any of the age groups tested, and that removal of these cues actually increases the sensitivity of the system to the remaining proprioceptive and vestibular cues. The slight reduction in latency of muscle responses and increased frequency of occurrence of monosynaptic reflexes in the two-three year olds when vision was removed could be evidence that vision is normally dominant in this age group, and that a shift occurs from the use of longer latency visual inputs with eyes open to shorter latency proprioceptive inputs with eyes closed.

6. THE DEVELOPMENT OF INTERSENSORY INTEGRATION

If we use platform *rotations* instead of *horizontal* translations to perturb balance we have a unique test for the ability to adapt postural responses to changing task conditions. Platform rotations, like translations, cause ankle rotations and stretch to the ankle joint musculature, but with neither a significant shift in the child's centre of mass nor significant body sway. Thus, ankle joint proprioceptive inputs associated with *horizontal* platform movements are congruent with visual and vestibular inputs in signalling moderate body sway, but ankle joint inputs associated with rotation are not congruent with visual and vestibular inputs, since the former indicate strong sway, while the latter inputs are only minimally activated, if at all. In adults, platform rotations produce postural responses in the stretched ankle muscles on initial trials. However, these muscle responses are *destabilising* under rotational conditions, and in the adult, the responses are attenuated to very low amplitudes within three to five trials (Nashner, 1976). Dorsiflexing ankle rotations can be used to test 1) the

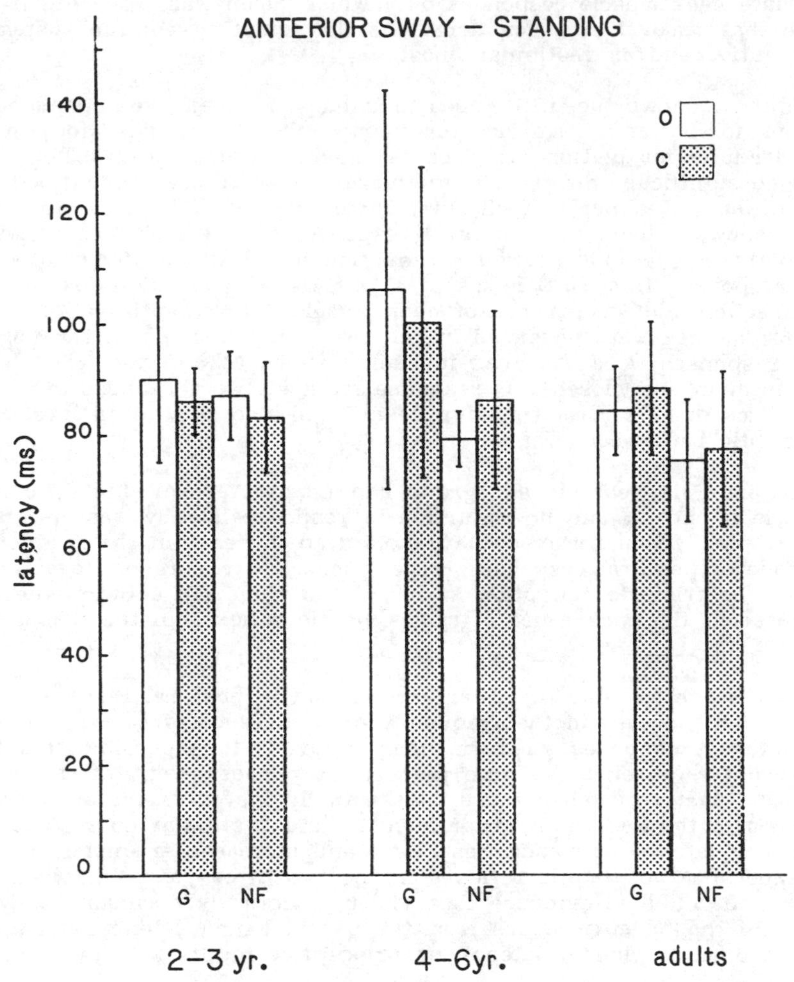

Fig. 4. Average response latency (± S.D.) of the appropriate neck (NF) and ankle (G) muscle in response to translations causing anterior sway. Responses are shown for conditions with vision present (O) and absent (C) for three age groups: 2-3 years, 4-6 years, and adults.

efficiency of ankle joint inputs in isolation in producing postural responses, and 2) the ability to attenuate postural response amplitudes, when they are inappropriate, due to changing task conditions.

We tested three children between 15 and 31 months with dorsiflexing rotational platform perturbations. Though monosynaptic reflexes were occasionally observed under these conditions, none of the children showed consistent longer latency postural responses in G and H (Shumway-Cook & Woollacott, 1985).

By three years of age the children exhibited normal longer latency

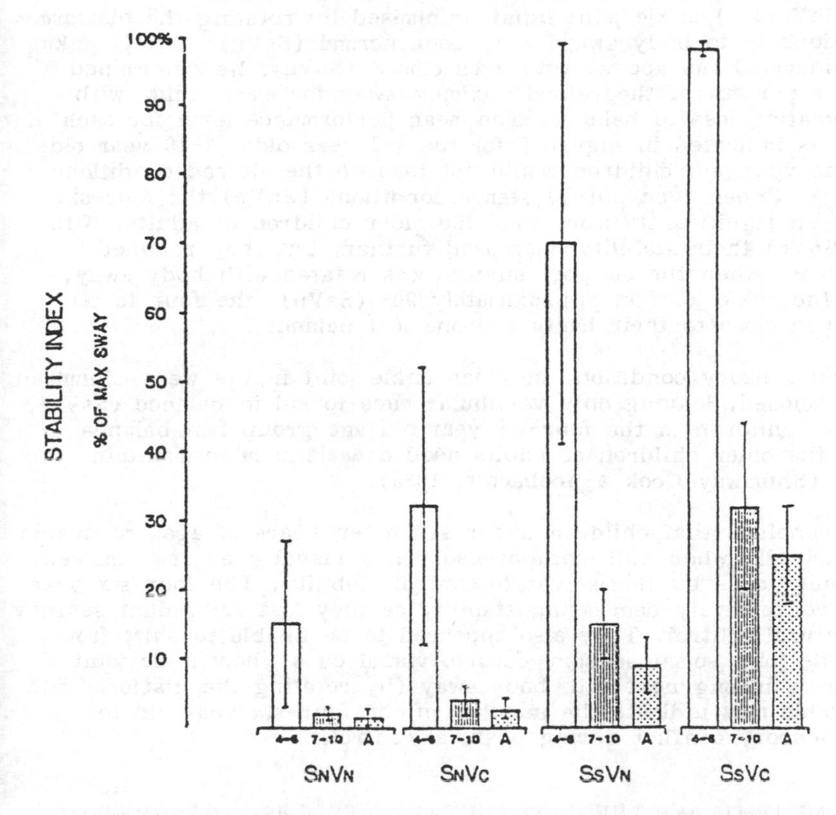

Fig. 5. Representation of body sway (as a percentage of maximum sway) under four sensory conditions, during 5 seconds of stance. SnVn: normal ankle joint somatosensory and normal visual inputs; SnVc: normal ankle joint somatosensory inputs with eyes closed; SsVn: ankle joint somatosensory inputs minimised, vision normal; SsVc: ankle joint somatosensory inputs minimised with eyes closed. Three age groups compared: 4-6 years, 7-10 years, and adults (from Shumway-Cook & Woollacott, 1985).

response synergies in leg muscles to platform rotations. The four-six year olds also exhibited these responses. In addition, two thirds of the four-six year old children tested showed *attenuation* of the amplitude of inappropriate rotational responses, but not within the three to five trials seen in the adult. They required, instead, the presentation of 10 to 15 trials before response amplitude attenuation occurred. Seven-ten year olds showed adult-like adaptation (Shumway-Cook & Woollacott, 1985).

We also used a second approach to test the ability of the children to adapt to altered sensory conditions. Children were asked to stand quietly for five seconds under four different sensory conditions which progressively decreased sensory inputs useful for balance control, until only vestibular inputs remained. The conditions were: 1) somatosensory ankle joint and visual inputs normal (SnVn); 2) somatosensory ankle joint inputs normal and eyes closed (SnVc); 3) ankle joint inputs minimised by rotating the platform in direct relationship to body sway, but vision normal (SsVn); and 4) ankle joint inputs minimised (as above) with eyes closed (SsVc). We determined body sway as a percent of theoretical maximum sway for each child, with 100% sway indicating loss of balance. The mean performance level for each of the conditions is indicated in Figure 5 for the 4-6 year olds, 7-10 year olds and adults (the youngest children would not tolerate the altered conditions without crying). Under even normal stance conditions (SnVn) the four-six year olds swayed significantly more than the older children or adults. With eyes closed (SnVc) their stability decreased further, but they retained balance. However, when the support surface was rotated with body sway, thus keeping the ankle joint at approximately 90° (SsVn), the four to six year olds swayed close to their limits and one lost balance.

In the last sensory condition, in which ankle joint inputs were minimised and eyes were closed, leaving only vestibular cues to aid in balance (SsVs), four of the five children in the four-six year old age group lost balance while none of the older children or adults needed assistance to maintain their stability (Shumway-Cook & Woollacott, 1985).

We thus conclude that children under seven-ten years of age are unable to balance efficiently when both somatosensory and visual cues are removed, leaving vestibular cues by themselves to control stability. The four-six year olds showed progressively decreasing stability as they lost redundant sensory inputs for postural control. They also appeared to be unable to shift from the use of ankle joint somatosensory cues to visual cues when ankle joint inputs were made incongruent with body sway (by rotating the platform with body sway). This may indicate the inability of the four-six year old to resolve inter-sensory conflict during postural control.

THE DEVELOPMENT OF POSTURAL-VOLUNTARY RESPONSE INTEGRATION

In order to analyse the manner in which postural and voluntary muscle responses are integrated in children, we asked children to perform a voluntary movement which required postural control. Standing children were asked to push or pull on a handle in response to the illumination of a set of brightly colored lights (Shumway-Cook, 1983). Muscle responses were recorded from the biceps (B) and triceps (T) muscles of the upper arm, as well as the gastrocnemius (G) and tibialis anterior (TA) muscles of the leg. Experiments on four normal adults with this apparatus confirmed previous findings (Cordo & Nashner, 1982) showing preparatory muscle activity in the postural G muscle *in advance* of activation of the prime-mover B muscle for all pull trials, and in TA prior to T for all push trials (see Figure 6). Four of the five children in the four-six year old group showed postural preparatory activity in all trials (Figure 6) while the last child showed preparatory activity in 80% of the trials. This implies that by four to six years of age, integration of the voluntary and postural systems is essentially mature, and characterised by a feedforward control process which anticipates instability associated with voluntary movement and minimises it by the use of preparatory postural responses.

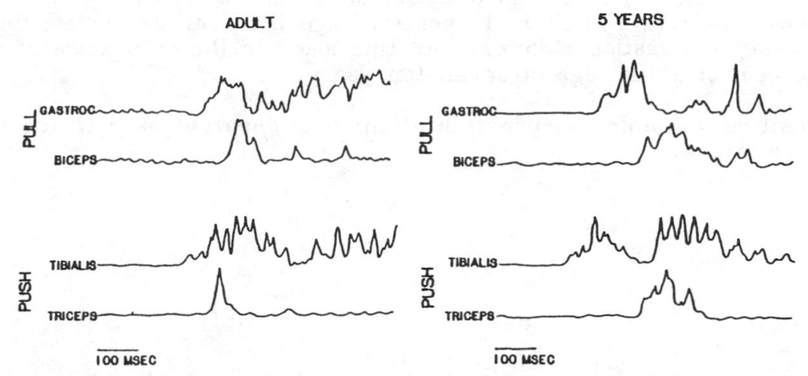

Fig. 6. Responses of leg and arm muscles during reaction time arm movements (push or pull) while standing. Note that postural activity in the leg precedes prime-mover activity in the arm, indicating feedforward postural control in both the 5 year old and adult (from Shumway-Cook, 1983).

7. SUMMARY

The results of our experiments exploring the development of children's postural responses indicate the coincident onset of voluntary control and postural reflexes. Monosynaptic proprioceptive reflexes are present early in the development of posture control, and thus may be genetically predetermined. However, it is interesting that these responses are suppressed when vision is present, and less organised visually elicited response patterns become apparent. It is possible that this is a time period during which visual and proprioceptive cues are integrated in the activation of postural responses. Learning periods are thus apparent and involve the fine tuning of balance control in the child beginning to sit and to stand. It is clear that vision is not required for the activation of postural responses in young children. In fact, responses are more frequent and often shorter in latency when vision is removed.

Postural responses, like voluntary responses, appear to develop in a cephalo-caudal direction, with neck muscle responses appearing first, as early as four months of age, followed by trunk muscle responses at 5-8 months, and leg muscle responses (in stance perturbations) at 10-14 months, coincident with the development of voluntary control in upper body muscles and stance control in leg muscles. When the child begins to stand independently, a new pattern emerges, and leg muscle responses develop effective organisation and strong activation levels prior to neck muscles.

An important transition period in the development of balance control appears at the age of four-six years. At this time responses become slower and more variable before attaining adult characteristics at the age of seven-ten years. We hypothesise that this variability in the four-six year olds' responses is due to their frequently shifting from one sensory input to another as they begin to learn to adapt responses to changing sensory conditions (Shumway-Cook & Woollacott, 1985). The four-six year old also shows the onset of the ability to adapt postural responses to changing task conditions. However, sensory integration abilities do not mature until the age of seven-ten years. It has been hypothesised (Shumway-Cook & Woollacott, 1985) that at four-six years of age the nervous system fine tunes intersensory integration abilities, and this leads to the emergence of mature posture control at the age of seven-ten years.

Postural-voluntary response integration is apparent as early as four-six years of age.

References

Belenkii, V.E., Gurfinkel, V.S. & Paltsev, R.I. (1967). On the elements of voluntary movement control. *Biofizika, 12,* 135-141.
Bower, T.G.R. (1972). Object perception in infants. *Perception, 1,* 15-30.
Bower, T.G.R. (1974). *Development in infancy.* San Francisco: W.H. Freeman.
Bower, T.G.R., Broughton, J.M. & Moore, M.K. (1970). The coordination of visual and tactual input in infants. *Perception and Psychophysics, 8,* 51-53.
Butterworth, G. (1982). The origins of auditory-visual perception and visual proprioception in human development. In R. Walk and H. Pick (Eds.), *Intersensory perception and sensory integration.* New York: Plenum Press.
Butterworth, G. & Hicks, L. (1977). Visual proprioception and postural stability in infancy: A developmental study. *Perception, 6,* 255-262.
Cordo, P.J. & Nashner, L.M. (1982). Properties of postural adjustments associated with rapid arm movements. *Journal Neurophysiology, 47,* 287-302.
Forssberg, H. & Nashner, L. (1982). Ontogenetic development of posture control in man: Adaptation to altered support and visual conditions during stance. *Journal of Neuroscience, 2,* 545-552.
Gahery, Y. & Massion, J. (1981). Coordination between posture and movement. *Trends in Neuroscience, 4,* 199-202.
Keogh, J. & Sugden, D. (1985). *Movement Skill Development.* New York: McMillan.
Lee, D.N. & Aronson, E. (1974). Visual proprioceptive control of standing in human infants. *Perception and Psychophysics, 15,* 529-532.
Nashner, L.M. (1976). Adapting reflexes controlling human posture. *Experimental Brain Research, 26,* 59-72.
Nashner, L.M. (1977). Fixed patterns of rapid postural responses among leg muscles during stance. *Experimental Brain Research, 30,* 13-24.
Nashner, L.M. & McCollum, G. (in press). The organization of human postural movements: A formal basis and experimental synthesis. *Brain and Behavior.*
Nashner, L.M. & Woollacott, M. (1979). The organization of rapid postural adjustments of standing humans: An experimental-conceptual model. In R.E. Talbot and D.R. Humphrey (Eds.), *Posture and Movement.* New York: Raven Press.
Shumway-Cook, A. (1983). *Developmental aspects of postural control in normal and Down's syndrome children.* Ph.D Thesis, University of Oregon.
Shumway-Cook, A. & Woollacott, M.H. (1985). The growth of stability: Postural control from a developmental perspective. *Journal of Motor Behavior, 17,* 131-147.
Thomas, J. (1984). *Motor Development during Childhood and Adolescence.* Minneapolis: Burgess.
Woollacott, M., Debu, B. & Shumway-Cook, A. (in press). Children's development of posture and balance control: changes in motor coordination and sensory integration. In D. Gould and M. Weiss (Eds.), *Advances in Pediatric Sport Sciences: Behavioral Issues.* Champaign, Illinois: Human Kinetics.
Woollacott, M., Debu, B. & Mowatt, M. (1985). The development of balance control in children: Sensorimotor integration. *Proceedings, NASPSA Meetings.*
Woollacott, M. & Keshner, E. (1984). Upper body responses to postural perturbations in man. *Neuroscience Abstracts, 10,* 635.
Yonas, A. (1981). Infants' responses to optical information for collision. In R. Aslin, J. Alberts and M. Petersen (Eds.), *Development of Perception: Vol. 2, The Visual System.* New York: Academic Press.

THE DEVELOPMENT OF PROPRIOCEPTIVE CONTROL

D.A. Sugden

INTRODUCTION

Investigation into any developmental process must ideally address itself to two issues: first what states do individuals pass through at different points in their development? Secondly, what are the agents or mechanism of this change process? Although, they appear to be separate questions, the first does lead to the second with accurate descriptions leading to propositions about the nature and mechanisms of change. It may be more realistic to view them as transactional in nature:

> ...explanations should proceed from the concerns identified in descriptions and they should lead to different levels and types of descriptions (Keogh and Sugden, 1985, p. v).

The concept of change underlies development but it must be remembered that there are different types of change, and these will be seen at different developmental stages only by examining a wide range of experimental paradigms. Flavell (1972) for example, identified five types of change processes in cognitive development: first, he specifies addition, in which behaviour XI starts and X2 is added: the two coexist as part of the child's repertoire providing diversity and alternative modes of response. Secondly, substitution is where X1 is gradually replaced by X2: they also coexist for a short period of time, but then X1 drops out. Thirdly, modification involves X1 becoming X2 providing the facility for differentiation, generalisation and stabilisation. Fourthly, inclusion is the use of X1 as a component of X2 to form higher orders of behaviour. Finally, mediation involves the use of X1 as a bridge to influence the formation of X2 without becoming a part of it. Thus a fundamental issue in development is change: what changes, what remains stable such that other changes can take place.

When we are examining the development, and thus change, in something as multifaceted as proprioception, then we are presented with many problems, not the least of which is definition of the term. Traditionally, proprioception is information obtained from receptor mechanisms associated with the muscles, tendons, joints and the vestibular system of the inner ear. These receptors signal force, velocity, acceleration, pressure and position of the body and its parts. This traditional concept is widened with the notion of visual proprioception (Gibson, 1966) which emerges from the idea that proprioception is not a special sense, classified on the basis of receptors, but is an overall function common to all systems. Here the stress is on vision providing information for and about our own movements, becoming a proprioceptive sense describing movements of our body in relation to the environment. Thus proprioceptive control involves information from mechanical, vestibular and visual receptors, all of which need to be coordinated in order for it to affect the precision and smoothness of a movement. It is important to recognise that the totality emerges from multiple inputs and this totality is used as a basis for action.

The situation is confused with many writers using kinaesthesis and proprioception interchangeably when they are referring to movement information that is not visual or auditory. In an effort to separate the terms, Smyth (1984) describes kinaesthesis as sensing the movement itself, while proprioception is the information about the position and movement of the body via mechanical, vestibular and visual receptors. Rather than clumsily switch terms, I will use proprioception throughout, distinguishing between proprioceptive control which is the total system linked to action, from proprioceptive perception which is the sensing of movement involving acuity and discrimination.

The variety of the types of change that are exhibited in the developmental process, together with the diverse nature of proprioception presents some selection problems when attempting to chart the developmental course. The approach here is to take samples of proprioceptive influence on motor control: first, an examination of neonate behaviour provides information not only about proprioception but more generally about the state of the newborn organism. Secondly, in early childhood, proprioceptive ability is refined, integrated and differentiated with different experimental designs examining its contribution to motor control. Finally, proprioception and motor control change when the organism does not pursue its normal course, with various handicapping conditions influencing the process of development.

ORIGINS AND EARLY DEVELOPMENT

At a fundamental level, proprioception is dependent upon the growth and development of the nervous system. Changeux (1985) notes that after 49 days in utero, the foetus responds to tactile stimulation of the lips; at five to seven months the sensory innervation of the fingers is practically completed. Vestibular apparatus starts to function between the 90th and 210th day, but without mature performance, and long after birth there is development characterised by a lowering of the sensitivity threshold. However, the major concern here is on proprioceptive functioning rather than on the development of structures. The relationship between function and structure is a complex one with a two way influence. Both Imbert (1985) and Parmelee and Sigman (1985) argue for early neural development following fairly rigid rules dictated primarily by genetic factors, the nervous system then developing to a level that allows it to be more interactive with environmental influences, with the normal structural and functional maturation of the brain depending to a large part on early experience.

An examination of proprioception early in life embodies the notion of it being an overall fucntion common to all systems. Questions that are raised about proprioception thus involve intersensory coordination and are usually concerned with the strength of the inferential data, methodology, and whether the results point to innate capacities. The review here is necessarily selective and includes those studies which I believe demonstrate that proprioception is being utilised for action very soon after birth. The stress on proprioception being the result of multiple inputs means that intra development of any one part will affect the inter development of the total system which is used for action.

FACIAL IMITATION

While even recent work disputes the presence of intersensory co-ordination in neonates (Bushell, 1981), work by Meltzoff and Moore (1977; 1983; 1985) would appear to point to neonates being competent in combining the senses for the picking up and utilisation of information. They use the action of facial imitation which involves intersensory matching with one perceptual system (vision) providing the model against which information from a different system (proprioception/motor) is compared. They asked the valid question about how the infant learns this correspondence when the perception of the object and the results of the production cannot be compared within the same modality. Their recent work (1983) involved 40 newborns all aged less than 72 hours with one only 42 minutes old. When the infants were alert, they were examined for imitation of mouth opening and tongue protrusion. Each infant was presented with two four-minute models, one for tongue protusion and the other for mouth opening, and the design involved examining the differential pattern of response. As was predicted, there were more tongue protrusions than mouth openings following the tongue protrusion presentation, with the results switched following the mouth opening presentation. The term convergence is used to explain the initial small approximations becoming more and more like adults over successive efforts.

The authors suggest that this early imitation reflects a process of active intermodel mapping in which the infants use the equivalences between visually and proprioceptively received body transformations as a basis for organising their response. It is not an exclusively visual or proprioceptive image, but appears to be a non-modality specific description of the event, and this internal representation constitutes the model that directs the infant's actions and against which he matches his motor performance. Metlzoff and Moore (1985) argue for a reciprocal relationship between acts seen and done, and not merely simple triggering of innately organised motor patterns. Thus intermodel matching, and representation, in this case vision and proprioception is a rather basic starting point for infant psychological development. This non-modality specific description of an event is very much akin to proprioceptive control, stressing function and utilising all the available resources. A problem does arise when the boundaries of what is called proprioceptive control becomes so wide and all embracing that a breakdown into parts not only is difficult but also artificial. In facial imitation for example, separating proprioceptive influence form efferent activity and control has not been attempted. The paradox here of course, is that in order to perform this separation, the event itself would be destroyed, thereby losing the natural functional properties of proprioception.

The picture that is emerging is one of crude intersensory connections being present at birth, with information being available, experienced and used, and it matters not whether it is heard, seen or touched and felt. Jones (1981) feels that at higher levels of the nervous system, space is represented by overlapping inputs from a number of different modalities rather than by independent visual, auditory and proprioceptive spaces. Proprioception at birth seems to be locked in to a multisensory description of an act; with development we shall see that it becomes differentiated in that proprioceptive information can be isolated, some would argue artificially, and yet with development, its links with other sensory systems, most notably vision, also improves. Whether the development of intersensory coordination can be explained by the individual development of each sensory modality, or is a true intersensory development is a debatable issue (Jones, 1981).

REACHING AND GRASPING

Reaching and grasping and postural control are two basic actions which develop during early infancy. They include proprioception and vision together with motor efference. In reaching and grasping, most studies have concentrated on the role of vision with proprioception examined incidentally by varying visual conditions. For example, Bower (1979) identified two reaching phases, with phase I being a single movement with no differentiation between reaching and grasping, and the total movement is visually elicited, but not visually controlled. Phase II is characterised by reaching and grasping being differentiated, with reaching being visually controlled, and the grasp is elicited by tactual contact with the object. While one is hesitant about advocating such discrete phases, there is evidence to suggest that the type of control is changing. Bower and Wishart (1972) for example, using a paradigm where babies were shown an object with the lights on and then turned off just before reaching was initiated, found 5 month old babies were more accurate than 7, 9 and 11 month olds. It seemed as though the younger ones did not need to use visual control for their reaching movements, and were possibly dominated by a combination of motor efference and proprioception.

Wishart, Bower and Dunkeld (1978) showed that up to 5 months there is no difference in success of an initial attempt at reaching to an object in the darkness or with the light on. However, by 7 months, success is higher with lights on. Lasky (1977) also found that babies after 5 months needed vision for reaching to progress in increasing accuracy. Babies, in conditions of hands in direct view or not seen, were successful at 5 and 6 months when vision was present, but with the hand not seen were no more successful than younger babies. In a series of studies, von Hofsten (1979; 1980; 1982; 1983) and von Hofsten and Lindhagen (1979) reported that babies can intercept a moving an object at around 4 months, and from that time, the type of reaching changes with the previous ballistic hand movement being replaced by a movement which has a short initial ballistic phase, followed by a second phase composed of small corrective movements as the hand nears the goal, suggesting the onset of visual control.

Early reaching seems not to require visual control; it is crude and inaccurate - appearing to rely on motor efference and proprioception. With development, vision is used more, accuracy improves, yet when the expected visual information is absent, confusion sets in and disruption can result. Proprioceptive information appears to be used early in reaching and grasping although the intersensory link with vision to produce full proprioceptive control is necessary for development to take its normal course.

POSTURAL CONTROL

Later in infancy, when the child is gaining postural control by sitting up or beginning to stand and walk, there is further opportunity to investigate this welding of proprioception and vision. Earlier, Gibson's (1966) term 'visual proprioception' was noted and is used to describe the role that vision plays in providing information for movement over and above proprioceptive cues given by the mechanical and vestibular systems. Gibson (1966) argued that information is available in the stimulus array to promote intersensory coordination. The refinement of this early established coordination is facilitated by feedback control which helps to explain the flexible recalibration with growth.

The well known studies of Lee and Aaronson (1974), Butterworth and Hicks (1977) and Butterworth and Ciccheti (1978) have demonstrated some of the properties of visual proprioception. Lee and Aaronson (1974), arguing that vision provides a proprioceptive function, examined standing in infants aged 13 - 16 months. Standing involves a continuous monitoring of feedback including compensatory adjustments of the musculature, with the classic view that information about body sway comes from receptors in the vestibular canals, joints, tendons and muscles, particularly of the ankles and hips. Their aim was to show that balance could be disturbed by visual stimulation in a direction specific to that stimulation, thus furnishing evidence that vision functions proprioceptively in standing. The infants stood on a stable floor in a 'movable room', comprising three walls and a ceiling which moved backwards and forwards. The infants did indeed sway, stagger and fall in the direction specified by the moving room. If the wall moved towards them, they fell backwards and vice versa. The question which arose and was taken up by Butterworth and HIcks (1977) was whether vision acquires its proprioceptive function as a consequence of motor activity and learning to stand. They examined infants at different developmental stages in different postural conditions. Infants who could sit and stand unsupported were compared with infants who could sit but who could not stand. The latter group who were younger were affected at least as much as those infants who could sit or stand without support, providing evidence that upright stance is not the catalyst for vision acquiring its proprioceptive function. Work with Down's Syndrome children provided further support for active locomotion not being a necessary condition for the visual proprioceptive influence (Butterworth & Ciccheti, 1978).

Proprioceptive control is so locked into other systems that different methodologies have been used to tease out and infer its presence in neonates and young infants. It does appear to be part of a multisensory description of an event, ripe for development both in the form of integration and differentiation. Flavell's (1972) processes of addition, substitution and modification are quite evident in this early period, examples being present in both reaching and postural adjustments. The processes of inclusion and mediation are more easily seen later in development.

REFINEMENT AND LATER DEVELOPMENT

During the early years of childhook, children modify their earlier achievements, leading to the development of a large repetoire of movement skills. The general achievement of children becomes less defined with age, and more detailed analyses of movement mechanics and components become important. For example, during infancy, major milestones are quite evident, with movements, like rolling over, standing and walking being quite distinct achievements. Beyond the infancy stage, milestones are still seen, such as hopping and skipping, but more often the child varies the movement or uses it in different ways, often in novel situations. The change processes of modification, inclusion and mediation can be teased out of the progressions seen, particularly in situations when the child is having to perform a skill in relation to a moving environment. Children are acquiring finer control over their own movement, and are learning how to control them in relation to moving others or objects. It would not be unreasonable to suggest that the development of proprioception is a necessary contributing factor to these changes.

PROPRIOCEPTIVE PERCEPTION: ACTIVITY AND MEMORY

The relationship between proprioceptive control by which I mean the multiple sensory inputs linked to action, and proprioceptive perception which is the sensing of movement, has largely been ignored in the developmental literature. In infancy we have little on proprioceptive perception, while in childhood the distinction between them has not often been made. Two basic abilities of proprioceptive perception are acuity and memory. Acuity is where the model or criterion is available throughout the testing situation, and the child is assessed for accuracy, and memory is involved if proprioceptive information is presented as a criterion and then removed before reproduction is required. The latter situation obviously demands more of the child's resources as mnemonic strategies can be employed in order to facilitate retention, which are in fact more cognitive rather than perceptual processes.

Proprioceptive acuity is measured by requiring individuals to detect differences or match quantities in location, distance, weight, force, time velocity and acceleration. These can be measured in active, passive or constrained modes. Changes with age in both acuity and memory have been measured in active and passive modes in children from 5 to 12 years of age and a group of young adults (Bairstow & Laszlo, 1981; Laszlo & Bairstow, 1980). The acuity assessment involved the individuals holding a car in each hand and simultaneously moving them up a runway. The two runways were set at different angles, and after the two cars had been moved up and down, the subjects had to indicate which car (or runway) went up higher. The results showed that children improved steadily until age 8 when they were approaching the adults mean performance, with even some 6 year olds performing at this level. The pattern of change was similar for active and passive modes with no difference between females and males. There is slightly better performance in the active condition when subject generated motor efference is available as well as proprioceptive feedback. On this task, the children were allowed time to make a decision the movement was slow and no time stress was present. In many motor control situations, fast decisions concerning limb position are required and it is possible that further developmental trends would be seen in these situations.

As soon as a delay is present between the presentation of proprioceptive information and its reproduction, performance will be affected by mnemonic strategies which we know are developmental in nature. Thus strategies such as rehearsal, organisation, naming, directed forgetting, visual imagery and logical search may be used depending upon the nature of the task and the developmental level of the child. Our research foundation is not wide in this area, but it is relatively consistent. Based on a series of studies of tactile and movement memory in blind and sighted children, Millar (1974; 1975 and 1978) concluded that movement memory is aided by mnemonic strategies and children's use of these strategies depends on their access to central processing space. Sugden (1980) noted that 6 year olds could not use the rehearsal strategy in a movement reproduction paradigm, but 9 and 12 year olds were able to improve performance when there was an opportunity to use rehearsal. The indication is clear; if a child has reached a developmental level where the adoption of mnemonic strategies is relatively spontaneous, and the task allows for these strategies to be utilised, then reproduction will be improved.

A major problem with comparing studies like these is that the experimental paradigms vary as to whether information is presented actively, passively, or in a constrained mode. We have very little information to determine how these interact with age.

In their second task Bairstow and Laszlo (1981) and Laszlo and Bairstow (1980) were able to compare active and passive modes for proprioceptive memory among children 5 through 12 years of age. This task was a pattern on a two-sided stencil and the children were required to remember this pattern. They first traced in the stencil, after which it was rotated and the children had to reorient the pattern back to its original position. Twelve patterns were available for use with different ages using different patterns, and error was measured in degrees. Children aged 5 and 6 years had such difficulty that they were tested on only four of the twelve stencil patterns. Mean error scores decreased from 7 through 12 but adults, tested only in the active mode had even lower scores. The general pattern for proprioceptive memory was a steady improvement with age through to the adult group, which was in contrast to proprioceptive acuity in which children by age 8 were approaching the adults' mean performance level. A rather strange result was that children performed significantly better for the passive compared to the active conditions. Laszlo and Bairstow (1985) explain this by noting:

> ...the need to control the movement places an attentional demand on the subject which seems to interfere with the perception and storage of the kinaesthetic input. This interference effect would be more pronounced in the physically handicapped child (p. 116).

This assertion rings true with additional information in the form of motor efference only being useful if the resources of the individual are capable of utilising it. Otherwise it will overload the processing capacity of the individual and subsequently interfere with the movement reproduction.

Many experimental paradigms involving proprioceptive acuity and memory have been examined with and without vision in an effort to detail intersensory coordination. Review articles by Jones (1981; 1982) have outlined the various controversies that have surrounded this area since the Birch and Lefford experiments (1967) and the Connolly and Jones account (1970).

POSTURAL CONTROL

Proprioceptive information clearly originates from vestibular, musculoskeletal and visual systems, and this tripartite nature can produce a confusing situation. The visual proprioception studies on infants demonstrated this (Butterworth & Ciccheti, 1978; Butterworth & Hicks, 1977; Lee & Aaronson, 1974), but is this effect seen in later childhood? Zernicke et al (1982) extended the visual proprioceptive studies of infants by using 7 and 11 year olds who performed five stances from normal two-footed with feet apart through to a one-foot stance, all with or without a target fixation which was a symmetrical cross with 5cm by 1cm arms placed at eye level. Lateral, anterior and posterior measurements were taken from force platforms recordings. Without exception the magnitude of the centre of pressure displacements - lateral, anterior and posterior - was lower for the older children than for the younger children, the average decrease being 35%. The order of difficulty of the balance tasks was the same for both groups. Developmental trends in the use of visual proprioception in balance became apparent during the more novel one foot stands. When the older children were allowed to focus on a target, significant reductions in the lateral sway fluctuations were found. However, the target did not similarly augment balance control for younger children. Neither group of children could use the static target to improve anterior posterior balance on one or two feet. This is an interesting finding as Lee and Lishman (1975) reported that adults were not only able to reduce lateral sway, but also anterior posterior trunk sway by focusing their gaze on a nearby stationary object as opposed to looking at more distant surrounds. In addition, Lee and Aaronson (1974) reported that with toddlers, anterior-posterior stability can be significantly influenced by a structured environment - the "swinging" room. A number of explanations are possible for these seemingly contradictory findings. It is possible that the optical stimulation was great enough for the toddlers, but in the Zernicke et al (1982) study was not powerful enough to affect a change in the anterior-posterior control of children. Adults, however, were able to use such stimulation. Another possibility is that there may be differences according to whether stability is being facilitated or impaired. It is possible that it is easier to impair stability by discrepant moving visual cues, than facilitate it by a stationary target.

We do seem to have some developmental progressions from infancy through adults involving the control of stance by visual proprioceptive information. Before standing behaviour is established, visual proprioceptive information causes alterations in posture: anterior-posterior swaying was quite severely affected. By 7 years of age, the young child can use visual proprioceptive information to his advantage, with lateral sway being reduced in two-footed stance positions. By 11 years of age, this information is now incorporated for aid in lateral stances during novel one-foot stances, and adults can use this information to improve anterior-posterior stances as well as lateral stances. This progression is made up from a very small number of experiments and more are required to confirm or modify this, and to make more fine grained analyses.

A wider age range of children was used by Shumay-Cook and Woollacott (in press) when they examined the developmental changes in the patterns of variability during the emergence of postural synergies in children under 10. These were studied together with age-related changes in visual versus mechanical sources in controlling postural stability, and the development of abilities to resolve intersensory conflicts. Children aged between 15 months and 10 years were placed on a stationary platform which could be perturbed in any direction. There were four sensory conditions: platform normal with eyes open; platform normal with eyes closed; eyes open, platform servoed so that it minimised mechanical proprioceptive perturbance and incongruent information was present to only visual and vestibular modes, eyes closed, platform servoed so that both visual and mechanical perturbance was minimised and incongruent informatin was present to only vestibular modes. Various EMG and stability measurements were taken. Response to platform perturbances in adults produced postural synergies appropriately specific to the direction of body sway. From 7 years of age, there was consistent, stereotypes and fine tuning as seen in dimunition of overall EMG activity over sequential trials. In infants 15 to 31 months of age, there was similar response, but no tuning over trials. From 4 to 6 years of age the children showed great variability of response. The authors suggest development in steps with the system remaining stable until dimensional changes reach a point where previous motor programmes are no longer effective. Thus there is change, transition, variability followed by a plateau of stability and the 4 to 6 year olds could be in a transition period thus evidencing variability. It is always puzzling when with increasing age children show a decrement in performance. There is a tendency to look within the child for the reason when in fact a closer examination of what the task does or does not do could maybe reveal the true state of affairs. In this particular task, the question to ask is what else were the children doing besides those actions being measured? It is realistic to see variability in one aspect of behaviour if the system in other areas is being refined, modified or even stabilised.

It is wise to remember that proprioception is only one part, albeit an important one, of the overall control process. Plateaus and even regressions may be evident in proprioception, yet the movement quality may be improving due to other factors, such as an increased ability to programme movements. Hay (1979) gives us an interesting example of the complexity of change and the inter-relationship between proprioception, visual feedback and programming. She noted three types of movements in fast reaching: at 5 years of age reaching movements were ballistic and open loop with no visual feedback control; this feedback control started to be used at age 7 and at first was a hindrance, and by age 9, children could move with smooth braking, coordinating the proprioceptive information of their hand with the visual information of the total spatial array. The change process here very much reflects that seen in infancy. In both instances, the initial reaching is ballistic, with vision being added which modifies the movement quality, and indeed in the first instance is not beneficial. Vision is then included naturally in the total act, proprioception and vision are coordinated to produce smooth adaptive movements.

PROPRIOCEPTIVE DEVELOPMENT IN HANDICAPPED INDIVIDUALS

An examination of children with different types of handicap can provide us with not only insight into their proprioceptive development, but also helps us understand the general role of proprioception in motor control. In handicapped conditions, various components of the motor control process are altered, arrested or absent. Thus in the blind population lack of vision adds responsibility to the proprioceptive system; in a group of mentally retarded individuals, inadequate cognitive strategies may alter the course of proprioceptive development; and cerebral palsied children may receive ambiguous proprioceptive feedback from muscle and joint linkages. All of these children, as groups, evidence certain types of motor control problems, and their proprioceptive ability may be a contributing factor.

PHYSICAL HANDICAP

Physically handicapped children are an obvious population group with poor motor control, and in the case of cerebral palsied children, neurological damage affecting motor efference is seen as a basic cause of this.

However, this is not the sole cause and proprioceptive influence has been demonstrated on more than one occasion.

Harrison (1975) described the role of afferent feedback in motor control noting that spindle action and other proprioceptors may give out signals that are so difficult to decipher in spastic children, that there is an inability to use them to judge success or otherwise of contraction, particularly if there are numerous simultaneous contractions. In a number of experiments she effectively demonstrated that spastic subjects were not able to match neuromuscular control shown by normal subjects. They were poor at repeating and ranking a set of responses yet they could increase or lower activity in the forearm flexors. That is, they were able to reproduce all tension levels required, but they were poor at repeating them. Thus motor activity could be produced to show all tension levels; yet proprioceptive processes were not efficient enough to give an accurate template of a particular tension level and the child was unable to reproduce it. They were particularly poor at repeating low tension levels which Harrison (1975) explains in signal detection theory terms, with gamma hyperactivity and the contraction of other muscle groups possibly producing a high level of 'noise' against which forearm flexor activity has to be detected. Thus low levels of afferent activity will be detected only rarely. The spastic children were poor at monitoring neuromuscular activity, poor at holding tension level constant and took longer to relax.

Harrison (1975) embarked upon a series of experiments using augmented feedback techniques to improve these abilities. After training, the subjects could relax more quickly, and showed some improvement in the ability to maintain specific levels of neuromuscular activity. They eventually achieved normal accuracy in producing high, low and medium levels of muscular activity and were also accurate in producing sequential and simultaneous patterns of activity in the biceps and forearm flexor muscles. We do not know if this increased ability involving contraction and relaxation led to any improvement of motor control in meaningful functional tasks.

The experimental apparatus and paradigm used by Shumway-Cook and Woollacott (in press) and described earlier, was originally devised by Nashner and his group, who used it with a number of different subject groups including cerebral palsied children (Nashner et al, 1983). They attempted to examine the interaction between central motor programmes and feedback mechanisms in children aged 7 to 9 years of age with clinical evaluation separating them into groups of pure ataxia, spastic hemiplegia, spastic diplegia or athetosis, rather than combinations of these problems. These experiments did tend to separate the cerebral palsied children into their sub-groups; for example, pure spastic hemiplegics had problems in muscle coordination, but were not destabilised by sensory conflicts as were the ataxia group. There appeared to be a breakdown in the structures fixing the temporal and spatial structures of action. The authors felt that the results were in conflict with our assumptions about the role of stretch reflex activity. For example, stretch reflexes in the gastrocnemius were judged elevated in the hemiplegic children and thus would have been unusually responsive to perturbation induced stretch during stance. But the responses of the gastrocnemius to stretch during antero-posterior sway preturbation were delayed (150m/secs compared to 95-110 m/secs in normals) allowing the synergist hamstrings to contract first thereby reversing the normal distal to proximal sequence of contraction. This was not attributed to elevated hamstring stretch responses and they were also a little delayed compared to normals. The authors conclude that pathological changes in stretch reflex machanisms are not the cause of poor movements of a spastic leg during stance but are a secondary symptom to central and spinal motor programmes which dictate the appropriate temporal and spatial structure upon motor activities in synergistic groups of muscles.

Like the Harrison (1975) series of experiments, the Nashner et al (1983) investigations provide some important findings with respect to proprioceptive ability in cerebral palsied children. The level of analysis is more fundamental than in many studies reported here and as such is difficult to compare with more functional investigations.

A final note in this section concerns so called clumsy children who are a group with no obvious constitutional problems, yet are usually defined in terms of their lack of ability on a number of motor tasks. Hulme (1982; 1984) has examined proprioception in a group of 10 year children identified as clumsy, and found them to be performing no better than 6 year old controls on intra and intersensory matching. Although limited in their scope, these studies are some of the few that try to relate proprioceptive perception to some funcitonal measure.

SENSORY LOSS

Loss of vision changes the way of knowing. There is a poverty of environmental description with a lessened knowledge of movements, and this increases processing requirements for other sensory perceptual systems. More attentional capacity is used to process poorer information with the net result of knowing less. In terms of motor control, proprioception takes on a dominant and isolated role, because an absence of vision not only deprives the individual of those resources that are peculiarly obtained from that source, but also prevents the important visual-proprioceptive link-up. In infancy proprioception is not enriched by the visual input and the non modality specific intersensory description of an event is incomplete. The results of this are evident in the delayed motor development of blind babies (Adelson & Fraiberg, 1974; 1976; Fraiberg, 1977; Freedman & Cannady, 1971; Gillman, 1973; Parmelee, 1955).

The stress on the proprioceptive system in blind individuals is not just a straight increase with one sensory system replacing the function of another. There is the overload on the proprioceptive system because of lack of redundancy, increased load on particular processes (short-term memory), inefficiences, selective attending (focusing or narrowing) and lack of anticipation including poorer interpretations and inferences (Shingledecker, 1978; 1981; 1983). Thus proprioceptive processes are over-loaded but how does this affect motor control? The lack of mobility and delayed development is evident, but are movements controlled differently?

Millar (1981) speculates that blind and sighted children on certain movement tasks adopted different processing strategies. In a task which required 3 age groups of children to trace a 5 sided display followed by a recall, there was a significant interaction between sighted status and recall (Millar, 1975). She suggests that blind children used proprioceptive memory which decays with time or is interfered with by subsequent movements. Sighted children who were blindfolded seemed to use visual imagery. Millar (1981) points out one model cannot account for all task and experimental conditions and all levels of processing by the organism. More importantly each model is usually explaining a different level of behaviour. She stresses that intersensory coordination depends on what information is available from vision and proprioception and how individuals code it.

In the blind population there is a lack of mobility with the remaining senses being unable to specify the environmental display in 'far space' as well as vision. the Millar studies suggest that movements in 'near space' are controlled differently with a greater stress on proprioception which is more susceptible to decay or interference. Lack of vision essentially downgrades proprioception as an overall function common to all systems and places greater stress on the other inputs contributing to this function.

COGNITIVE LIMITATIONS

Children with cognitive limitations are a varied lot, with a range of involvement and a diversity of characteristics. As a general guide, the more limited the cognitive ability, the poorer are the motor skills, and it is obvious that proprioception is not the only process that has determined this lower ability. Yet proprioceptive acuity and memory have been seen as such real contributors to motor control, that it was a natural progression for researchers to investigate these processes in the mentally retarded.

By definition these children have poorer cognitive skills than their non-retarded counterparts, and a reasonable prediction would be that as tasks allowed for more cognitive processes, the deficit between the two groups would increase. Indeed a point made by Henderson (1985) about proprioception is that many studies require conceptual decisions rather than solely perceptual discriminations, and this would obviously put the mentally retarded at a disadvantage. Proprioceptive acuity is thought to represent reasonably pure perceptual discriminations and to examine this Sugden and Wann (in preparation) tested two groups of children with moderate learning difficulties on the Laszlo and Bairstow Kinaesthetic sensitivity test. On the acuity task, only 3 out of 31 8-year olds and 4 out of 33 12-year olds reached the mean level score from the normative data. Scores were low, but trends were similar to the normal sample in that there was not much improvement after 7 years of age. When the children were tested on the kinaesthetic perception and memory, it was expected that scores would be correspondingly lower than on the acuity task, because of the greater conceptual demand. This was not the case, with 11 8-year olds out of 31, and 7 12-year olds out of 33 reaching the mean level score from the normative sample. Again developmental trends were similar to the normal sample with improvement between ages 7 and 12.

I would argue that both acuity and memory tasks in these experiments require processing strategies, involving attention and memory. We have sound information in the verbal area for both of these processes being poorer in the mentally retarded, and information in the motor area on memorary skills (Belmont & Butterfield, 1969; Brown & Campione, 1981; Campione & Brown, 1977; Krupski, 1980, for reviews).

Proprioceptive memory was examined by Kelso et al (1979) in 6 and 9 year old mentally retarded children. They found no evidence of a rehearsal strategy over a 15-second retention interval, yet in two further experiments, the children were allowed to preselect their movements with the result that rehearsal was present over a seven second unfilled interval, with the suggestion that some rehearsal may have been continuing over the 15 second unfilled interval. Sugden (1978) examined visual motor memory in mentally retarded children with mental ages of 6, 9 and 12 years, with little evidence of rehearsal being used in any condition at any age. These discrepant findings are not so surprising as Sugden (1978) used vision as well as proprioceptive cues but the movement was constrained. Kelso et al (1979) on the other hand only allowed proprioceptive cues, but individuals could actively preselect their own movements. Reid (1980a) using older mentally retarded individuals (13.8 years to 20.3 years) and again the results confirmed the lack of spontaneous strategy production my mentally retarded subjects. In general, studies indicate that mentally retarded individuals' performance on proprioceptive memory tasks is inhibited by a lack of spontaneous mnemonic strategies. When these strategies are not available, differences between the mentally retarded and non-retarded are minimal. Anwar (1983), for example, reports that Down's Syndrome individuals were better at drawing a shape after it had been presented proprioceptively than visually, but as Henderson (1985) points out the children's fingers were physically guided around the shape which of course places some order on the formation which is not present in the visual condition. The experimenter, actually gave the children the strategy of 'logical search' with the possibility that they may have used the more inefficient 'random exploration' if left on their own. Training has produced some promising results (Reid, 1980b), suggesting that when a strategy is produced, mediation can take place. Flavell (1970) has distinguished between mediational and production deficiences with the former involving strategic behaviour but to no effect, while the latter is when the strategy is not produced in the first place.

Mediation is one of the change processes that Flavell (1972) described as making up the developmental progression. Children spontaneously begin to utilise behaviour X1 as a bridge to influence the formation of X2 without necessarily becoming part of it. Thus certain mnemonic strategies will influence proprioceptive memory and when there is an absence of them, training encourages the use of strategic behaviour which in turn facilitates memory performance. An extension of these training studies encompassing generalisation have been used in the verbal domain but not with proprioceptive memory. This would involve the training of a strategy on one class of movements and determining whether its usefulness is seen in another class.

Down's Syndrome children are a group of mentally retarded individuals with known chromosomal abnormalities and their motor performance is low in comparison to normative data (see Henderson, 1985 for a review). When proprioception has been examined with either vision or motor efference. Vision acting as a proprioceptive function for posture appears to follow a dissimilar course in DS individuals than in normal infants. The DS children in the Butterworth and Ciccheti (1978) study were less responsive to the movement of the room than the normal controls when both groups were seated, but the DS children who had just learned to stand were more responsive. They differed in the way they responded to it in the two positions. The authors argue for postural control being dependent on congruence between mechanical-vestibular and visual indices of posture, and stability is related to the amount of discrepancy tolerated by the system. It was suggested that DS children have a higher threshold for detecting any discrepancy between internal and external sources of perceptual information. The work of Shumway-Cook and Woollacott (in press) confer and expand these findings with their platform perturbation experiments. When the platform was perturbed, the onset latencies of postural muscles of Down's Syndrome children were significantly slower than normal children, and they swayed more, particularly the older group which performed no better than a younger group. The 22-month old were poorly organised, inconsistent and slow in their sway responses, and the authors conclude that equilibrium problems found in Downs Syndrome children are not just delayed normal development, but represent a difference in the evolution and development of postural control.

A final note on proprioceptive ability in Down's Syndrome individuals is provided by Davis and Kelso (1982) when they examined the possibility that muscles are constrained to act as a unit qualitatively similar to a mass spring system. This is a simple model of control with the motor system not needing to know the starting position of a limb, as the muscles will move back to some equilibrium point after being innervated no matter what the amount of direction of the innervation, and this equilibrium point depends upon the stiffness of the flexor and extensor muscles acting on a limb. Using DS individuals and non-retarded controls, they instructed the subjects to hold their fingers against a resistance, and told them not to interfere with finger movement if the load on the finger changed. For both groups of subjects, the joint angle curves looked identical with the results from both groups supporting the notion of muscles constrained as a unit behaving like a mass spring system. The underlying movement organisation was basically the same, with both populations being capable of specifying stiffness and equilibrium length, the system parameters that may determine movement at the joint. There were however, some qualitative differences between the two groups. The DS subjects took longer to reach the target angle and were less able to maintain a steady position once they had reached the target. There was also greater overshoot of fluctuation about the equilibrium point following unloading of the resistance. This is taken as an index of the damping parameter and the DS subjects were underdamped, a position that is characterised by fluctuation about the equilibrium position and for most purposes is unstable. In a second experiment, the task was identical except the subjects were required to maintain their original position when the resistance changed. The DS subjects were able to increase a stiffness parameter voluntarily when asked to tense their muscles against a load change. There were wide individual differences in both groups but in general the non-retarded controls increased stiffness to a greater extent than the DS subjects.

CONCLUDING COMMENTS

The preceding section on mentally retarded children presents most of the issues that can be raised when examining the development of proprioceptive control. The range of paradigms and concepts embraced by proprioception make it difficult to pull out developmental threads. However, a starting point is the relationship between proprioceptive perception, and proprioceptive control. When Sugden and Wann (in preparation) measured proprioceptive perception (acuity and memory) in children with learning difficulties, there was a very low correlation and poor prediction between that and motor impairment as measured by a standardised test. But why should we expect any relationship? In one situation, we have a test assessing static measures of acuity and memory with few time constraints, drawing on a limited number of structures, while in the second we have a global measure of motor impairment requiring numerous abilities often having to be performed spontaneously and with severe time constraints. It does suggest that when we are investigating skilled actions, proprioceptive control would seem the more useful variable to measure.

Another issue in proprioceptive control is the role that cognition plays. The paradigms of the 1970s involving short term memory often investigated various so called cognitive strategies, couched within information processing terms. There were many attempts to use strategies from the verbal domain and investigate them in the motor area. Proprioceptive memory provided the vehicle for these investigations, with the suggestion that many of the strategies could be conscious in nature. On the other hand proprioceptive control is often studied in situations where fast natural responses are required and the role of cognitive strategies is minimised. Indeed this difference has reflected the change in research directions from cognitive and processing involvement in motor control to the study of action, with the emphasis on motor systems rather than cognitions. Our teasing out of individual components suggesting processing capacities and strategies has given us more detail about an act, but we have often lost the totality of the act itself. It would appear to be more fruitful for research in this area to be more action oriented, with less emphasis on static measures and cognitions. The studies on reaching, grasping and catching, facial imitations and postural controls are models for the future.

References

Alderson, E. & Fraiberg, S. (1974). Gross motor development in infants blind from birth. *Child Development, 45,* 126-144.

Adelson, E. & Fraiberg, S. (1976). Sensory deficit and motor development in infants blind from birth. In Z.S. Jastrzembska (Ed.), *On the effects of blindness and other impairments on early development.* New York: American Foundation for the Blind.

Anwar, F. (1983). The role of sensory modality for the reproduction of shape by the severely retarded. *British Journal of Developmental Psychology,* 317-327.

Belmont, J.M. & Butterfield, E.C. (1969). The relation of short term memory to development and intelligence. In L.C. Lipsitt and H.W. Reese (Eds.), *Advances in child development and behavior.* Vol. 4. New York: Academic Press.

Bairstow, P.J. & Laszlo, J.I. (1981). Kinaesthetic sensitivity to passive movements and its relationship to motor development and motor control. *Developmental Medicine & Child Neurology, 23,* 606-616.

Birch, H.G. & Lefford, A. (1964). Intersensory development in children. *Monographs of the Society for Research in Child Development, 32,* (2, serial no. 110).

Bower, T.G.R. (1977). *A Primer of infant development.* San Francisco: Freeman.

Bower, T.G.R. & Wishart, J.G. (1972). The effects of motor skill on object permanence. *Cognition 1,* 165-172.

Brown, A.D. & Campione, J.C. (1981). Inducing flexible thinking: the problem of access. In M.P. Freidman, J.P. Das and N. O'Connor (Eds.), *Intelligence and learning.* New York: Plenum Press.

Bushell, E.W. (1981). The ontogency of intermodal relations: vision and touch in infancy. In R.D. Walk and H.L. Pick (Ed.), *Intersensory perception and sensory integration.* New York: Plenum Press.

Butterworth, G.e. & Ciccheti, D. (1978). Visual calibration of posture in normal and motor retarded Down's Syndrome infants. *Perception, 7,* 513-525.

Butterworth, G.E. & Hicks, L. (1977). Visual proprioception and postural stability in infants: a developmental study. *Perception, 6,* 255-262.

Campione, J.C. & Brown, A.L. (1977). Memory and metamemory development in educable retarded children. In R.V. Kail and J.w. Hagen (Eds.), *Perspectives on the development of memory and cognition.* Hillsdale, N.Y.: Lawrence Erlbaum Associates.

Changeux, J.P. (1985). Remarks on the complexity of the nervous system and its ontogenesis. In J. Mehler and R. Fox (Eds.), *Neonate cognition: beyond the blooming buzzing-confusion.* Hillsdale, N.J.: Erlbaum.

Connolly, K. & Jones, B. (1970). A developmental study of afferent - reafferent integration. *British Journal of Psychology, 61,22,* 259-266.

Davis, W.E. & Kelso, J.A.S. (1982). Analysis of "invariant characteristics" in the motor control of Down's Syndrome and normal subjects. *Journal of Motor Behavior, 14, 3,* 194-213.

Flavell, J.H. (1970). Developmental studies of mediated memory. In H.W. Reese and L.P. Lipsitte (Eds.), *Advances in child development and behavior.* New York: Academic Press.

Flavell, J.H. (1972). An analysis of cognitive-development sequences. *Genetic Psychology Monographs, 86,* 279-350.

Fraiberg, S. (1977). *Insights from the blind.* New York: Basic Books.

Freedman, D.A. & Cannady, C. (1971). Delayed emergence of prone locomotion. *Journal of Mental and Nervous Diseases, 153,* 108-117.

Gibson, J.J. (1966). *The senses considered as perceptual systems.* Boston: Houghton-Mifflin.
Gillman, A.A. (1973). Handicaps and cognition: visual deprevation and the rate of motor development in infants. *New Outlook for the Blind, 67,* 309-314.
Harrison, A. (1975). Studies of neuromuscular control in normal and plastic individuals. In K. Holt (Ed.), *Movement and child development.* London: Heinemann Medical.
Hay, L. (1979). Spatial-temporal analysis of movements in children: Motor programs versus feedback in the development of reaching. *Journal of Motor Behavior, 11,* 189-200.
Henderson, S.E. (1985). Motor skill development in Down's Syndrome. In D. Lane and B. Stratford (Eds.), *Current approaches to Down's Syndrome.* Eastbourne: Holt Saunders.
Hofsten, C. von (1979). Development of visually directed reaching: the approach phase. *Journal of Human Movement Studies, 5,* 160-178.
Hofsten, C. von (1980). Predictive reaching for moving objects by human infants. *Journal of Experimental Child Psychology, 1, 30,* 369-382.
Hofsten, C. von (1982). Eye hand coordination in the newborn. *Developmental Psychology, 18,* 450-467.
Hofsten, C. von (1983). Catching skills in infancy. *Journal of Experimental Psychology: Human Perception and Performance, 9,* 75-85.
Hofsten, C. von & Lindhagen, C. (1979). Observations on the development of reaching for moving objccts. *Journal of Experimental Child Psychology, 28,* 158-173.
Hulme, C., Biggerstaff, A., Moran, G. & McKinlay, I. (1984). Visual kinaesthetic and cross modal judgements of length by clumsy children: a comparison with young normal children. *Child Care & Health Development, 10, 2,* 117-125.
Imbert, M. (1985). Physiological underpinnings of perceptual development. In J. Mehler and R. Fox (Eds.), *Neonate cognition: beyond the blooming buzzing confusion.* Hillsdale, N.Y.: Lawrence Erlbaum Associates.
Jones, B. (1981). The developmental significance of cross modal matching. In R.D. Walk and H.L. Pick (Eds.), *Intersensory perception and sensory integration.* New York: Plenum Press.
Jones, B. (1982). The development of intermodal coordination and motor control. In J.A.S. Kelso and J.E. Clark (Eds.), *The development of movement control and coordination.* New York: Wiley.
Kelso, J.A.S., Goodman, D., Stamm, C.L. & Hayes, C. (1979). Movement coding and memory in retarded children. *American Journal of Mental Deficiency, 83,* 601-611.
Keogh, J.F. & Sugden, D.A. (1985). *Movement skill development.* New York: MacMillan.
Krupski, A. (1980). Attention processes: research, theory, and implications for special education. In B.K. Keogh (Ed.), *Advance in special education. Vol. 1.* Greenwich, Connecticut: J.A.I. Press.
Lasky, R.E. (1977). The effect of visual feedback of the hand on the reaching and retrieval behaviour of young infants. *Child Development, 48,* 112-117.
Laszlo, J.I. & Bairstow, P.J. (1980). The measurement of kinaesthetic sensitivity in children and adults. *Developmental Medicine and Child Neurology, 22,* 454-464.
Laszlo, J.I. & Bairstow, P.J. (1985). *Perceptual-motor behaviour: developmental assessment and therapy.* London: Holt, Rinehart & Winston.
Lee, D.N. & Aaronson, E. (1974). Visual proprioceptive control of standing in human infants. *Perception and Psychophysics, 15,* 529-532.
Lee, D.N. & Lishman, J.R. (1975). Visual proprioceptive control of stance. *Journal of Human Movement Studies, 1,* 87-95.

Meltzoff, A.N. & Moore, M.K. (1977). Imitation of facial and manual gestures by human neonates. *Science, 198,* 75-78.
Meltzoff, A.N. & Moorem M.K. (1983). The origins of imitation in infancy: Paradigm, phenomena and theories. In L.P. Lipsitt and C.K. Rouvee-Collier (Eds.), *Advances in Infancy research.* Norwood, N.J.: Ablex.
Meltzoff, A.N. & Moore, M.K. (1985). cognitive foundations and social functions of imitation and intermodal representation in infancy. In J. Mehler and R. Fox (Eds.), *Neonate cognition: beyond the blooming buzzing confusion.* Hillsdale, N.J.: Erlbaum.
Millar, S. (1974). Tactile short term memory by blind and sighted children. *British Journal of Psychology, 65,* 253-263.
Millar, S. (1975). Effects of input conditions on intramodal and cross modal usual and kinaesthetic matches by children. *Journal of Experimental Child Psychology, 19,* 63-78.
Millar, S. (1975). Spatial memory by blind and sighted children. *British Journal of Psychology, 56,* 449-459.
Millar, S. (1978). Short-term serial tactual recall: effects of grouping on tactually probed recall of Braille letters and nonsense shapes by blind children. *British Journal of Psychology, 66,* 17-24.
Millar, S. (1981). Cross modal and intersensory perception and the blind. In R.D. Walk and H.L. Pick (Eds.), *Intersensory perception and sensory integration.* New York: Plenum Press, 1981.
Nashner, L.M., Shumway- Cook, A. & Marin, O. (1983). Stance posture control in select groups of children with cerebral palsy: deficits in sensory organisation and muscular condition. *Experimental Brain Research, 49,* 393-409.
Parmelee, A.H. (1955). The developmental evaluation of the blind premature infant. *American Journal of Diseases of Children, 90,* 135-140.
Parmelee, A.H. (1966). Developmental studies of blind children: I. *New Outlook for the Blind, 60,* 177-179.
Parmelee, A.H. & Sigman, M. (1983). Perinatal brain development and behaviour. In M. Haith and J. Campos (Eds.), *Biology and infancy.* New York: Wiley.
Reid, G. (1980). The effects of memory strategy instruction in the short motor memory of the mentally retarded. *Journal of Motor Behavior, 12,* 221-227.
Reid, G. (1980). Overt and covert rehearsal in short term motor memory of mentally retarded and non-retarded persons. *American Journal of Mental Deficiency, 85,* 66-77.
Shingledecker, C.A. (1978). The effects of anticipationon performance and processing load in blind mobility. *Ergonomics, 21,* 355-371.
Shingledecker, C.A. (1981). Handicap and human skill. In D.H. Holding (Ed.), *Human skills.* New York: Wiley.
Shingledecker, C.A. (1983). Measuring the mental effort of blind mobility. *Journal of Visual Impairment and blindness, 77.*
Shumway-Cook, A. & Woollacott, M.H. (in press). The growth of stability: postural control from a developmental perspective.
Shumway-Cook, A. & Woollacott, M.H. (in press). Dynamics of postural control in the child with Down's Syndrome.
Smyth, M.M. (1984). Perception and action. In M.M. Smyth and A.M. Wing (Eds.), *The Psychology of human movement.* London: Academic Press.
Sugden, D.A. (1978). Visual motor memory in educationally subnormal boys. *British Journal of Educational Psychology, 48,* 330-339.
Sugden, D.A. (1980). Developmental strategies in motor and visual motor short term memory. *Perceptual and Motor Skills, 51,* 146.

Sugden, D.A. & Wann, C. (Manuscript in preparation). Assessment of motor performance in children with moderate learning difficulties.

Wishart, J.G., Bower, T.G.R. & Dunkeld, J. (1978). Reaching in the dark. *Perception, 7,* 507-512.

Zernicke, R.F., Gregor, R.J. & Cratty (1982). Balance and visual proprioception in children. *Journal of Human Movement Studies, 8,* 1-13.

POSTURAL CONTROL

P.J. Bairstow

1. INTRODUCTION

The term "postural control" means different things to different people. Clinical workers when speaking of patients with poor postural control often are referring to self-prescribed postures, and abnormalities of function that are apparent when a patient is standing or seated in his usual way. Figure 1a shows a 10 year old child with a neuropathy attempting to stand, and Figure 1b a 12 year old boy with cerebral palsy in a distorted standing posture; both are in a posture of their own prescription.

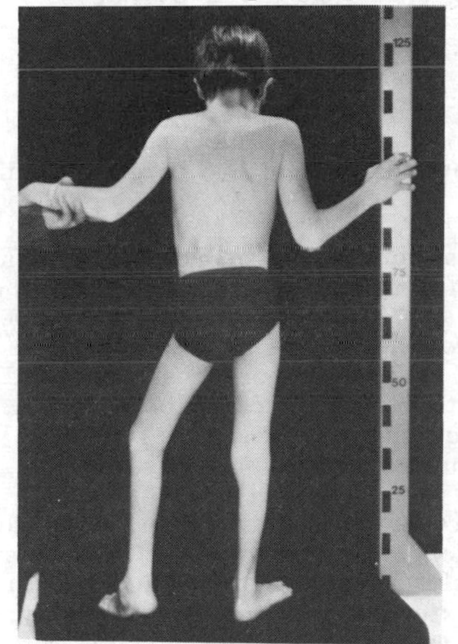

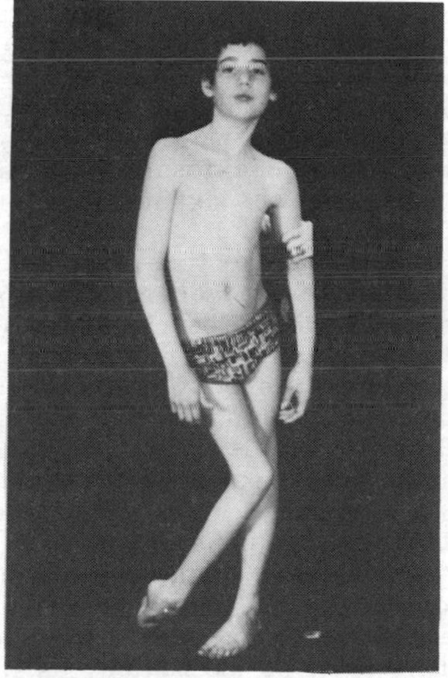

Fig. 1. Children with abnormal motor functioning, in standing postures of their own prescription.
LEFT: 10 year old child with a neuropathy
RIGHT: 12 year old boy with cerebral palsy.

When teachers of dance speak of pupils with good or bad postural control they can be referring to the ability to achieve and maintain a posture in accordance with an external prescription. Figure 2 shows a 7 year old girl attempting to copy a posture given by the teacher.

Research workers who talk about studies on postural control are usually

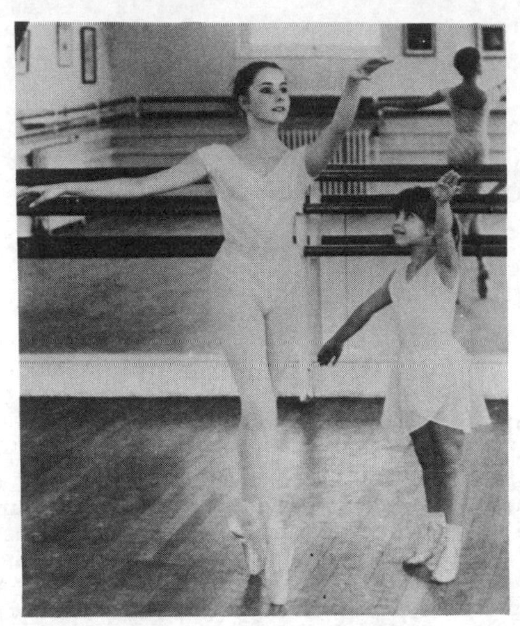

Fig. 2. A 7 year old girl copying a posture given by her dancing teacher.

talking about the ability to maintain a basic posture when one part of the body is voluntarily moved (e.g., staying upright while reaching out with an arm), or when an external force is applied to the body (e.g., standing still when someone leans against you).

From the above it is apparent that four types of motor functioning can be listed under the general heading of postural control: (1) achieving and maintaining a self-prescribed posture and (2) an externally-prescribed posture, and (3) maintaining a posture when there is a self-induced change in one part of the body and (4) when there is an externally induced change This multiple meaning of the term postural control could be somewhat worrying. However, while each type of functioning has its own literature, on reflection, they depend on a common underlying system of control.

The present paper grew from a review of, in the main, physiological literature relevant to the above functions. The review lead to the development of a unifying construct which helps tie together publications in a number of areas, and which may be extended for thinking about dynamic situations such as locomotion, as well as motor development and motor disorders. No attempt is made to place the construct within the context of existing theories or models relating to any of the above four types of functions. Rather, the construct was developed "from scratch", from a detailed consideration of the first type of postural control, and with the intention of subsequently bringing together the other types in a single framework.

2. SELF-PRESCRIBED POSTURES

People take up postures for particular situations and needs - postures that are sometimes characteristic of the individual. Figure 3 is a drawing of

Suzie watching television; she habitually sits in this position for rather long periods of time (!).

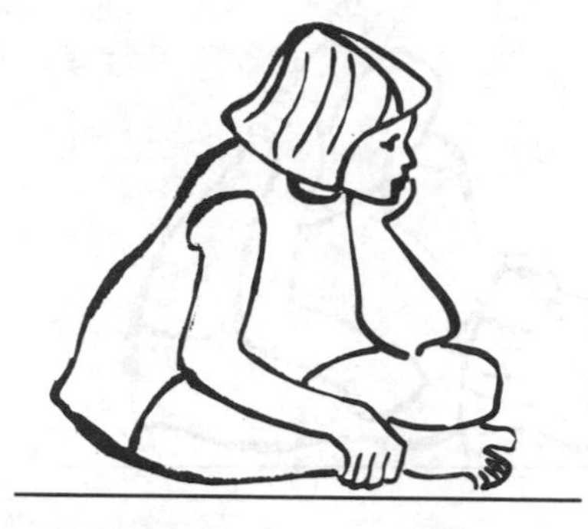

Fig. 3. A drawing of Suzie in a characteristic self-prescribed posture.

I want to consider this posture in some detail, to elaborate concepts that will be central for later sections. I shall begin with a logical analysis and a discussion of the physical and physiological specification of this posture - not how Suzie got herself into this shape, but to describe the nature of her present condition.

The posture can be described in terms of a combination of joint angles; one could bend a wire model into this shape and the combination of angles defines this geometric shape and no other shape. A joint angle causes stretching of muscles, tendons and ligaments. Kinaesthetic receptors (Burgess, Wei, Clark & Simon, 1982), have different inputs for different angles. All the angles making up this posture generate a pattern of kinaesthetic input for this shape.

But there is more to specifying this posture than the pattern of joint angles. Various segments of the body are in mutual contact. One could have the situation of nearly identical joint angles, but with body surfaces separated by part of a millimetre. In the present case, however, areas of the skin are in mutual contact. This mutual contact generates a pattern of input from receptors in the skin - the cutaneous receptors (e.g., Lamb, 1983). Hence, the kinaesthetic pattern of input from joint angles has a coexisting cutaneous pattern of input from the skin-to-skin contact.

There is still more to defining this posture; Suzie could probably get herself into the position shown in Figure 4 - or something close to it. There would be a similar pattern of joint angles and a similar pattern of skin-to-skin contact, as before, but the different orientation has different sensory and motor characteristics. Going back to Figure 3, this orientation generates specific input from the vestibular apparatus (e.g., Parker, 1980), from the eyes, and input from the cutaneous receptors in the skin at the floor surface. One must now add to the specification, a coexisting pattern of vestibular, visual and additional cutaneous input.

Suzie is actively maintaining her posture; if she didn't she would collapse. Forces that are passively generated by gravity acting on the body and by visco-elastic properties of muscles, by themselves, make this shape - made up as it is of mobile segments - unstable. This pattern of forces

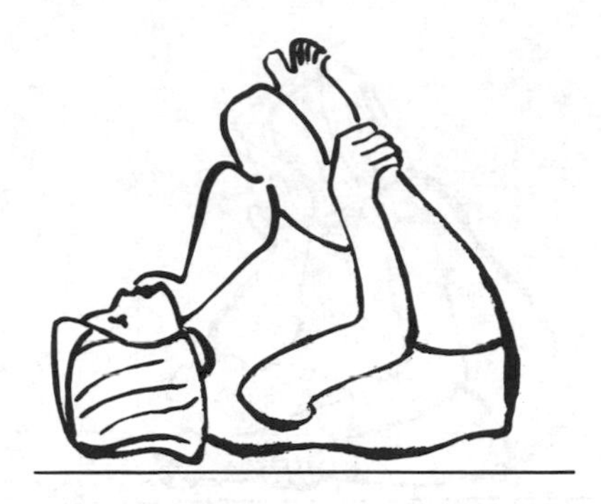

Fig. 4. An alternative orientation of the same shaped posture shown in Figure 3.

depends on the dimensions and construction (e.g., muscle mass) of the body, the shape of the posture, and the body's orientation with respect to gravity. A counteracting and stabilising pattern of forces is actively generated by way of a pattern of motor commands to muscles all over the body which pull on the segments. The pattern of passively and actively generated forces in combination, generate a pattern of input from kinaesthetic and cutaneous receptors.

In summary, Suzie's current postural state can be physically described as a body of particular physical dimensions, with mobile segments under the influence of forces, being maintained in a configuration of joint angles, skin-to-skin contact, and orientation. The posture is physiologically specified according to the above physical descriptions. Hence, the motor output pattern is determined by all of the above physical factors in combination; a different body dimension, joint angle, orientation, or mutual contact, would necessitate a different motor output pattern. The kinaesthetic input pattern is determined by the joint angles and the motor output pattern, in combination. The cutaneous input pattern is determined by the combination of orientation, mutual skin contact, and the motor output pattern. Visual and vestibular input is determined by orientation.

The above five physiological factors are shown in Figure 5a and I shall often refer to them as sets. Any one of these sets is insufficient to specify the posture. For example, the pattern of motor output cannot be specified unless joint angles, and orientation are taken into account; the pattern of kinaesthetic input relevant to joint angles is insufficient if there is not a pattern of motor output to maintain the angles; the pattern of input from cutaneous receptors at the floor surface is common to a large number of other postures. The first point I wish to make is that all of these physiological patterns or sets, in combination, specify this posture. This notion is visualised in Figure 5b. The shaded area is to be called a conjoint set; it is a conjoint set of sensory and motor patterns which is a posture's specification.

The sets shown in Figure 5b are not completely superimposed because I wish to imply that some of them separately, may be present in other conditions as well. Getting oneself into a familiar posture involves setting up such a conjoint set of sensory and motor patterns. Once in the posture, we

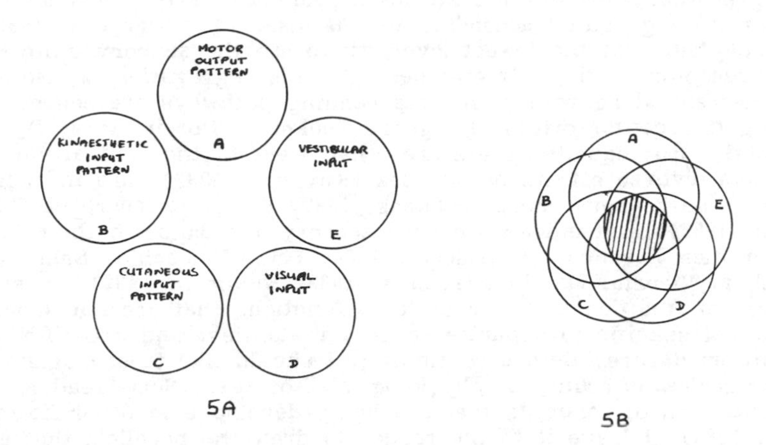

Fig. 5. A diagramatic representation of the different sensory and motor physiological patterns of neural activity associated with a posture.
5a: the individual patterns of activity
5b: the combination of patterns which physiologically specify a posture. The shaded area is termed a conjoint set of sensory and motor patterns (see text).

generally recognise it as being appropriate in global terms. We should all be familiar with the everyday experience of being in a favourite and comfortable posture, and recognising it, without being aware of the separate patterns making up the posture (e.g., sitting at ones desk).

2.1. Evidence for conjoint sensory and motor functioning

Now I would like to move on to physiological data, to consider why it is necessary to talk in terms of patterns of motor output, patterns of sensory input, and conjoint sets of patterns. What is the physiological evidence for this notion of sensory and motor conjoint specification and recognition of a posture?

I should begin with some discussion of what I will be referring to when using the term "pattern". Briefly, I will mean patterns of neural activity within the central nervous system; patterns which are both spatial (activity distributed across groups of neurons at given points in time) and temporal (patterns of activity extending across time within a group of neurons). While the basic idea of motor and sensory functioning depending on patterns of neural activity is hardly a point of controversy, I shall be developing the notion perhaps further than usual. There is a growing realisation among physiologists that future modelling of sensory and motor functioning will have to take account of the rules by which patterns of neural activity arising from different sources are combined into new patterns within the central nervous system. This direction of thinking is a distinct move away from traditional research which has focussed on segregated functions. Separate sensory and motor structures, pathways, centres and functions have been well documented. On the motor side, at the lowest level, there are the motor units (Burke, 1980) - discrete motor nerves with their own muscle fibres.

This segregation is maintained within the central nervous system; descending pathways are segregated according to muscles (e.g., Kuypers, 1982). On the sensory side, at the lowest level, there are the sensory units - discrete sensory receptors with their own nerves. This segregation is also maintained within the central nervous system; ascending pathways are segregated according to receptor origin (Burgess, Tuckett & Horch, 1984; Dykes, 1983; Kaas, 1983). But equally, there are other areas of the central nervous system which have diverse effects on muscles (Kuypers, 1982), are influenced by more than one sensory receptor (Kaas, 1982; Kang, Herman, MacGillis & Zarzechi, 1985), and indeed are both sensory and motor in their functional characteristics (Asanuma & Arissian, 1984; Fetz, Finocchio, Baker & Soso, 1980; Ghez, Vicario, Martin & Yumiya, 1983; Kuypers, 1982). In such areas specificity of function is subordinate to functions that are not specific to muscles, not specific to separate sensory modalities, and are both sensory and motor in nature. Before continuing, I should like to say again that the following review is mainly of physiological literature. Some readers may be aware of echoes of concepts that are being developed in other literature (e.g., Whiting, 1984). I leave it to the reader to draw the parallels that exist between current thinking in physiological and psychological work on motor skills.

2.1.1. Conjoint motor functioning

I will first take each of the patterns shown in Figure 5a individually, beginning with the motor pattern; I will discuss why it is necessary to think in terms of patterns of motor output, and put forward the notion that the total pattern is, itself, a conjoint set made up of motor subsets.

While motor units are discrete, there is nothing specific in the way they are employed in motor activities. Take as an example one motor nerve to the biceps muscle; it may be active during elbow flexion, a lengthening contraction (extension), forearm supination, shoulder flexion, and elbow fixation. (As an aid to understanding this point, it is useful to place a hand on your biceps and feel that it is active during all of these actions). One motor action cannot be distinguished from another according to whether a particular motor nerve is active, because a single nerve is employed in many actions. The effect of activity in a given nerve on the state of a limb, depends on the context in which it is active (Desmedt, 1980). So, in our example, activity in a motor nerve to the biceps will be associated with elbow fixation if the total force generated by the biceps is balanced by other forces; elbow movement will occur if the forces are not in balance, and whether the movement is flexion, extension or supination, will depend on what other muscles are simultaneously active. It is the pattern of activation of the total population of motor nerves to all the muscles of the arm which is an important determinant of what will happen at the elbow joint. This pattern can be thought as one motor subset. A similar description can be made of other joints involved in an action - there are many other motor subsets. One can go further in building a picture of patterns of motor output associated with separate body segments, combining into a conjoint set for the whole body; each subset can be found in other actions, and only the total combined pattern fully describes the motor component of a body posture.

While it is necessary to think in terms of a pattern of output to muscles, it is quite another matter to explain how these patterns are generated. How are the motor nerves to different muscles, functionally combined to cooperate in a unitary action? There is no clear answer to this question, but there is physiological data which is beginning to define the picture. Organised patterns of neural activity which ultimately shape the pattern of activity in the population of nerves going to the muscles, can be found at many levels of the central nervous system (Murphy, Wong & Kwan, 1985). For example, Georgopoulos, Kalaska, Caminiti and Massey (1982) and Georgopoulos, Caminiti, Kalaska and Massey (1983) recorded the activity of cells within the motor cortex of monkeys as movements were made in different directions with an upper limb. It was found that individual cells in the cortex are active for more than one particular direction and force of a limb response. Individual cells are broadly "tuned" - they are maximally active for one direction but have a lower level of activity for neighbouring directions as well. It was suggested that the population discharge of all the directionally tuned cortical cells generates a response in a certain direction with a certain force. It is evident that there are functions high in the motor system which generate patterns of activity in ensembles of neurones; these patterns, effectively, combine or functionally conjoin separate motor nerves, to serve a common purpose.

The notion that different muscles operate conjointly and in a functional unit can be found in other studies which report a degree of functional linkage or combined action of different body parts engaged in a single activity (Baldissera, Cavallari & Civaschi, 1982; Corcos, 1984; Gielen, Vanden Heuvel and Van Gisbergen, 1984).

2.1.2. Conjoint sensory functioning

Turning to the input patterns, there is a wealth of literature supporting the notion that individual sensory receptors do not usually have isolated effects. Moreover, isolated input is ambiguous and only has "meaning" for an animal when taken along with a total pattern.

The kinaesthetic modality provides a clear illustration of this point. In the previous section there is a discussion of the multifunctional nature of motor units and muscles. Just as muscles are multifunctional so their receptors respond in more than one joint position, more than one direction of a limb response, and under more than one condition of active and passive force. Receptor physiologists (e.g., Simon, Wei, Randic & Burgess, 1984) have come to the conclusion that individual kinaesthetic receptors give input that is ambiguous in terms of what is happening at a joint. The receptors are broadly "tuned" in regard to the limb actions which activate them, yet accurate information about what is going on at a joint is somehow available for perceptual and motor systems. It has been suggested that the total pattern of input from the population of kinaesthetic receptors in someway defines what is happening, although the exact nature of this pattern, and the method by which it is interpreted by the central nervous system has yet to be defined.

A broadly similar story - of sensory function depending on a pattern of responses in a group of sensory nerves - has been proposed for other sensory modalities. Erikson (1982, 1984) has formulated an across fibre pattern theory, in which individual sensory nerves lack specificity of function; the internal code for a particular sensory stimulus is not activity in specialised neurones, but rather the ratio or relative amounts of activity in several parallel nerves. The total pattern of activity in the sensory system is the internal code for a particular stimulus condition.

I now move on to consider the combining of neural patterns relevant to separate sensory modalities. Just as activity in a single sensory nerve gives ambiguous information, so also the pattern of activity within a modality very often only has use in the context of input received from other modalities.

It is very common to be in a situation of receiving multimodality input; Suzie's television posture is one such example (Figure 3). The sensory system operates in such a way to combine input from separate sources, and perception, for example, frequently involves the coalescence of input provided by different modalities. It is not difficult to find data showing the combined action at many levels, of vestibular and visual inputs (Jouen, 1984; Miles, 1984), kinaesthetic and cutaneous inputs (Craske, Kenny & Kieth, 1984), kinaesthetic and vestibular inputs (Lund & Broberg, 1983), visual and kinaesthetic inputs (Lackner & Levine, 1978, 1979; Lackner & Taublieb, 1984; Mather & Lackner, 1980). In a physiological study, Zarzecki and Wiggin (1982) reported on the convergence of sensory inputs upon neurons of the somatosensory cortex, and concluded that the cortex of the awake, behaving animal receives afferent information not in the form of impulses from one or another peripheral nerve or receptive field, but rather in the form of constellations of inputs from a variety of receptors in many different locations in the body. Another study on the somatosensory cortex was reported by Jennings, Lamour, Solis and Fromm (1983). Monkeys were trained to maintain postural stability of the forearm in various positions against various loads. The activity of single neurons was recorded and it was concluded that it was activity in the population of neurons as a whole that signalled uniquely the steady posture of the limb and the force exerted by the limb. While the cortex is the focus of convergence of many different inputs, exactly how the inputs are combined into new central patterns of activity, and the rules for combination, have yet to be fully established.

At a functional level, Ryan (1940) in his paper on the interrelations of the sensory systems in perception, developed a notion of a dynamic interplay between sensory stems, such that one system cooperates with another for the perception of a total meaningful situation; perceptions transcend the sensory pattern of a single mode, and exist in a single spatial frame which is continuous from one modality to another.

2.1.3. Conjoint sensory-motor functioning

Turning now to evidence for a conjoint functioning of sensory and motor systems, there is a wealth of physiological data which shows that motor centres have a direct effect on sensory input, and sensory input has a direct effect on motor centres. An action of the body can be conceived of, only in terms of conjoint patterns of sensory and motor activity.

Figure 6 is taken from Wiesendanger (1969), and gives an example of how motor commands affect the transmission and processing of sensory input. The pyramidal tract, sending motor commands down to the spinal cord, also has collaterals going to the sensorimotor cortex, thalamic nuclei, reticular formation, dorsal column nuclei, etc. All these recipients of collaterals are centres for the transmission and processing of sensory input. This means that at least part of sensory input cannot ascend to any level of the central nervous system in a pure form; as it ascends, it is combined with motor commands responsible for current muscle activity. Certainly the pattern of input received at the cerebral cortex when an individual is actively controlling his musculature is a blend of sensory and motor patterns. (See also Angel & Malenka, 1982; Chapin & Woodward, 1982; Coulter, 1974; Humphrey

& Corrie, 1978; Tsumoto, Nakamura & Iwana, 1975; Zarzecki & Wiggin, 1982).

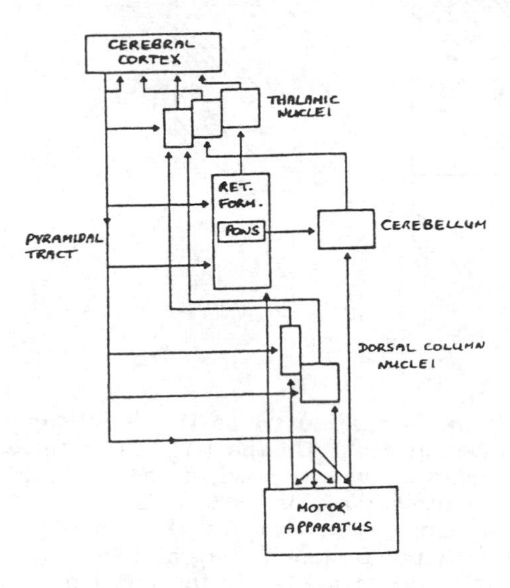

Fig. 6. The pyramidal tract, originates in the sensorimotor cortex and terminates close to motor nerves. The tract sends off collaterals to areas of the central nervous system concerned with the transmission and processing of sensory input. Ascending patterns of input are modified by descending patterns of motor output (Redrawn from Wiesendanger, 1969).

There is some highly suggestive behavioural evidence for this blending of motor and sensory patterns. Bairstow and Laszlo (1980) reported experiments in which blindfolded subjects moved around previously unseen stencil patterns. The patterns were arbitrary, curved, closed shapes and two families of stencils were constructed; one in which the interior of the shape was raised above the level of the backing board, the other in which the interior of the shape was recessed. The blindfolded subjects held a stylus in the hand, and moved around the raised edge. The construction of the stencils imposed a directional bias in the motor commands; for one set the subjects had to move toward the inside of the pattern, for the other set toward the outside. While the actual movements around the two sets were identical in shape and size, subjects perceived, tracked, and recalled the patterns with directional biases in size depending on the direction in which the movement was commanded (see Figure 7). In other studies of the perception of limb position, Feldman and Latash (1982) write that the perception and control of joint angle are closely interrelated processes, and the perception of joint positions is a combined function of sensory and motor activity.

In a similar way to motor patterns combining with sensory patterns in sensory systems, sensory patterns combine with motor patterns in the motor system. Very briefly, motor nerves in the spinal cord are the focus of

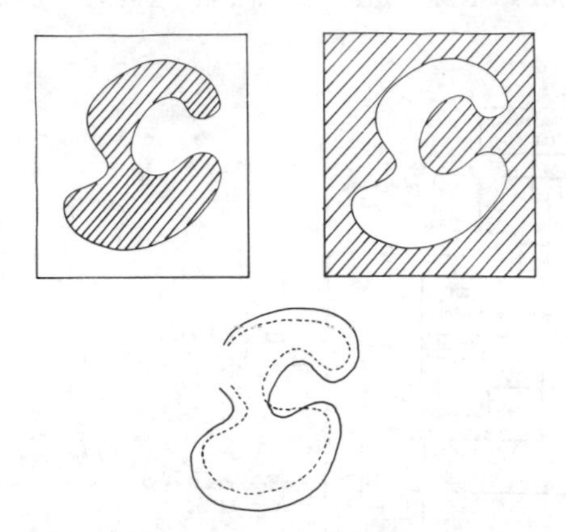

Fig. 7. The top part of the figure illustrates the construction of two sets of stencil patterns. On the left, the interior of the pattern is raised above the level of the backing board; on the right, the interior of the pattern is recessed. The lower part of the figure shows the result of a tracking task performed with these stencils. Right hand movements around the stencils were tracked by the left hand. The left hand movement showed systematic biases depending on how the right hand movement was commanded (Redrawn from Bairstow & Laszlo, 1980).

convergence of commands from within the central nervous system, along with activity from sensory receptors (Andreassen & Rosenfalck, 1980; Behrends, Schomburg & Steffens, 1983). At the level of the motor cortex, neurones are under the constant influence of sensory inputs. Asanuma and Arissian (1984) reported experiments on the functional role of peripheral input to the motor cortex during voluntary movements in the monkey, and concluded that sensory input functions by selectively changing the excitability of cortical efferent zones before and during the execution of voluntary movements. In a similar way Georgopoulos, Kalaska, Caminiti and Massey (1983), from exepriments on monkeys, concluded that motor cortical commands subserving arm movements are processes which can be affected in the course of their formation and/or execution, by changes in afferent controlling inputs. In short, motor activity at many levels of the central nervous system is a blend of motor and sensory patterns.

2.2. Representation of conjoint sensory and motor patterns

In the previous sections, discussion has centered on the coexistence and blending of sensory and motor patterns of neural activity which specify a posture. I will now consider the point that we can readily take up a characteristic posture, and we immediately have a sense of it being appropriate. A familiar example is when we are preparing to go to sleep; many of us curl up in a similar way night after night (see Figure 8). Another example for anyone who has done yoga, is how quickly a posture can be taken up, and how immediately familar it can feel. How can one explain the rapid taking up of a stereotyped or characteristic posture?

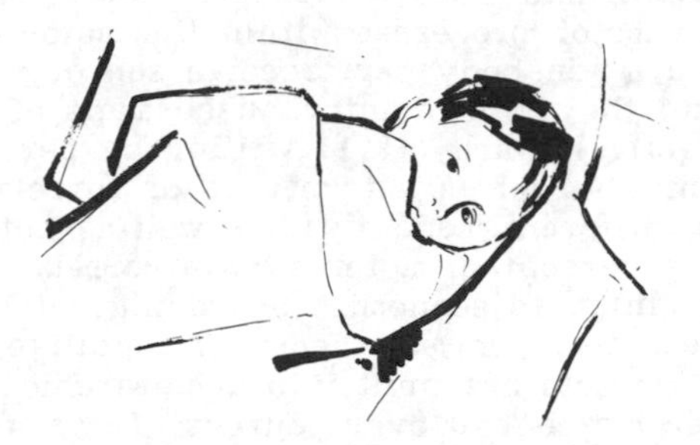

Fig. 8. A drawing of a child preparing for sleep. We can readily take up a characteristic posture, and we immediately have a sense of it being appropriate in global terms.

There is a suggestion in the writings of some authors that after repeated experiences with a given motor action, functional links are forged between coexisting or related sensory and motor factors. Figure 9, taken from Laszlo and Bairstow (1985) is one illustration of this kind of notion. I refer to it here, not because the concept it encapsulates is novel (see Buckingham, 1984; Mandler, 1962; Smith, 1984), but rather because an explicit diagram can help to focus an idea and make it easier to communicate. During any action, there are a large number of discrete sensory and motor events registered as focii of activity within the central nervous system. These events either co-exist at given points in time, or are related across time. With repeated experiences, links are forged between the discrete events; these links are depicted as the double-headed arrows, forming an internalised structure for the action.

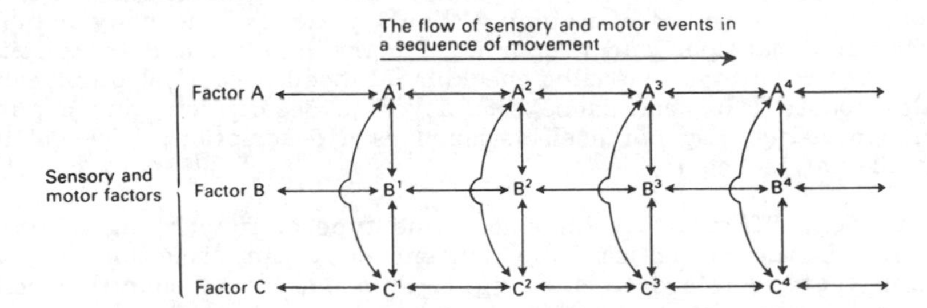

Fig. 9. Diagram illustrating links between sensory and motor events. The numbered letters (eg, A1, A2, A3) represent discrete sensory and motor events at different points in time. Vertical arrows represent relationships at particular points in time between neural inputs to different sensory receptors ,between neural outputs to different muscle groups, and between input and output. Horizontal arrows represent relationships across time between events. An internalised structure for an action emerges from the repeated experience of inter-related events, and this is visualised as a grid of arrows. (Redrawn from Laszlo & Bairstow, 1985).

Ghez, Vicario, Martin and Yumiya (1983) reviewed electrophysiological studies on sensory and motor processes within the motor cortex. Regions of the cortex controlling a given body part receive sensory input from closely related body parts, and they talk of internalised maps of correspondence between input and output. Howard (1971) writing on perceptual learning and adaptation said that animals seek out invariants or correlations within modalities and between different modalities, as well as between motor output and sensory input. The perceptual motor system correlates what it can in order to reduce uncertainty, to economise on coding, and to coordinate action. Fischer (1980) has presented a formal theory of cognitive development in which linked sensory and motor sets are built into a hierarchical knowledge structure which allows us to exercise control over sources of variation in our own behaviour.

Returning to the conjoint sensory and motor set defining a posture (Figure 5), over many experiences, the set comes to exist as a unit. Getting oneself into a self-prescribed and familiar posture, involves calling up such a unit, which is in effect, a set of associated sensory and motor patterns of activity.

3. EXTERNALLY PRESCRIBED POSTURES

I will now use this construct of a conjoint set of sensory and motor patterns defining a posture, in a discussion of the other types of motor functioning which come under the heading of postural control.

To my way of thinking, the ability to achieve an externally prescribed posture (Figure 2) is a most remarkable albeit common place ability; furthermore, it is an ability I find rather difficult to discuss. The pupil in Figure 2 has her eyes on the teacher, she takes in a certain visual input of the teacher's posture, and puts her own body into a similar shape. This behaviour is not a matter of matching visual patterns; the body being copied has different dimensions and proportions to the pupil's, and the pupil gets into the posture without visually checking. Indeed a capable pupil can generate a posture in accordance with a verbal description, and a pupil with a lot of experience may not need as much as a description; a verbal label may be all that is needed.

It is very difficult to think about this type of functioning in physiological terms. What is the mechanism by which one body can mimic another, via intervening patterns (a pattern of light, or a pattern of sound) which have nothing in common with the conjoint sensory and motor set being taken up? I don't believe it is possible - as yet - to be explicit, and the best I can do is talk around the issue. One thing seems certain, there is an inborn predisposition to imitate the actions of others. Babies in the first month demonstrate the ability to imitate facial movements made by mother (Meltzoff, 1981) although the capability to accurately imitate an action undergoes a long developmental progression (the child in Figure 2 is recognisably copying the teacher, but with errors). Perhaps there is a need to invoke two factors, the first of which is a higher level map of the body and the space it occupies; a map that is spatial in nature but not specific to any sensory or motor factor. This map is different to the conjoint set of sensory and motor patterns; it is a superordinate abstract representation. (An attempt to visualise this notion is given in Figure 10). It exists separate from what might be called the concrete sensory-motor set. It is invoked to account for the notion that regardless of the current postural state, we have a more generalised representation of the structure of the body, and the spatial distribution and potential mobility of it's parts. This abstract representation is none-the-less related to the conjoint sensory-motor set defining a posture; it may exist as a result of previous attempts at producing postures, and a visual pattern, a verbal description or a verbal label is translated into a conjoint sensory-motor pattern through its' mediation. It is an intervening factor between sensory patterns which are the external specification of a posture, and the sensory-motor patterns which are the internal specification of a posture.

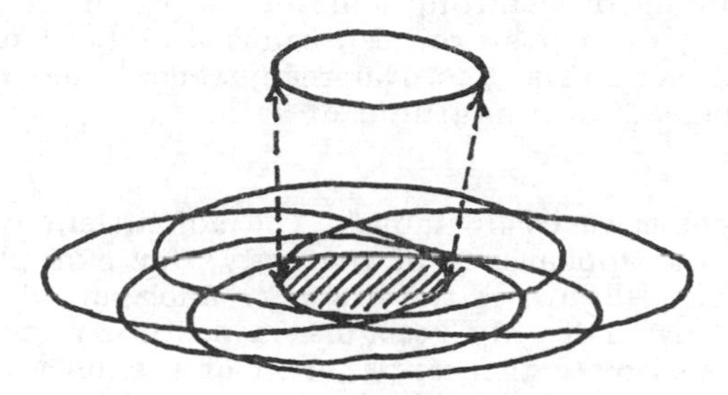

Fig. 10. An attempt to visualise the relationship between an abstract representation of the body, and the concrete sensory-motor conjoint set specifying the postural state of the body.

The second factor that one needs to invoke is some kind of modelling or searching process. The abstract map of the body may be shaped from postural experiences, but one cannot think in terms of an automatic mapping of the abstract onto the concrete representation of a posture. Indeed, one can observe, especially in children, a short sequence of adjustments as the body is progressively brought to a shape that the child evaluates as an accurate imitation of a model.

4. MAINTAINING A POSTURE WHEN ONE PART OF THE BODY IS VOLUNTARILY ADJUSTED

I shall move on now to discuss postural adjustments. As was argued earlier, defining any one subset of the conjoint set of sensory and motor patterns is insufficient to specify a posture. Changing one of the subsets however will often induce or necessitate a change or an adjustment in other subsets. An isolated change can bring about a new conjoint set, defining an essentially new posture. This notion is visualised in Figure 11, as a "shuffling" of sets; one set is shifted, and others shift in an overlapping configuration.

I shall first discuss the effect of voluntarily shifting part of the motor pattern; a change that induces change in the pattern of internal and external forces operating on the body, and subsequently to other parts of the motor pattern, and the sensory patterns. There are two illustrative examples. Firstly, after we have been in one posture for sometime, it is common to feel uncomfortable. We may be placing pressure on a focal area of the body surface, we may be causing stretching and tension in a group of muscles or ligaments, or the posture may be demanding a high level of output to a group of muscles which is fatiguing. After some time, we usually effect an adjustment

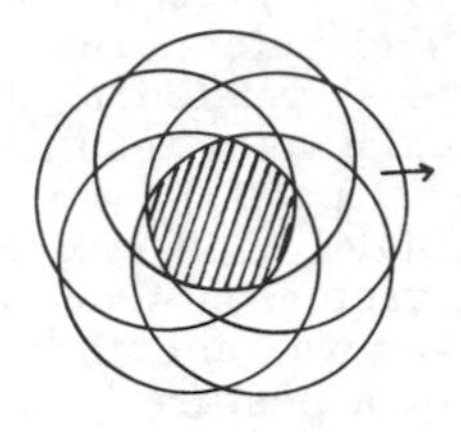
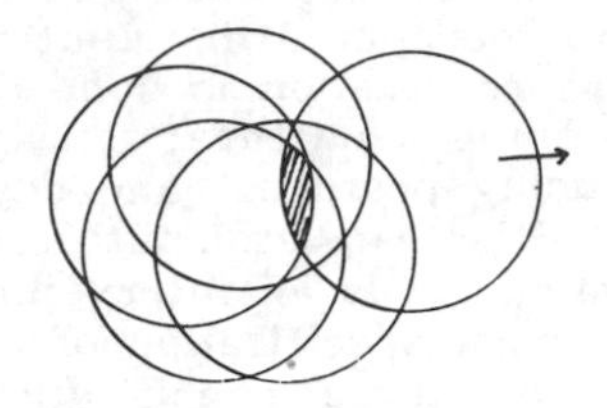
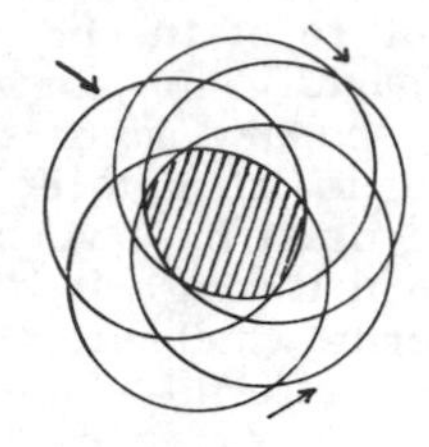

Fig. 11. Changing or "shifting" one of the motor or sensory sets specifying a posture, can cause a shift in one or more other sets. The postural readjustment that occurs, is visualised as a shuffling of sets.

in posture - we "get more comfortable". The adjustment may only be slight with no change in the appearance of the body; for example, tensing or arching the back in a slightly different way. Such an adjustment indicates two things. (1) We can not only recognise a posture in terms of a conjoint set, but we can also isolate the contribution of a subset to the total - that is, is the discomfort associated with the kinaesthetic pattern, the cutaneous pattern, or the motor output pattern? (2) The motor pattern is itself made up of subsets (a point made in the discussion of conjoint motor functioning). We can shift a subset, and specify a new motor pattern. Other changes in motor and sensory patterns follow the initial (focal) change, and a new conjoint set is the outcome. A second illustrative example is the situation in which we need to reach out with an arm to obtain an object. Our basic posture remains the same, but the act of shifting the arm causes a shift in the centre of gravity which necessitates a widespread change in output to other muscle groups in order to maintain the posture. The motor changes, in turn, cause a change in the patterns of tensions and pressures; a new conjoint sensory and motor set is the outcome.

A number of workers have looked into the kinds of secondary adjustments which take place when one part of the motor pattern is altered. (See later references). It is clear that some of the motor adjustments to the voluntary shift are induced as a response to the primary change, while others are induced by higher centres in anticipation of the need to make an adjustment. The "reflexive" mechanisms have been rather well documented. If the load on a muscle is increased (in the present case by a motor action somewhere else in the body), the muscle will stretch unless there is an increase in the strength of contraction. Likewise, if a muscle is unloaded, it will shorten unless there is a decrease in the strength of contraction. If there is no adjustment for a change in load, movement or a shift in body segments will occur which will change the posture and may well cause the body to become unbalanced. An increase in load causing muscle stretching, results in a spinal reflexive excitation of motor nerves to that muscle, which tends to strengthen the force of contraction to overcome the effect of the load; the reverse occurs for a decrease in load. Transcortical, reflexive type responses to a change in load have also been demonstrated. The stiffness of muscles - their resistance to the effect of a change in load, mediated by such reflexive responses - can be controlled from high levels of the central nervous system. It is not possible to go into further detail on these mechanically (Kinaesthetically) driven adjustments to the motor pattern, but the following references will provide a useful introduction to the topic: Allum, Mauritz and

Vogele (1981), Burke (1978, 1980), Burke, Hagbarth and Lofstedt (1978), Conrad and Meyer-Lohman (1980), Gottlieb and Agarwal (1979), Gottlieb, Agarwal and Jaeger (1983), Vincken, Gielen and Vander Gon (1983), Vincken, Gielen, Vander Gon and Terharr Romeny (1982).

Higher anticipatory mechanisms for motor adjustments have also been documented (Hugon, Massion & Wiesendanger, 1982). For example, Bouisset and Zattara (1981) had standing subjects voluntarily elevate their upper limb. They found that movement of the upper limb was preceded by postural adjustments in the lower limbs and pelvis. These postural pre-adjustments were organised in a consistant pattern and tended to counteract the imbalance that would have occurred due to a shift in the body's centre of gravity. In a similar vein, Horak, Esselman, Anderson and Lynch (1984) studied the activation times for trunk and leg muscles in subjects who raised their right arms at different speeds. Activity in the lower postural muscles preceded arm displacement, and the muscles were activated in a similar sequence during all types of rapid movement; the postural adjustments provided stability for the ensuing movement. The widespread adjustments that occur in advance of a voluntary change to part of the conjoint motor set, shows that not only can part of the conjoint set be isolated and adjusted, but a pattern of necessary adjustments in other parts of the body can be specified in anticipation and without the subject necessarily being aware of them. Referring back to Figure 11, changes in sensory patterns result from these anticipatory and reflexive changes in the total motor pattern; which sensory patterns and the degree to which they are readjusted depends, of course, on the nature and the extent of the motor change. The outcome is a new conjoint sensory and motor set.

5. MAINTAINING A POSTURE DURING EXTERNALLY INDUCED CHANGES

I shall now turn to the effect of changing a sensory set. As an illustration, consider the situation of someone standing still, and another person coming and learning against him; the first person does not fall over, but stands his ground. Another example is someone standing with arms out, preparing to receive a package. When it is placed in his arms he doesn't fall forward, but maintains his posture. In both examples, a primary change in the kinaesthetic sensory subset, induces a change in the motor pattern, and there are changes in the pattern of cutaneous input. Changes in other sensory subsets also induce postural adjustments; for example tilting a platform to cause change in the kinaesthetic subset at the ankle joint, tilting the whole body causing changes to the vestibular and visual subsets, or certain types of shifts in the visual input pattern like moving the entire field (eg., Aiello, Rosati, Serra, Tugnoli & Manca, 1983; Allum, 1983; Diener, Bootz, Dichgans & Bruzek, 1983; Diener, Dichgans, Bootz & Bacher, 1984; Diener, Dichgans, Guschlbauer & Mau, 1984; Gottlieb & Agarwal, 1979; Gottlieb, Agarwal & Jaeger, 1983; Jouen, 1984; Paulus, Straube & Brandt, 1984; Shumway-Cook & Woollacott, 1984). In their various ways, these studies seek to elucidate the effect of changing the kinaesthetic, vestibular or visual sensory subsets, alone or in combination, on the readjustments to the conjoint set that is necessitated by the change. From these and other studies it is clear that the different sensory systems have different functional ranges (Diener et al, 1984; Paulus et al, 1984; Shumway-Cook & Woollacott, 1984); that is, some subsets have to be shifted further or more rapidly than others, in order to induce a readjustment to the conjoint set of the type visualised in Figure 11. Studies also show that the effect of a shift in a sensory subset depends on the prevailing conditions - that is, on the exact nature of the conjoint set existing at the time of the shift (Belanger & Patla, 1984; Diener et al, 1983, 1984; Ghez & Vicario, 1978; Nashner, 1980, 1982). For example, a push against the shoulder induces a completely different set of postural adjustments when one is seated compared to standing.

A paper by Marsden, Merton and Morton (1981) gives particularly valuable insights into postural adjustment mechanisms. They studied the effect of a shift in the kinaesthetic subset, and revealed a highly sensitive and complicated system, reacting to stimuli below the subjects perceptual threshold. An externally induced change at one part of the body, causing a change in part of the kinaesthetic subset, induces local reflexive adjustments to the motor pattern (see previous section), but also adjustments to the motor pattern of distant muscles. Distant muscles react very quickly, and distant parts of the body are braced before they have been mechanically affected by the external agent. The muscles which contract or relax are only those able to assist with posture. It was suggested that high level control mechanisms use afferent signals in an automatic though not stereotyped way. They generate a complex and specific set of adjustments to the output of widely separated muscles of the body. Again, the story is one of local change in one part of the conjoint set, inducing local changes to the output of muscles, as well as other widespread patterns of change directed by higher centres - a re-shuffle occurs and a new conjoint motor and sensory set is formed (Figure 11).

6. COMPLICATING ISSUES

I shall move on now to consider two characteristics of the conjoint sensory-motor set defining a posture (Figure 5b) which I have not specifically addressed, and which make the postural control system immeasurably more mysterious and complicated than I have indicated.

When a posture is being maintained, we have a sense of it being unchanged. On the other hand, we can readily detect small changes in the pattern of input. Furthermore, if there is a small change of a particular type in one of the subsets, the system as a whole can respond to it in a highly sensitive way. The sensitivity of the system is remarkable, even more so given that the pattern of activity within the sensory and motor subsets is anything but constant during a steady posture. There are continual changes in the exact firing pattern of the population of motor nerves, as muscle fibres fatigue and new motor units are recruited. This results in changes in the sample of kinaesthetic receptors being activated, because there is a direct link between which motor nerves are active and which muscle spindles and tendon organs are stimulated (eg., Crago, Houk & Rymer, 1982). In addition, there are spontaneous changes in the input from kinaesthetic and crutaneous receptors as they adapt and change their level of activity. And there certainly isn't anything constant about input from the visual receptors as we sit in one place and move our eyes about. However, we perceive ourselves as being still, while the sensory and motor patterns are constantly changing. This is not to say that our perception of posture doesn't shift from the veridical - this shift can be revealed with appropriate experiments (Gross & Melzack, 1978) - but we do not normally sense a shift. The question is, how do inexact and changing ("fuzzy") individual sets of sensory and motor patterns combine into a conjoint set giving the familiar sense of stillness? What are the characteristics of a change that will be detected, that is significa for the postural control system, and which will induce a shift in the conjoint s Such questions have yet to be systematically addressed.

The second characteristic I wish to mention concerns the nature of the conjoint set which is almost certainly different from what might be predicted from the nature of the parts. The individual sensory and motor sets defining a posture, not only coexist, not only exist as a blend or as a conjoint set, but they also impinge on, and bias one other. To visualise this, one may imagine the sets in Figure 5a being "elastic". When they combine (Figure 5b) they change their nature due to multiple influences, and the shaded conjoint set is affected accordingly. In fact, the subsets making up the total are highly interactive - a point that has been ably made by Werness and Anderson (1984). They write that human postural regulation is a complex motor function, dependent upon the integration of information from several modalities, and upon the properties of subsystems at the spinal and higher levels of the central nervous system. They quote Simon as giving a definition of a complex system as follows: "Roughly, by a complex system I mean one made up of a large number of parts that interact in a non-simple way. In such systems, the whole is more than the sum of parts...in the important pragmatic sense that, given the properties of the parts and the laws of their interaction, it is not a trivial matter to infer the properties of the whole" (p. 155). There is a wealth of literature on the interactions that occur within sensory systems (Craske, 1977; Lackner & Levine, 1979; Roll & Vedell, 1982; Ryan, 1940; Tardy-Gervet, 1984; Welch & Warren, 1980). There is a dynamic interplay between the systems, such that one sensory system can influence the specific qualities or functions of another. Similarly, motor and sensory systems directly influence and bias each other (Angel & Malenka, 1982; Bairstow & Laszlo, 1980; Chapin & Woodward, 1982; Coulter, 1974; Lund & Broberg, 1983; Nashner, 1982), and superordinate representations of sensory and motor patterns (Figure 10) can influence the way the conjoint set is recognised (Alloy & Tabachnik, 1984). When one adds to the fact that the individual subsets specifying a posture are in a constant flux, the additional factor that the subsets have a pull on each other, it becomes even more difficult to imagine how the parts coalesce into a conjoint set specifying a posture.

7. A SUMMARY

(a) A posture is specified and recognised as a conjoint set of sensory and motor patterns; defining any one subset or component is insufficient for defining a posture.

(b) After repeated experiences of a posture, the conjoint set of sensory and motor patterns specifying the posture, is represented as a unit within the central nervous system.

(c) It may be ncessary to invoke a superordinate abstract representation within the central nervous system of the space occupied by the body. This representation is the interface between sensory patterns which are the external specification of a posture, and the (sometimes) different sensory and motor patterns which are the internal specifications of a posture.

(d) We can not only recognise and specify a conjoint set for a current posture, but also isolate the contribution that a single sensory or motor subset makes to the total.

(e) A change in one sensory or motor subset often induces or necessitates a change or an adjustment in other subsets, and a new conjoint set is formed, defining a new posture. Whether a shift occurs in the combination of sets depends on which subset is being shifted, how rapidly and by how much, and also on the exact nature of the existing conjoint set. The postural control system can somehow specify what adjustments will be needed, because while part of the shuffling of sets is a direct response to a change, other parts can be directed from higher centres in anticipation of the need for a re-shuffle. Whether in response, or in anticipation, many of the adjustments occur automatically with the subject scarely being aware of them.

(f) The postural control system is a highly sensitive and complex system, consisting of a large number of parts that interact in non-simple ways.

8. FUTURE RESEARCH DIRECTIONS

I wish to suggest that we are some way from being able to propose a comprehensive model for postural control - a model that takes into account the physical properties of a body with mobile segments under the influence of forces, and the physiological properties of the body's sensory receptors, nerves, neural circuitry, and muscles, in an explanation of such questions as: how the motor nerves come to be functionally linked in a cooperative action; how the input from discrete sensory units are combined in sensory systems; the rules by which sensory and motor patterns are combined; how mechanisms determining higher anticipatory control over postural adjustments cooperate with reflexive mechanisms; how we effect control against the background of spontaneous changes in sensory and motor patterns, and complex interactions between different factors. Much work is being done on isolated factors, and combinations of some factors, but the ultimate challenge, surely, is to describe the total, and all the laws of interaction. The intention is not to give an impression of overwhelming complexity and confusion, but rather to make the point that progress towards a comprehensive model requires the combined disciplines of physics, physiology, psychology and mathematics.

In the interim, the venn diagram construct put forward in the present chapter, may usefully unify the literature, and may be extended to guide thinking in three other areas. Consider first, locomotion, which involves continuing dynamic postural adjustments. All the factors operating in the static postural situation, are also operating in the dynamic situation, and figure 11 can be used to visualise changes underlying this complex activity. At the "leading edge" is a voluntary shift in a subset of the total motor pattern; which subset, depends on the phase of the locomotor cycle. A focal change in the motor pattern brings about changes in the patterns of internal and external forces operating on the body, changes in other parts of the motor pattern - some reflexive, and some driven by higher centres - and changes in sensory patterns. A continual "shuffling" of sensory and motor sets can be visualised. A different conjoint set exists at successive moments in time, with all the attendent biases and interactions between the components. It will be very difficult to specify the transition from one conjoint set to another, until the rules of a single state are known, along with the interactions between a changing subset and the existing conjoint set. A useful line of research is likely to be one in which the effect of a particular sensory or motor change is investigated at varying points in the cycle of locomotion. Further investigation along these lines (Belanger & Patla, 1984; Nashner, 1980; Prohazka, Sontag & Ward, 1978) would help elucidate the laws of interaction between sensory and motor patterns in a dynamic situation.

A second area is that of development. There is a long developmental progression in the ability to achieve self-prescribed and externally prescribed postures, and to maintain a posture when one part of the motor or sensory pattern is altered (eg., Clark & Watkins, 1984; Shumway-Cooke & Woollacott, 1984). A venn diagram construct (Figure 5) can help focus attention on research areas that will lead to a full description of the aetiology of the development of control. During development, the body with its mobile segments, is changing in dimensions, mass, and physical makeup. The effect of forces that are passively generated by gravity and the viscoelastic properties of tissues are therefore changing, as are the requirements for counteracting actively generated forces. Hence, a given posture actively maintained by a five year old child, is specified by a different conjoint set of sensory and motor patterns, than an outwardly identical posture maintained by a 10 year old. One must add to this class of developmental change, other changes to do with mechanisms that functionally combine motor nerves to cooperate in a unitary action (Thelen & Fisher, 1983), mechanisms for the combining of sensory and motor patterns (eg., Butterworth, 1981; Jouen, 1984), and the gradual development of representations, both concrete and abstract, of conjoint sensory and motor patterns. The latter type of development can be illustrated with an intriguing observation. Figure 12a shows an eleven year old boy accurately imitating a posture prescribed by a toy model; Figure 12b shows a six year old girl attempting the same task. Along with other children of this age, she is doing a very curious thing; she has curled herself up, convinced that she has got herself into the correct shape. These illustrations are taken from a test which aims at measuring the ability of children to accurately sense the position of their limbs (Laszlo & Bairstow, 1985); the requirement to copy a two dimensional posture in the supine position would eliminate the effect of destabilising forces generated by gravity, eliminate the need to generate controlled patterns of motor output, and allow the child to focus attention on kinaesthetically sensing the position of the limbs. One interpretation of the poor performance shown in Figure 12b is that children aged 6 years have an inaccurate kinaesthetic sense. Another interpretation centres on the role of an abstract representation of the space occupied by the body (see Section 3). It could be argued that it is more usual for children to imitate postures and movements in the upright orientation (rather than the supine), producing patterns of motor output to counter the effect of passive forces generated by gravity (see Section 2). In the supine position, the limbs have to be actively placed in an unusual context of forces, while the final correct posture does not require the continuous generation of a motor pattern. The fact that the child in Figure 12b has taken up a posture that does require the continuous generation of a motor pattern, may be an indication that she is trying to produce the concrete sensory motor conditions that are more usual for this kind of imitation task. The present supine condition may make demands on a higher order abstract map of the space occupied by the body, that is as yet undeveloped. A productive line of research is likely to be one investigating how various factors involved in postural control, combine and operate depending on the age of a child, and the orientation of the body with respect to gravity.

Finally, I would like to refer back to Figure 1 which shows two children with neurological disorders, in distorted standing postures. The notion of a conjoint sensory and motor specification of an action can assist in the understanding of abnormal development, and the (sometimes) intractable nature of motor disorders. A lesion high in the central nervous system, in addition to affecting postural adjustments to external changes (Dietz & Berger, 1984; Nashner et al, 1983) can alter the pattern of motor output in the static situation. Certain groups of muscles can have an excessively large or excessively small contribution to the total motor pattern; in terms of Figure 11, pathology causes a shift in a subset of the motor pattern. During subsequent development, a particular conjoint sensory and motor set for a

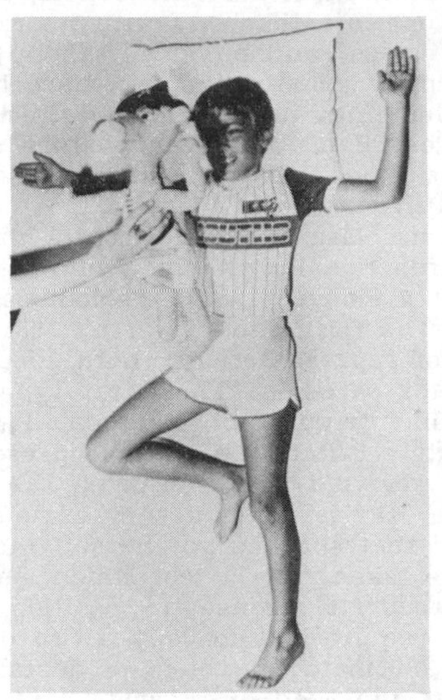
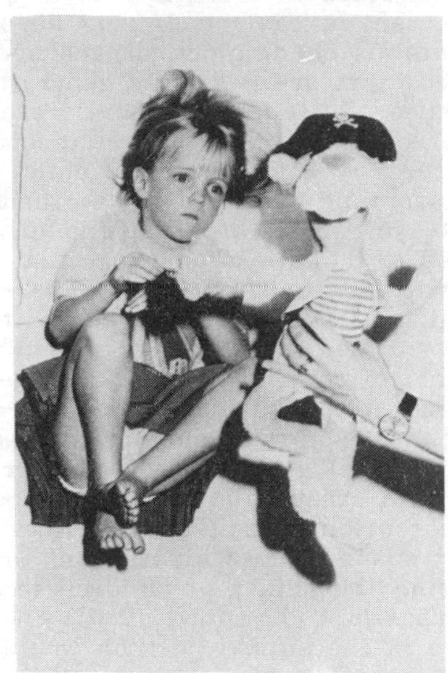

Fig. 12. An illustration of the development in ability to imitate a posture.
LEFT: an 11 year old boy accurately imitating a posture prescribed by a toy model.
RIGHT: a 6 year old girl attempting the same task and producing an incorrect posture that requires the continuous generation of a motor pattern.

standing posture (for example) will result from a focal motor change - it flows from the initial conditions as naturally as the case of a "normal" child. A posture becomes globally specified and recognised, and a cerebral palsied child will be no more aware of a sensory or motor component of the total, than a child without pathology. Such a notion can help in understanding why physiotherapists have such a difficult time trying to correct postures. They are, in effect, attempting to bring about a complete re-specification of a posture, and it is no easier for the cerebral palsied child to take up a new posture, than it would be for the therapist to take up the abnormal posture, with its different and singular motor and sensory patterns. It can also help in understanding why the effects of surgery are so hard to predict. Orthopaedic surgeons operate on muscles to change their mechanical properties, and the once familiar relationship between patterns of motor output and patterns of sensory input are altered. The cerebral palsied child has to adjust to the new conditions - become recalibrated - and has to acquire new representations of conjoint sensory and motor sets. It will be difficult to predict the effects that flow from a focal change in the mechanical properties of muscles, until we have a comprehensive model of postural control of the type alluded to it at the beginning of this section. On the other hand, the careful study of the effects of surgical interventions, would help to elucidate the dynamic interplay between the physical properties of a body, and the physiological properties of evolving motor and sensory patterns that underlie· the development of postural control.

ACKNOWLEDGEMENTS

I wish to acknowledge the work of George Laszlo, the artist who drew the figure of Suzie (Figure 3 and 4) and also Figure 8. My thanks go to George Butterworth, Sheila Henderson, Judith Laszlo and Mary Smyth, who helped a great deal with comments on drafts of this chapter, and to Mandi Clark for typing the drafts. The chapter was prepared while the author was in receipt of a grant from the Medical Research Council (UK).

References

Aiello, I., Rosati, G., Serra, G., Tugnoli, V. & Manca, M. (1983). Static vestibulospinal influences in relation to different body tilts in man. *Experimental Neurology, 79,* 18-26.

Alloy, L.B. & Tabachnik, N. (1984). Assessment of covariation by humans and animals: the joint influence of prior expectations and current information. *Psychological Review, 91,* 112-149.

Allum, J.H.J.(1983). Organization of stabilizing reflex responses in tibialis anterior muscles following ankle flexion perturbations of standing man. *Brain Research, 264,* 297-301.

Allum, J.H.J., Mauritz, K.H. & Vogele, H. (1982). The mechanical effectiveness of short latency reflexes in human triceps surae muscles revealed by ischaemia and vibration. *Experimental Brain Research, 48,* 153-156.

Andreassen, S. & Rosenfalck, A. (1980). Regulation of the firing pattern of single motor units. *Journal of Neurology, Neurosurgery and Psychiatry, 43,* 897-906.

Angel, R.W. & Malenka, R.C. (1982). Velocity-dependent suppression of cutaneous sensitivity during movement. *Experimental Neurology, 77,* 266-274.

Asanuma, H. & Arissian, K. (1984). Experiments on functional role of peripheral input to motor cortex during voluntary movements in the monkey. *Journal of Neurophysiology, 52,* 212-227.

Bairstow, P.J. & Laszlo, J.I. (1980). Motor commands and the perception of movement patterns. *Journal of Experimental Psychology: Human Perception and Performance, 6,* 1-12.

Baldissera, F., Cavallari, P. & Civaschi, P. (1982). Preferential coupling between voluntary movements of ipsilateral limbs. *Neuroscience Letters, 34,* 95-100.

Behrends, T., Schomburg, E.D. & Steffens, H. (1983). Group II muscle and low threshold mechanoreceptive skin afferents converging onto interneurons in a common reflex pathway to motoneurons. *Brain Research, 265,* 125-128.

Belanger, M. & Patla, A.E. (1984). Corrective responses to perturbation applied during walking in humans. *Neuroscience Letters, 49,* 291-295.

Bouisset, S. & Zattara, M. (1981). A sequence of postural movements precedes voluntary movement. *Neuroscience Letters, 22,* 263-270.

Buckingham, H.W. (1984). Early development of association theory in psychology as a forerunner to connection theory. *Brain and Cognition, 3,* 19-34.

Burgess, P.R., Tuckett, P.R. & Horch, K.W. (1984). Topographic and non-topographic mapping of spatial sensory information. Predictions from Boring's formulation. In L. Bolis, R.D. Keynes and S.H.P. Madrell (Eds.), *Comparative physiology of sensory systems.* Cambridge: University Press.

Burgess, P.R., Wei, J.Y., Clark, F.J. & Simon, J. (1982). Signalling of kinaesthetic information by peripheral sensory receptors. *Annual Review of Neuroscience, 5,* 171-187.

Burke, D. (1978). The fusimotor innervation of muscle spindle endings in man. *Trends in Neurosciences, 1,* 89-92.

Burke, D. (1980) Muscle spindle function during movement. *Trends in Neurosciences, 3,* 251-253.

Burke, D., Hagbarth, K.E. & Lofstedt, L. (1978). Muscle spindle responses in man to change in load during accurate position maintenance. *Journal of Physiology, 276,* 159-164.

Burke, R.E. (1980). Motor unit types: functional specialization in motor control. *Trends in Neurosciences, 3,* 255-258.

Butterworth, G. (1981). The origins of auditory-visual perception and visual proprioception in human development. In R.D. Walk and H.L. Pick (Eds.), *Intersensory perception and sensory integration*. New York: Plenum Press.

Chapin, J.K. & Woodward, D.J. (1982). Somatic sensory transmission to the cortex during movement: gating of single cell responses to touch. *Experimental Neurology, 78,* 654-669.

Clark, J.E. & Watkins, D.L. (1984). Static balance in young children. *Child Development, 55,* 854-857.

Conrad, B. & Meyer-Lohman, J. (1980). The long-loop transcortical load compensatory reflex. *Trends in Neurosciences, 3,* 269-272.

Corcos, D.M. (1984). Two-handed movement control. *Research Quarterly, 55,* 117-122.

Coulter, J.D. (1974). Sensory transmission through lemniscal pathways during voluntary movement in the cat. *Journal of Neurophysiology, 37,* 831-845.

Crago, P.E., Houk, J.C. & Rymer, W.Z. (1982). Sampling of total muscle force by tendon organs. *Journal of Neurophysiology, 47,* 1069-1083.

Craske, B. (1977). Perception of impossible limb positions induced by tendon vibration. *Science, 196,* 71-73.

Craske, B., Kenny, F.T. & Keith, D. (1984). Modifying an underlying component of perceived arm length: adaptation of tactile location induced by spatial discordance. *Journal of Experimental Psychology: Human Perception and Performance, 10,* 307-317.

Desmedt, J.E. (1980). Patterns of motor commands during various types of voluntary movement of man. *Trends in Neurosciences, 3,* 265-268.

Diener, H.C., Boots, F., Dichgans, J. & Bruzek, W. (1983). Variability of postural "reflexes" in humans. *Experimental Brain Research, 52,* 423-428.

Diener, H.C., Dichgans, J., Bootz, F. & Bacher, M. (1984). Early stabilization of human posture after a sudden disturbance: influence of rate and amplitude of displacement. *Experimental Brain Research, 56,* 126-134.

Diener, H.C., Dichgans, J., Guschlbauer, B. & Mau, H. (1984). The significance of peoprioception on postural stabilization as assessed by ischaemia. *Brain Research, 296,* 103-109.

Dietz, V. & Berger, W. (1984). Interlimb coordination of posture in patients with spastic paresis. *Brain, 107,* 965-978.

Dykes, R.W. (1983). Parallel processing of somatosensory information: a theory. *Brain Research Reviews, 6,* 47-115.

Erickson, R.P. (1982). The across-fiber pattern theory: an organizing principle for molar neural function. *Contributions to Sensory Physiology, 6,* 79-108.

Erickson, R.P. (1984). On the neural bases of behaviour. *American Scientist, 72,* 233-241.

Feldman, A.G. & Latash, M.L. (1982). Afferent and efferent components of joint position sense: interpretation of kinaesthetic illusion. *Biological Cybernetics, 42,* 205-214.

Fetz, E.E., Finocchio, D.V., Baker, M.A. & Soso, M.J. (1980). .Sensory and motor responses of precentral cortex cells during comparable passive and active joint movements. *Journal of Neurophysiology, 43,* 1070-1089.

Fischer, K.W. (1980). A theory of cognitive development: the control and construction of hierarchies of skills. *Psychological Review, 87,* 477-531.

Georgopoulos, A.P., Caminiti, R., Kalaska, J.F. & Massey, J.T. (1983). Spatial coding of movement: a hypothesis concerning the coding of movement direction by motor cortical populations. *Exp. Brain Res., 7,* 327-336.

Georgopoulos, A.P., Kalaska, J.F., Caminiti, R. & Massey, J.T. (1982). On the relations between the direction of two-dimensional arm movements and cell discharge in primate motor cortex. *J. of Neurosci., 2,* 1527-1537.

Georgopoulos, A.P., Kalaska, J.F., Caminiti, R. & Massey, J.T. (1983). Interruption of motor cortical discharge subserving aimed arm movements. *Experimental Brain Research, 49,* 327-340.

Ghez, C. & Vicario, D. (1978). The control of rapid limb movement in the cat: scaling of isometric force adjustment. *Experimental Brain Research, 33,* 191-202.

Ghez, C., Vicario, D., Martin, J.H. & Yumiya, H. (1983). Sensory motor processing of target movements in motor cortex. In J.E. Desmedt (Ed.), *Motor control mechanisms in health and disease.* New York: Raven Press.

Gielen, C.C.A.M., Vanden Heuvel, P.J.M. & Van Gisbergen, J.A.M. (1984). Coordination of fast eye and arm movements in a tracking task. *Experimental Brain Research, 56,* 154-161.

Gottlieb, G.L. & Agarwal, G.C. (1979). Response to sudden torques about ankle in man: myotatic reflex. *Journal of Neurophysiology, 42,* 91-106.

Gottlieb, G.L., Agarwal, G.C. & Jaeger, R.J. (1983). Response to sudden torques about ankle in man: effects of peripheral ischaemia. *Journal of Neurophysiology, 50,* 297-312.

Gross, Y. & Melzack, R. (1978). Body image: dissociation of real and perceived limbs by pressure-cuff ischaemia. *Experimental Neurology, 61,* 680-688.

Horak, F.B., Esselman, P., Anderson, M.E. & Lynch, M.K. (1984). The effects of movement velocity, mass displaced, and task uncertainty on associated postural adjustments made by normal and hemiplegic patients. *Journal of Neurology, Neurosurgery, and Psychiatry, 47,* 1020-1028.

Howard, I.P. (1971). Perceptual leaning and adaptation. *British Medical Bulletin, 27,* 248-252.

Hugon, M., Massion, J. & Wiesendanger, M. (1982). Anticipatory postural changes induced by active unloading and comparison with passive unloading in man. *Pflugers Archives, 393,* 292-296.

Humphrey, D.R. & Corrie, W.S. (1978). Properties of pyramidal tract neuron system within a functionally defined subregion of primate motor cortex. *Journal of Neurophysiology, 41,* 216-243.

Jennings, A., Lamour, Y., Solis, H. & Fromm, C. (1983). Somatosensory cortex activity related to position and force. *Journal of Neurophysiology, 49,* 1216-1229.

Jouen, F. (1984). Visual-vestibular interactions in infancy. *Infant Behaviour and Development, 7,* 135-146.

Kass, J.H. (1982). The segregation of function in the nervous system: why do sensory systems have so many subdivisions? *Contributions to Sensory Physiology, 7,* 201-240.

Kass, J.H. (1983). What, if anything, is SI? Organisation of first somatosensory area of cortex. *Physiological Reviews, 63,* 206-231.

Kang, R., Herman, D., MacGillis, M. & Zarzechi, P. (1985). Convergence of sensory inputs in somatosensory cortex: interactions from separate afferent sources. *Experimental Brain Research, 57,* 271-278.

Kuypers, H.G.J.M. (1982). A new look at the organization of the motor system In H.G.J.M. Kuypers and G.F. Martin (Eds.), *Descending pathways to the spinal cord; Progress in brain research, vol. 57.* Elsevier: Biomedical Press.

Lackner, J.R. & Levine, M.S. (1978). Visual direction depends on the operation of spatial constancy mechanisms: the oculobrachial illusion. *Neuroscience Letters, 7,* 207-212.

Lackner, J.R. & Levine, M.S. (1979). Changes in apparent body orientation and sensory localization induced by vibration of postural muscles: vibratory myesthetic illustions. *Aviation Space, and Environmental Medicine, 50,* 346-354.

Lackner, J.R. & Taublieb, A.B. (1984). Influence of vision on vibration-induced illusions of limb movement. *Experimental Neurology, 85,* 97-106.

Lamb, G.D. (1983). Tactile discrimination of textured surfaces: peripheral neural coding in the monkey. *Journal of Physiology, 338,* 567-587.

Laszlo, J.I. & Bairstow, P.J. (1985). *Perceptual-motor behaviour: developmental assessment and therapy.* London: Holt, Rinehart & Winston.

Lund, S. & Broberg, C. (1983). Effects of different head positions on postural sway in man induced by a reproducible vestibular error signal. *Acta Physiologica Scandinavica, 117,* 307-309.

Mandler, G. (1962). From association to structure. *Psychological Review, 69,* 415-427.

Marsden, C.D., Merton, P.A. & Morton, H.B. (1981). Human postural responses. *Brain, 104,* 513-534.

Mather, J.A. & Lackner, J.R. (1980). Adaptation to visual displacement with active and passive limb movements: effect of movement frequency and predictability of movement. *Quarterly Journal of Experimental Psychology, 32,* 317-323.

Meltzoff, A.N. (1981). Imitation, intermodal co-ordination and representation in early infancy. In G. Butterworth (Ed.), *Infancy and epistemology.* Brighton: Harvester Press.

Miles, F.A. (1984). Sensing self-motion: visual and vestibular mechanisms share the same frame of reference. *Trends in Neurosciences, 7,* 303-305.

Murphy, J.T., Wong, Y.C. & Kwan, H.C. (1985). Sequential activation of neurons in primate motor cortex during unrestrained forelimb movement. *Journal of Neurophysiology, 53,* 435-445.

Nashner, L.M. (1980). Balance adjustments of humans perturbed while walking. *Journal of Neurophysiology, 44,* 650-664.

Nashner, L.M. (1982). Adaptation of human movement to altered environments. *Trends in Neurosciences, 5,* 358-361.

Nashner, L.M., Shumway-Cook, A. & Marin, O. (1983). Stance posture control in select groups of children with cerebral palsy: deficits in sensory organization and muscular coordination. *Brain Research, 49,* 393-409.

Parker, D.E. (1980). The vestibular apparatus. *Scientific American, 243,* 118-137.

Paulus, W.H., Straube, A. & Brandt, T. (1984). Visual stabilization of posture. Physiological stimulus characteristics and clinical aspects. *Brain, 107,* 1143-1163.

Prohazka, A., Sontag, K.H. & Ward, P. (1978). Motor reactions to perturbations of gait: proprioceptive and somaesthetic involvement. *Neuroscience Letters, 7,* 35-39.

Roll, J.P. & Vedel, J.P. (1982). Kineasthetic role of muscle afferents in man, studied by tendon vibration and microneurography. *Experimental Brain Research, 47,* 177-190.

Ryan, T.A. (1940). Interrelations of the sensory systems in perception. *Psychological Bulletin, 37,* 659-698.

Shumway-Cook, A. & Woollacott, M.H. (1984). The growth of stability: postural control from a developmental perceptive. Manuscript.

Simon, J., Wei, J.Y., Randic, M. & Burgess, P.A. (1984). Signalling of ankle joint position by receptors in different muscles. *Somatosensory Research, 2,* 127-147.

Smith, P.H. (1984). Five-month-old infant recall and utilization of temporal organisation. *Journal of Experimental Child Psychology, 38,* 400-414.

Tardy-Gervet, M.F., Gilhodes, J.C. & Roll, J.P. (1984). Perceptual and motor effects elicited by a moving visual stimulus below the forearm: an example of segmentary vection. *Behavioural Brain Research, 11,* 171-184.

Thelen, E. & Fisher, D.M. (1983). From spontaneous to instrumental behaviour: kinematic analysis of movement changes during very early learning. *Child Development, 54,* 129-140.

Tsumoto, T., Nakamura, S. & Iwana, K. (1975). Pyramidal tract control over cutaneous and kinaesthetic sensory transmission in the cat thalamus. *Experimental Brain Research, 22,* 281-294.

Vincken, M.H., Gielen, C.C.A.M. & Vander Gon, J.J.D. (1983). Intrinsic and afferent components in apparent muscle stiffness in man. *Neuroscience, 9,* 529-534.

Vincken, M.H., Gielen, C.C.A.M., Vander Gon, J.J.R. & Terharr Romeny, B.M. (1982). Afferent contributions to postural tasks. In R. Huiskes, D. Van Campen and J. de Wijn (Eds.), *Biomechanics: principles and applications.* London: Nijhoff.

Welch, R.B. & Warren, D.H. (1980). Immediate perceptual response to intersensory discrepancy. *Psychological Bulletin, 88,* 638-667.

Werness, S.A.S. & Anderson, D.J. (1984). Parametric analysis of dynamic postural responses. *Biological Cybernetics, 51,* 155-168.

Whiting, H.T.A. (Ed.), (1984). *Human Motor Actions: Bernstein Reassessed.* Amsterdam: North Holland Publishing Co.

Wiesendanger, M. (1969). The pyramidal tract. Recent investigations on its morphology and function. *Ergebnisse der Physiologie Biologischen Chemie and Experimentellen Pharmakologie, 61,* 72-136.

Zarzecki, P. & Wiggin, D.M. (1982). Convergence of sensory inputs upon projection neurons of somatosensory cortex. *Experimental Brain Research, 48,* 28-42.

SECTION 2

SKILL DEVELOPMENT AND LEARNING DISABILITIES

SOME ASPECTS OF THE DEVELOPMENT OF MOTOR CONTROL IN DOWN'S SYNDROME

S.E. Henderson

There are two reasons for studying abnormal behaviour. The first is that the form taken by abnormality is interesting in its own right. The second reason stems from the belief that it can tell us something about normal processes. Currently, the testing of models of normal processes with regard to abnormalities in adult performance is very much in vogue. An obvious example can be found in work on skilled reading. The pattern of co-occurrence of symptoms in the acquired dyslexias is believed by many to cast light on the processes involved in normal reading (e.g., Coltheart, Patterson & Marshall, 1980). Proponents of this approach within the field of motor control are rapidly increasing in number (e.g., Nashner, Shumway-Cook & Marin, 1983; Roy, 1985; Wing, 1984).

When we consider the question of whether studies of normality and of pathology in children can likewise be seen as mutually informative, we are faced with a number of problems, some of which are present but less acute when we study abnormality in adults. As many of the issues have been dealt with in depth elsewhere (e.g. Sameroff & Chandler, 1975; Connolly & Prechtl, 1981), I will mention only one or two examples here. Perhaps the most obvious is that developmental disorders rarely take the definite form that has attracted attention to some adult acquired disorders, especially in the realms of perception and language. One reason for this is that damage to the immature system is often more structurally diffuse than it is in adults. Another reason is that any damage, however specific initially, tends to have more diffuse consequences in a developing system. It is now well known that environmental factors may act to alter the course of development quite radically. Whether the altered course of development can inform us in any way about the normal course is a difficult question. Another problem which follows closely on the last concerns the significance of the strategies we observe in children who have managed to compensate for their impairment. Even though the atypical child may reach the same goal as the normal child, it may be that the way he accomplishes this bears little relationship to the normal process. What is really at issue in this case is whether what we are observing is the product of a "reduced set of normal processes" or a compensatory invention. Consider, for example, Kopp and Shaperman's (1973) work on thalidomide children. What they demonstrated was that crucial aspects of cognitive development, often thought to be dependent on the manipulation of objects, can occur without the use of the hands, obviously an important finding. However, the next question that one might ask, is how did these children acquire the cognitive skills under debate? Were we to establish the answer to that question, what we are not at liberty to conclude is that the way a thalidomide child achieves success necessarily tells us anything about how normal children accomplish the same thing. Such are the kinds of problem which confront those who study pathology in children with a view to understanding either the course of the disorder or its implications for normal development.

The development of Down's syndrome children is often considered separately from that of the general population of those suffering intellectual retardation. The argument which is usually used to justify the separate study of this particular syndrome is that more progress has been made in identifying the aetiology than has been made for other types of mental retardation. At a chromosomal level at least, the description of what has gone wrong is fairly clear and although there are several variants of the aberration, one form, Trisomy 21, is far more common than any other. That this circumscribed aetiology has led to a search for homogeneity in the behavioural outcome is perhaps not surprising. However, the question of what sort of homogeneity in behavioural terms might result from a distinct, and in this case, genetically preprogrammed, defect is more complex than might at first be supposed. Perhaps the most obvious possibility is that inter-individual variability might be reduced. To some extent this is true. At least ninety per cent of Down's syndrome children can be identified at birth on the basis of physical signs alone. Hypotonia, to which we return later, occurs in virtually all cases. A very high proportion of D.S. infants are born prematurely. In contrast, there are other features of the disorder which vary considerably from one individual to another. Even within the Trisomy 21 karyotype IQ may range from severely subnormal to almost normal. Consistency of developmental progression is also low within the syndrome. For example, although most Down's syndrome children attain the standard motor milestones such as sitting, walking, or talking later than normal, for many such milestones the *range* in age of acquisition actually exceeds that of normal children (see Table 1).

Despite the fact that there is considerable between - subject variability on most behavioural characteristics within the Down's syndrome population there remains the question of whether any homogeneity or cohesion can be identified within the symptom pattern. If the pattern of symptoms within individuals exhibits some cohesion then the questions we might ask about the syndrome as a whole are probably easier to formulate than if the symptoms appear totally unrelated to each other. A relationship between short stubby fingers, slanting eyes and hypotonia is not immediately apparent but hypotonia, slowness and poor balance form a more promising set. A model which is capable of encompassing at least the majority of symptoms characteristic of a syndrome would not only increase our understanding of the syndrome, it is also more likely to tell us more about how normal processes operate. It might be useful to note at this point, however, that our notion of what symptoms might or might not "hang together" is, itself, theoretically derived. Starting from a model of how a system might work we try to predict what effects particular deficits might have, which in turn leads us back to a consideration of the cohesion of the observed symptom set. This process, although at first sight rather circular would work well if pathological conditions actually manifested themselves in a neat and orderly way. However, it is unfortunately the case that intra-individual cohesion in the symptom pattern is often lower than we might expect. A good example of this sort of problem is evident in the study of Parkinson's Disease in adults, a condition in which the neuro-anatomical basis has been fairly fully described. It has often been suggested that one of the cardinal signs of P.D. is slowness of movement, particularly ballistic movements. An obvious question one might ask is whether the locus of the slowness is in the processes underlying the planning of movement or in the processes underlying execution. Now, there are well researched paradigms which enable us to partition total response time into initiation and execution components. When Parkinson's patients are tested on tasks of this type, however, a constant patterns of performance across individuals is not apparent. Whereas some show a pattern of slowness in the time taken to begin a movement, with normal execution time, others show the opposite pattern or are slow in both components (Evarts, Teravainen & Calne, 1981). The point to note here is that even though slow initiation time and slow movement times have quite different theoretical bases, the global "slowness" observed clinically doesn't seem to be reliably tied to one or the other. Thus the idea that there is a homogeneous set of behavioural symptoms which can be identified as characteristic of that particular pathological condition, and which is associated with a fairly specific type of damage to the brain is open to question. Rather similar problems have confronted those who have suggested that there might be some cohesion in the pattern of symptoms (or problems) which seem to occur in the development of motor control in Down's syndrome individuals.

It has frequently been suggested that the pattern of motor development in Down's syndrome is unique and cannot be viewed simply as part and parcel of a general lowering of functional ability, such as is characteristic of undifferentiated mentally retarded individuals (e.g. Laveck & Laveck, 1977; Cunningham, 1979). Before considering some of the reasons for believing this to be the case, it might be useful to describe briefly what we find if we take a very general look at motor performance in Down's syndrome children.

Much of what we know about the course of development in the early years derives from clinical or psychometric studies which employ tests such as those of Gesell and Armatruda (1941), Bayley (1969) and Griffiths (1954). Criticisms of these tests are now well documented (e.g. Yang, 1979; Gaussen, 1984). Suffice it to note here that there is little cohesion in the item content of these scales and the composite scores which emerge tend to conceal the specific features of the competences or deficits being expressed by a particular individual or group of individuals and, therefore, do not help us to form hypotheses about the precise nature of the problem. Despite such difficulties, however, the following general observations can be made:

(1) At any age, the Down's syndrome child will tend to be less motorically competent than his or her normal peer (e.g. Fishler, Share & Koch, 1964; Dicks-Mireaux, 1972; Carr, 1970, 75) (See Table 1). Though early intervention studies have sometimes demonstrated impressive short term effects these have not been shown to be long lasting and there is as yet little support for the view that the delays in development can be fully compensated for.
(2) Though Down's syndrome children do make progress in motor development and eventually acquire a basic repertoire of functional skills, as they grow older they seem to fall further and further behind normal children (See Table 1).
(3) On certain movement tasks, Down's syndrome children seem to be even less competent than *other retarded children* of the same chronological and mental age. e.g. they often complete a task more slowly than their intellectually retarded peers. Support for this finding comes from numerous experimental studies, some of which will be mentioned later (see Henderson, 1985 for a review).
(4) When detailed analyses are made of performance on the component items of tests such as the Bayley Scales (1969), qualitative as well as quantitative differences emerge between Down's syndrome infants and

Table 1. Developmental milestones for children with Down's syndrome

	Children with Down's Syndrome		'Normal' Children	
	Average age (months)	Range (months)	Average age (months)	Range (months)
Gross motor activities				
Holds head steady and balanced	5	3 - 9	3	1 - 4
Rolls over	8	4 - 12	5	2 - 10
Sits without support for 1 min or more	9	6 - 16	7	5 - 9
Pulls to stand using furniture	15	8 - 26	8	7 - 12
Walks with support	16	6 - 30	10	7 - 12
Stands alone	18	12 - 38	11	9 - 16
Walks alone	19	13 - 48	12	9 - 17
Walks up stairs with help	30	20 - 48	17	12 - 24
Walks down stairs with help	36	24 - 60+	17	13 - 24
Fine motor activities				
Follows objects with eyes, in circle	3	1.5- 6	1.5	1 - 3
Grasps danging ring	6	4 - 11	4	2 - 6
Passes objects from hand to hand	8	6 - 12	5.5	4 - 8
Pulls string to attain toy	11.5	7 - 17	7	5 - 10
Finds objects hidden under cloth	13	9 - 21	8	6 - 12
Puts 3 or more objects into cup or box	19	12 - 34	12	9 - 18
Builds a tower of two-inch cubes	20	14 - 32	14	10 - 19
Completes a simple three-shape jigsaw	33	20 - 48	22	16 - 30+
Copies a circle	48	36 - 60+	30	24 - 40
Personal/social/self-help activities				
Smiles when touched and talked to	2	1.5- 4	1	1 - 2
Smiles spontaneously	3	2 - 6	2	1.5 - 5
Takes solids well	8	5 - 18	7	4 - 12
Feeds self with biscuit	10	6 - 14	5	4 - 10
Plays pat-a-cake, peep-bo games	11	9 - 16	8	5 - 13
Drinks from cup	20	12 - 30	12	9 - 17
Uses spoon or fork	20	12 - 36	13	8 - 20
Undresses	38	24 - 60+	30	20 - 40
Feeds self fully	30	20 - 48	24	18 - 36

Adapted from Henderson (1985).

their normal peers (e.g. Cunningham, 1979; Hogg & Moss, 1983). For example, they may attain the same total score but have passed a different set of items.

(5) Down's syndrome children show a pattern of developmental progression which is unlike that of any other group of handicapped children. As with normal children, there are plateaux in their development but these seem to occur at different times and last much longer than they do in normal children. An example of this, given by Cunningham (1979), occurs at the transition from the simple activity of sucking and banging objects to searching for hidden objects. The Down's syndrome infants he studied remained at the banging stage for a very long time.

Before proceeding further, it might be useful to note the inadequacy of the term 'delayed' as a description of the course of motor development in Down's syndrome children. More appropriate is the term 'deviant', since it draws attention to the need to account for those differences noted above which cannot be readily explained in terms of "normal but slow" development. Different kinds of explanation have been offered to account for various aspects of the deviant trajectory but at present no single explanation adequately encompasses all features of it.

Perhaps the most puzzling aspect of the data yielded by psychometric studies of young Down's syndrome children is the apparent decline in performance with increasing age. (This is true of IQ measures in general as well as composite motor scores). One attempt to account for this outcome does so by proposing that the effects are artefactual. Two points are often made. One is that, in the early months, the test items used are such that subtle sensory motor deficits in populations of handicapped infants are not identified. There is no doubt that this is true and that this tends to produce a deceptively high measure of competence in the first months. Cowie's (1970) work on the early development of reflexive behaviour in Down's infants is an excellent example of how different the Down's baby actually is from his normal peer. Yet, in many studies the Down's syndrome infant gains scores approaching normal. However, even if some account is taken of this problem either by adjusting scores or ignoring that portion of the curve, the decline is still present. The second point that has been considered is that the decline can be attributed to the increased cognitive and verbal complexity of later items in the tests. While this sounds plausible it is not borne out in the data of several studies. For example, Carr (1975) found the greatest decline in scores took place between 6 weeks and 10 months before items requiring verbal competence appear. Analysing overall developmental quotients rather than just motor quotients, Carr (1975) removed the verbal items from the scores between 10 and 24 months and showed that the decline increased rather than decreased. In sum, attempts to dismiss the decline in scores as an artefact are not satisfactory. Nonetheless, Carr (1975) clings to the view that the psychometric pattern misrepresents the situation. Her clinical impression of the Down's syndrome child is not one of "ever diminishing powers".

A completely different kind of explanation of the deviant trajectory of performance may be found in the proposition that Down's syndrome is a progressive disorder manifesting itself in continuous neurological deterioration. This is a very controversial viewpoint. It is true that a proportion of Down's syndrome individuals exhibit signs of an Alzheimer-like condition remarkably early in life (e.g. Ball & Nuttall, 1980; Price et al, 1983) but though early, this does not occur until adulthood and hence cannot contribute much to our understanding of why the childhood pattern of development should take the form it does. (It is worth noting that the hypothesis of a degenerative component brings with it particularly pessimistic implications for the view that an understanding of motor development in D.S. will illuminate the normal course of motor development).

With regard to the plateaux that occur in the measurement of development of Down's syndrome infants, attempts have been made to dismiss these, too, as artefactual. This view is based on the indisputable fact that global developmental tests designed for and standardised on normal populations are insensitive to small changes and therefore fail to register slow rates of change. Consequently, artificial plateaux may be created. That some plateaux are real and not artefactual, however, seems to be attested to by Cunningham's (1979) observation work in which he found that qualitative differences between Down's syndrome and normal infants accounted for the extended plateaux (See below for further discussion).

These are two other notions which present themselves in discussions of the peculiar nature of development in Down's syndrome. Both seem to me intuitively appealing. The first is that the behavioural disability is "biologicall; emergent" and that anomalies associated with the syndrome do not become fully manifest until the relevant stages of development are reached. (This view requires to be carefully distinguished from the degenerative hypothesis mentioned above). For example, we might speculate about the role of the cerebellum in the control of movement and the notion that defects in cerebellar functioning might not become evident until the child begins to sit or stand. The second is that the Down's syndrome infant suffers a self-perpetuating form of sensory-motor deprivation sparked off by an inbuilt passivity and disinclination to move.

At this stage it is not possible to adjudicate between these various hypotheses, so what I propose to do now is less ambitious. I shall simply describe briefly some of what we know about Down's syndrome that goes beyond global psychometric measures. I will also impose an organisation on the material which I hope will indicate how I think we might proceed in this area. I shall start with what I have called the neuromotor machinery - for want of a better term.

NEUROMOTOR MACHINERY

When considering what factors might limit motor competence in a condition such as Down's syndrome one place to start might be the integrity of the neuromotor system. There is little doubt that the basic machinery with which the Down's syndrome child is endowed is not as efficient as that of the normal child. When we begin to ask questions about exactly how the system is deficient, however, what faces us is a tangled mass of facts which, though linked by the thinnest of threads, bears otherwise little resemblance to the beautifully organised form of the spider's web. What facts can we isolate from this mass - and how can we tie them together?

1) Brain weight:

First, there is anatomical evidence of a selective effect of the genetic anomaly on the parts of the brain known to be intimately involved in the control of movement. Crome, Cowie, and Slater (1966) have shown that whereas the brain as a whole in Down's syndrome is reduced on average to 76% of its normal weight the cerebellum and brain stem are only 66% of normal. What are we to make of such a fact? The weight of brain tissue is no more transparently related to the efficiency of motor function than it is to intellectual function. The weight of a neural structure is as difficult to interpret as it is simple to measure and far from providing us with an insight into the process disturbance underlying poor performance it actually offers an even more undifferentiated view than does behaviour itself.

2) Hypotonia:

Numerous authors have proposed a relationship between the brain weight findings and the presence of hypotonia in D.S. (Kirman, 1951; Crome, Cowie & Slater, 1966) but so far the mechanism whereby the low cerebellar weight and hypotonia might be linked to the genetic aberration remains unexplicated (Dubowitz, 1980). As a behavioural feature, however, hypotonia is one of the most common signs. It is almost universally present in very young Down's syndrome infants and though it often diminishes considerably in severity, it remains detectable in many older individuals. In a longitudinal study of 67 D.S. infants between birth and 48 weeks, Cowie (1970) noted hypotonia in every one throughout that period. In the first two weeks 44% were "extremely hypotonic" 53% "markedly hypotonic" and 3% "moderately so". By the end of the year, these proportions had changed but no child was yet rated as normal. These findings are consistent with those of McIntire and Dutch (1964) who reported normal tone in only two of 86 D.S. children under six years. The picture we have after the first few years, however, is less clear. Some studies report the persistence of hypotonia, without mentioning individual differences (e.g. Morris, Vaughan & Vaccaro, 1982) whereas others report a change in incidence, with the number of individuals exhibiting the symptoms diminishing with age (Loesch-Mdzewska, 1968). A major problem with the most of these studies is that hypotonia is defined in terms of a composite score derived from the clinical judgement of a number of quite disparate factors, such as joint mobility and resistance to passive movement. While this may be adequate for some purposes, it is essential that we move beyond such undifferentiated judgements if we are to understand what the consequences of hypotonia are for voluntary motor control. Recently, Davis and Kelso (1982) made a rather important contribution to this area of enquiry by examining the biomechanical properties of the muscle-joint system in Down's syndrome males. What they found was that at a gross level of analysis the Down's syndrome subjects' responses were similar to those of normal subjects. However, a more detailed inspection of their data revealed some interesting differences. First, the Down's syndrome subjects took much longer to move their fingers to a visually specified target position. Second, when a load placed on the finger was removed, without the subject resisting, the finger oscillated much more around the enw position before coming to rest. Finally, when the subjects were instructed to resist the change in load the Down's syndrome subjects were less able to do so. In summarising their findings, Davis and Kelso suggest that damping and stiffness regulation may be related to and, indeed, considered as a sensitive measure of hypotonia in Down's syndrome. By so doing they invest a passive measure (tonus) with possible functional significance.

In a slightly different, but not unrelated, study Davis and Sinning (1985) explored the possibility that strength training might alter the damping and stiffness characteristics of the muscle-joint system in Down's syndrome and other mentally retarded subjects. Because the training did not have the requisite effect the main hypotheses could not be tested. However, an incidental finding of considerable interest emerged. In the Down's syndrome group, the magnitude of maximum voluntary contraction per unit of muscle tissue was significantly lower than in either normal or other mentally retarded subjects. Davis and Sinning (1985) tentatively suggest that this finding supports the view that Down's syndrome individuals are less capable of muscle activation than retarded persons.

To complement these studies there are others which have attempted to increase muscle tone by the administration of drugs, notably 5-Hydroxytriptophan (e.g. Bazelon, Paine, Cowie, Hunt, Houck & Mahanand, 1967; Coleman, 1975). The rationale for the use of this particular drug is related to the fact that children with Down's syndrome are known to have low levels of serotonin (5-Hydroxytryptamine) in their blood. Serotonin, a protein enzyme, is known to cross the blood-brain barrier and is believed to play an important role in neural transmission and muscle contraction (Ahlman, Grillner & Udo, 1971). Consequently, it was suggested that elevation of the level of serotonin might have an effect on the muscle tone as well as on other aspects of performance. However, although some studies have claimed to demonstrate improvements in muscle tone (e.g. Airaksinen, 1974) none have shown any concomitant effects on motor functioning. As an incidental practical matter, long term administration has been contra indicated (Coleman, 1975).

3) The Early "Reflex" Repertoire:

In addition to the presence of hypotonia, one of the most frequently noted characteristics of the Down's syndrome infant is the weakness of expression of many of the so-called "primitive reflexes" and the extent of the delay in their emergence and dissolution. A study of this aspect of development in Down's syndrome infants by Cowie in 1970 provided some excellent data on some of the most commonly studied of these reflexes. At an intuitive level many of the atypical features of the responses seem to be attributable to the presence of hypotonia. For example, the traction response, the plantar and palmar grasp responses and Moro responses are often weak or even absent initially. In ventral suspension the baby is unable to lift its head or legs and simply hangs like a banana. However, other aspects such as the persistence of a response once it has emerged fully are not explicable in terms of the presence or absence of low tone, suggesting that the cause of these various problems is not unitary. Though there is much debate about the relationship between these early "reflex" responses and the emergence of voluntary control over the neuromotor system, what does seem to be clear is that deviations from normal may either prevent the attainment of normal patterns of movement or delay their acquisition. In contrast to what we know of the early reflexes which typically disappear in the first few months of life, relatively little information is available on the emergence of the postural adjustment reactions which follow. Molnar (1981) has recently demonstrated a close relationship between the emergence of these reactions and the achievement of significant motor milestones in an undifferentiated group of mentally retarded children but unfortunately Down's syndrome children were specifically excluded from the sample. A replication of Molnar's study on Down's syndrome children would be of considerable value. It is also a pity that we know little about other aspects of the motor repertoire of the Down's infant. For example, Thelen's elegant studies of "spontaneous" movements in normal infants have no parallel in the literature on Down's syndrome children (Thelen & Fisher, 1983a and b; Thelen, this volume).

4) Postural Control:

The development and maintenance of stability is a salient feature of the young child's motor repertoire. Being able to sit or stand upright paves the way for the acquisition of a whole range of new skills and locomotor ability leads to a systematic change in an infants exploratory and social behaviour (Gustafson, 1984). On average, the Down's syndrome child attains these milestones considerably later than the normal child. For example, estimates for standing without support converge on a figure of 18 months and some may do so as late as three years. Over the last 10 years a great deal of effort has gone into the investigation of the involuntary processes which underlie this component of motor performance in normal individuals (e.g. Lee & Aaronson, 1974; Lee & Lishman, 1975; Nashner & McCollum, 1982; Nashner & Woollacott, 1979). The basic paradigms and findings on normal children have already been reported in detail and are summarised by Butterworth and

Woollacott in this volume.

The first study to compare Down's syndrome infants with their normal peers was that of Butterworth and Cicchetti (1978). Adopting the methodology described by Lee and Aaronson (1974) they explored the effects of discrepant visual and proprioceptive input on the Down's syndrome child's ability to maintain stability while sitting or standing. four groups of infants were included, two normal and two with Down's syndrome. Two groups were matched on the amount of time that had elapsed since they had acquired the ability to sit and two on the ability to stand unsupported. (Obviously, there were considerable differences in chronological age between the infants in each group. For example, the D.S. infants who had been standing for one month or so were approximately 30 months old whereas the normal children were only 14 months). As the results for the sitting position were difficult to interpret I will not include them in this discussion. In the standing position, however, the results were intuitively consistent with the clinical observation that Down's syndrome children have considerable difficulty with balance tasks well into childhood. Though the groups seemed equally stable under normal conditions the D.S. children were nevertheless much more influenced by the discrepant visual and proprioceptive input than the normals. They fell over much more frequently and swayed more. In addition, whereas falls became rare in normal infants after 3 months of standing experience it took 7-12 months for the Down's infants to acquire the same degree of stability. In considering the implications of their findings Butterworth and Cicchetti suggest that it takes much longer for the mechanical-vestibular system of the Down's syndrome child to be "calibrated" against vision.

Turning now to the work of Shumway-Cook and Woollacott (1985), we come to a study which examines the dynamics of postural control in Down's syndrome children in more detail. As is customary in the experiments of this group, both biomechanical analysis and electromyography are used to determine the characteristics of postural adjustments under normal conditions and in situations where inter-sensory conflict is present. Their findings were generally in accord with those of Butterworth and Cicchetti (1978) but expand the picture in a number of ways. Six Down's syndrome children were studied, the first four in the age range 3-6 years, the remaining two between 15 and 31 months. When the 3-6 year old D.S. children were compared to their normal peers in a condition which involved the floor surface simply moving forward and backwards, their responses were generally similar in that they were directionally appropriate and the muscles responded in the same sequence. However, the Down's syndrome children were considerably more variable than the normal subjects and were much slower to respond. As far as the younger children were concerned, the differences between the groups was greatly exaggerated. The Down's syndrome children's adjustment responses were very poorly organised and on half the trials were absent i.e. the child simply fell over. When exposed to conditions involving reduced or conflicting sensory information the Down's syndrome children were much less able to cope than their normal peers. At this point, Shumway-Cook and Woollacott note a similarity between their findings on Down's children and those on adults with cerebellar pathology. When they finally compared the overall pattern of performance for the Down's group with that of normal children they suggest that "possibly the equilibrium problems of the Down's syndrome child are not just the result of delayed, albeit normal, development but in fact represent a difference in the evolution and development of postural control".

5) Speed:

Any discussion of the possible deficits in the neuromotor system of Down's syndrome individuals would be incomplete without some mention of the apparent slowness with which they move. Slowness, however, can have its origin in numerous different components of the processing chain and at present the data on Down's does not allow us to get very far in specifying its locus. Slowness in unpaced movement, (Hogg & Moss, 1983), in reaction time tasks, (e.g. Berkson, 1960a,b,c; Belmont, 1971) in tapping tasks, (Frith & Frith, 1974; Seyfort & Spreen, 1979) and in tracking tasks (Frith & Frith, 1974; Henderson, Morris & Frith, 1981) are all fairly clearly demonstrated but in many of these there are obvious cognitive elements which might make as much contribution to slowness as problems located in the neuromuscular machinery itself.

There are few studies which have systematically analysed the relative contribution of different factors to the overall picture of slowness in Down's syndrome. Those which have, have tended to focus on the manipulation of cognitive complexity. However, there are two recent studies which attempt a more detailed analysis of the "motor" end of the response (Saqi, 1981; Davis, Ward & Sparrow, 1985). In the first, Saqi (1981) separates initiation time from movement time and, in the second Davis et al (1985) further separate initiation time into premotor and motor components. Saqi reports two experiments involving Down's syndrome and other retarded controls of the same chronological and mental age. A simple and a choice reaction time task were included. No differences at all were found on the movement time component of the response, indicating that once the Down's subject had actually begun to move they were just as fast as the controls. However, there was a difference in the decision time component of the response. The more detailed study by Davis et al (1985), compared the performance of Down's, other retarded and normal subjects. As has been frequently demonstrated the normal subjects were faster than their retarded peers on all measures taken. The differences between the Down's and the other retarded subjects, however, were more interesting. The data on movement time were consistent with those of Saqi (1981) in that no difference emerged on movement time, confirming that, once a movement has begun, it can be executed at a similar speed by both groups, albeit much more slowly than by their normal peers. As far as the initiation time component was concerned the results supported the view that Down's subjects are slower than other retarded individuals. When Davis et al examined the pre-motor and motor components of the initiation time separately, they found in both that the difference between the two retarded groups was significant. If, as they suggest, the pre-motor and motor components of RT are independent of each other and can be influenced by different factors, then experiments must be planned to replicate and extend these findings. By so doing, we will begin to accumulate information which specifies more exactly the origin of the slowness in Down's subjects. In summarising these results Davis is careful to point out that he sees an enormous gulf between the finds he obtained with Kelso noted earlier (Davis & Kelso, 1982) and those he reports in the reaction times study and warns against loosely drawing together the concepts of slowness and hypotonia as has been done in the past.

So far I have dealt with five topics of study - brain weight, hypotonia, early reflex behaviour, the control of upright posture and speed. All of the studies considered under these headings document ways in which Down's

Syndrome individuals differ significantly from their normal peers and in some instances ways in which they also differ from other retarded individuals of similar mental and chronological age. What we have achieved, therefore, is an inventory of attributes that clearly differentiate Down's Syndrome from other conditions within the motor domain. There is something consoling about being able to produce such a list but its contribution should not be over-estimated. Clearly, these five lines of enquiry differ in many respects. What they have in common is that their findings have been interpreted as signs of the state of the neuromotor machinery. There are two sorts of problems, however. First, there is the question of how exactly these signs do map onto the state of the neuromotor machinery. Perhaps the most obvious area where there is quite a wide gap between the discovery of a deficit and postulating an underlying cause is in the study of response speed. The measures taken in such studies are behavioural measures from which we make inferences about possible underlying neurological deficiencies, (save for brain weight which might be regarded as a putative cause in search of a behavioural effect). Whether such a disparate set of findings can eventually be woven into a coherent pattern, therefore, remains to be seen. The second problem concerns the mapping between the neuromotor state, of which these signs are taken to be diagnostic, and performance in the real world. So far we have dealt with either laboratory based studies or studies which are not concerned with voluntary motor behaviour. How these identified deficits manifest themselves in every day life situations, remains unexplored. It is to this kind of study of Down's syndrome children that we now turn.

Before dealing with specific aspects of the purposive behaviour of the Down's syndrome child, however, it might be useful to note the multiplicity of developmental problems such children face. Most people are aware that Down's syndrome children look different from their peers, that they are intellectually retarded and that they walk in an odd way. Much less well known are things like the raised incidence of heart conditions and susceptibility to respiratory infection, the metabolic disorders and tendency towards obesity, the more subtle anatomical differences, and so on. Though it is unlikely that factors such as these play a primary role in altering developmental progress in the motor domain, as secondary factors they must be entered into the reckoning.

Despite the fact that deviant motor development is so frequently documented in the clinical and psychometric literature it is depressing how few studies there are which examine directly the development of motor skills in the context of object manipulation or interaction with people. In what follows, I have taken these two topics, the handling of objects and interacting with people and attempted to select studies which are specific in their attempt to examine the "motor" elements of the actions involved.

THE WORLD OF OBJECTS

Over the last decade the conceptualisation of the human infant as a uniformly helpless, passive organism has been continuously eroded. Normal babies possess much more sophisticated perceptual abilities than was once thought and are capable of exercising more control over their eyes, hands and arms than was previously believed possible (see Von Hofsten, 1983 for a review). For example, the normal neonate will follow an attractive moving object with his eyes (Aslin, 1981) will turn towards a target introduced into the periphery of the visual field (Aslin & Salapatek, 1975) and will turn towards a sound. Moreover, even though they do not grasp successfully, infants will reach out for objects which appear in front of them (either stationary or moving) with some accuracy. It is, of course, some time before infants can truly be said to handle objects efficiently and many changes take place before the movements of the hand and eye are co-ordinated in a stable pattern. Many of these changes have now been documented with considerable precision (e.g. Von Hofsten, 1979, 1980, 1982). Consequently, we have available a rich source of information against which the difficulties of handicapped children can be judged.

Although the picture is a fragmented one, what we know of the development of manipulative skills in the Down's syndrome child contrasts sharply with our impression of ever increasing competence in the normal child. The simple acts of looking at objects and reaching towards them do not appear until much later than in normal children. The way Down's syndrome infants explore objects sometimes differs considerably from normal. Drawing a simple shape or colouring a picture may prove difficult for the Down's syndrome child long after he has begun to attend school. Even though most eventually do master the skills of fastening buttons, handling a spoon and using a pencil, the way they do so often remains clumsy and slow. In fact, some authors single out fine motor skills as being particularly impaired in Down's syndrome children (e.g. Hogg & Moss, 1983). In this paper, I will consider in detail a few studies which focus on the early stages of the development of manipulative skills.

Surprisingly, there seems to be only one study which traces the development of reaching and grasping behaviour in Down's syndrome infants, that of Cunningham (1979). Twelve Down's syndrome infants and ten normal infants of similar chronological age and social background participated. Starting when the infants were about four weeks of age, Cunningham made a videotape once every two weeks,of each child's response to the presence of a succession of attractive objects. To begin with a brightly coloured ball suspended on a stick was placed at eye level in front of the child. Whenever the child could reach out and touch the ball with the palm of the hand (not necessarily grasp it) a new task was introduced. A cube was then placed on a table in front of the infant and observation continued until it was successfully picked up in one hand. Following completion of the data collection various measures of eye, hand and arm movements were taken from the videotapes.

As predicted the Down's Syndrome subjects took longer than their normal peers to achieve success on both tasks. Of more interest, however, was the fact that the delay in acquisition on the later developing task was much greater than on the early one. On the visually directed reaching task the average delay was some seven weeks whereas on the manipulative task the corresponding delay was 18 weeks and some of the Down's syndrome children had not yet acquired the skill when the study ended. This finding is, of course, in accord with the general view noted earlier that Down's syndrome infants fall progressively further and further behind their peers.

What sets Cunningham's study apart from others, however, is the more detailed analysis of what happened *before* the infants acquired the skills in question. As space is limited I will attempt to summarise only that relating to the reaching task. Cunningham's data on the normal infants was in accord with that of many others. For example, they reached more often when the object was present than when it was absent and also reached more accurately when they were looking at the object than when they were looking away or had their eyes closed. By twelve weeks of age they were also leaning forward and making mouthing movements at the object, giving the impression that they wanted to obtain it. In contrast, the Down's syndrome infants behaved rather differently in the presence of the object. Though the pattern of looking behaviour was quite similar for the two groups what they did with their hands and arms was not at all the same. At first the Down's syndrome infants reached out for the object but when they did so the trajectory was much less accurate and there was little evidence of corrective movements being made. Over the weeks the frequency of arm extensions gradually reduced and the infants were observed fingering their clothing, clasping their hands and sucking their fingers much more than the normal children. At about 20 weeks, however, the Down's infants began to indicate their desire to obtain the object by leaning forward and making the same mouthing movements as the normal infants had done much earlier. Finally by about twenty four weeks the skill was attained.

In passing Cunningham makes a very interesting observation concerning the differences between the two groups in their response to the introduction of the second of the tasks set for them. When the form and location of the object changed from a ball suspended at face level to a cube placed on a table at about waist height the normal infants exhibited immediate transfer of reaching whereas the Down's syndrome infants did not. For some it took six weeks before they began to reach for the new object.

It is not easy to find an explanation which adequately encompasses all aspects of Cunningham's results and he himself remains rather speculative. One of his suggestions is that there are two rather different processes at work. First, he proposes that the atypical form of the relationship between looking and reaching behaviour in the Down's syndrome infants provides support for the hypothesis that the deficits associated with the syndrome are "biologically emergent". Whereas the visual behaviour normally associated with reaching for objects emerges appropriately, the corresponding motor activity seems to emerge as deficient. In addition, he argues that the lack of success and possible frustration which accompanies the child's early efforts might reduce interest in the task and contribute generally to the frequently noted "defect in exploratory drive". Here, therefore, Cunningham seems to be suggesting that lack of motivation to explore the environment is a secondary consequence of initial failure, whereas elsewhere he and others have commented on passivity and apparent lack of desire to move as being evident from rather earlier in life.

Another study which equals that of Cunningham in its attention to detail is that of Hogg and Moss (1983), who focus their attention on the manipulative skill of Down's syndrome children in the age range 15-44 months. The children's task in this investigation was a simple one - to place different sized wooden rods in appropriately sized holes. As only one rod and one hole were presented simultaneously, the task did not involve working out which rod fitted into which hole. All that was required was that a sequence of movements be planned to meet the spatial constraints of a task which increased progressively in difficulty as the rods and holes became smaller. Although the infant was not aware of a time factor, two aspects of the time taken to complete the task were measured (1) the time from when the child actually grasped the rod to when it was brought into contact with the plate in which the hole was located, and (2) the time between touching the plate and successfully inserting the rod. In addition, a description of the grip used to hold each rod was recorded.

The results of the study were as follows. With respect to prehension, the two groups of children did not differ either in the way they gripped the rods in one hand or in the number of times they used two hands to pick them up. Adopting Connolly's (1973) suggestion that grips might be viewed as "sub-routines" from which specific manipulative actions are constructed, Hogg and Moss conclude that by 15 months of age Down's syndrome infants possess the same repertoire of "sub-routines" as their normal peers.

When the timing measures were considered, however, the picture was rather different. The Down's syndrome infants were slower both at picking up the rods and at inserting them in the holes. Thus, despite having the necessary movements available, they found it more difficult both to select a response which met the spatial constraints placed upon them and to make the appropriate movement once it had been selected.

Taking the movement pattern and timing results together, Hogg and Moss suggest that the manipulative difficulties experienced by Down's children are due, not to a failure to produce movements of a given topography but in organising them as efficiently as their non-handicapped peers.

As an incidental matter, the differences in speed of movement which Hogg and Moss observed between the two groups of subjects were actually predictable from the outset of the study. When the profiles of performance exhibited by the two groups were examined, it was evident that the Down's syndrome and normal children had arrived at the same total score by a different route. The Down's syndrome children were significantly poorer on items requiring fine motor co-ordination and better on items involving language. A useful aspect of this study was, therefore, to highlight the pitfalls of matching children on overall developmental quotients.

A rather different aspect of the Down's syndrome child's difficulty in using their hands efficiently is apparent in how they handle objects which they cannot see. Though it might be argued that trying to identify objects while blindfolded is a rather artificial task, difficult to equate with anything we do in the real world, it remains the case that normal children can do this reasonably well whereas mentally retarded children cannot. Moreover, several authors have found that Down's syndrome individuals are significantly worse than other retarded individuals of the same intellectual ability (e.g. O'Connor & Hermelin, 1961). This is quite a well documented finding and the problem is nearly always attributed to a deficiency in proprioceptive perception. In fact this view has become so entrenched that Lewis and Bryant (1982) claim "This (the tactual deficit) is probably the most reliable *perceptual* anomaly ever demonstrated within any kind of mental subnormality". However, I think this proposition requires some revision. I do not think that the existing studies allow us to conclude that there is anything basically wrong with the Down's child's ability to perceive information received through non-visual channels. What I think is a more parsimonious explanation is that they do not "know" how to organise their movements to collect meaningful information about objects.

Consider the following experiment by Lewis and Bryant (1982) in which Down's syndrome and normal infants are compared. There are two conditions, one involving visual - visual matching the other involving haptic - visual matching. In the visual - visual conditions, the infant is shown two objects:

one is then made to bleep while the other remains silent. The two objects are then placed in front of the child and the experimenter notes which one is reached for. In the haptic - visual condition, a noisy object is placed in the infant's hand without it being visible, then the two objects are placed on the table as before. Reaching for the noisy object is obviously taken as recognition of it. Whereas most of the normal infants could do both tasks the Down's children performed accurately only in the visual - visual matching tasks but failed when the first object was presented in the hand. It does seem therefore that even at this early age, Down's children have some difficulty with non-visual information. However, this finding does not allow us to conclude that they suffer some defect in the transmission of such information. Lewis and Bryant present no data on how their subjects handled the objects placed in their hands so the question of how the haptic information was dealt with is not answered. One might ask, for example, were the Down's infants seeking haptic information systematically but not receiving it, or was the strategy they adopted to obtain it so unsystematic that what was available was simply not integrated into a usable scheme or image of the object?

In a second experiment, Lewis and Bryant complicate the picture even further by showing that there were differences not only in the amount of time Down's syndrome and normal children spent touching the objects but also in the amount of time they spent looking at them. Although the Down's syndrome infants seemed to realise that objects were touchable, the extent to which they exercised their visual and manual exploratory skills seemed to be limited. As a result of this second experiment Lewis and Bryant (1982) note that a specific deficit limited to the processing of haptic information does not adequately account for their data. To the haptic deficit must be added a visual deficit.

As indicated above, however, it seems to me that there is another hypothesis one might consider in the context of experiments of this type. It relates to the way a child's knowledge about the properties of objects might influence the efficiency with which they are handled. From a very early age, we deduce that a normal child "knows" that objects are solid, have corners, are smooth and so on, at least in part from the way he acts upon them. It seems reasonable to assume, therefore, that when an object is not visible a child's knowledge of the properties of objects "directs" his haptic exploration of them. Perhaps, this is where the problems lie in the Down's syndrome child. Tangential support for this notion comes from two studies. First Anwar (1983) has demonstrated that under certain conditions Down's Syndrome children are quite capable of using non-visual sources of information. For example, if the child's hand is guided round the shape by the experimenter, then his ability to use that information is as good as that of his mentally retarded peers. (though both remain less accurate than normal). Second, Davidson, Pine, Wiles Kettenmann and Appelle (1980) have shown that the strategies used by retarded children to explore objects was highly correlated with their success in recognising them. Though they do not provide statistical support for this, they particularly note that the Down's syndrome subjects in their sample were disorganised in this regard.

It is perhaps injudicious to attempt a premature synthesis of so little data, but there does seem to me to be some support in these studies for the notion that it takes a long time for the Down's syndrome child's spatial representation of the world to become mapped on to the neuromotor system. This would, of course, draw together the findings on postural control and those on hand-eye co-ordination, but still leaves other elements such as the failure of transfer and slowness requiring explanation. For these elements it seems necessary to appeal to other sorts of explanations which are not "motor" in the simple sense but which affect action in the motor domain.

THE WORLD OF PEOPLE

As Trevarthen (this volume) points out, the motor skills of human communication are among the most intricately programmed and finely regulated skills that humans possess. They include not only the oral and manual expression of language but also many facets of the expression of emotion such as the regulation of prosody, the signalling of feeling through expressive gesture, the regulation of eye contact and so on. Recently, a wealth of information has accumulated showing that the normal infant is capable of producing and interpreting many of these communicative actions from a very early age (e.g. Dunn, 1981; Trevarthen, 1984). At the same time, there has been a growing awareness that in many instances biologically impaired infants do not engage in the same type of frequency of interactions which normally occur between infants and their caregivers. As noted above, however, the specific role that "motor" deficiencies might play in disrupting the interaction between infant and caretaker is rarely evaluated.

The mothers and caretakers of Down's syndrome infants often describe them as "good" babies. They are passive, undemanding and cry little. At first sight this might seem like a description of an ideal baby. However, there are negative aspects of this early developmental picture too. A floppy, inactive baby is difficult to handle. It is not uncommon for parents of Down's syndrome infants to perceive them as weak or delicate. Consequently, they are afraid to handle them as they would a normal child and, therefore, miss the naturally occuring opportunities such as bathtime to encourage more vigorous movement in the infant. Floppy infants are often difficult to breast feed too, not only because they may suck weakly but also because they fail to seek out the nipple and do not "actively" mould themselves into positions that are comfortable to both mother and child. Carr (1975) noted a variety of feeding difficulties in her group of Down's syndrome infants studied from birth to age four and recorded a persistence of problems for a considerable length of time in some.

Perhaps the most salient feature of any adult's interaction with an infant is the exchange of a smile. There are two studies which have reported delays in the onset of smiling behaviour in Down's syndrome infants (Cicchetti & Srouffe, 1976; Emde, Katz & Thorpe, 1978), the first of which demonstrates an association between degree of hypotonia and the capacity to express positive emotions by smiling or laughing. Cicchetti and Srouffe's (1976) study involved a detailed comparison of the responses of Down's and normal infants to a series of 30 stimuli ranging from simple cooing or tickling to more cognitively demanding items involving the covering and uncovering of a favourite toy. The results showed that, although the Down's syndrome infants responded to the groups of items in the same order as the normal children, the process was generally delayed. For example, the median age of onset of laughter was 10 months, compared to age 3-4 months for normal infants. Of most interest to this discussion, however, was the finding that the more hypotonic the infant the greater the lag. In addition, the intensity of the affective responses was consistently more muted in the Down's syndrome infants - they rarely laughed vigorously - and the latency between the onset of the eliciting stimuli and the response was longer than for the non-handicapped children. While it is clear that these results might be accounted for in other ways, the hypothesis that the "motor" deficit might be a major factor seems not unreasonable. The other study which draws attention to differences between Down's and non-handicapped infants in smiling behaviour is that of Emde, Katz and Thorpe (1978). In a discussion of the impact of these differences on adults, they point to similarities between their own observations and those of Fraiberg (1977) on blind children and their caretakers. Fraiberg described a feeling of disappointment experienced by the parents of blind children as they lean over the crib to find their infant sober and non-reactive rather than smiling and responsive.

When we consider the reasons why the pattern of eye contact between a child and his caretakers or siblings might develop abnormally, inability to control the movement of the eyes does not emerge as a highly probable explanation. However, that such failure may be a contributory factor has recently been suggested by Berger and Cunningham (1981) who systematically compared the development of eye contact between Down's syndrome infants and their mothers and normal infants and their mothers, over a six month period. Recording was begun at about six weeks of age and continued at weekly intervals until the infants were 24 weeks old. Analysis of the temporal aspects of the eye contact between the mothers and their infants revealed several differences in the development of such interactions. First, the onset of eye contact between mother and child was delayed in the Down's syndrome group. Second, the length of time contact was maintained in any one interaction was initially much shorter in the Down's syndrome group and took a long time to build up to the maximum duration exhibited by the normal infants at seven weeks of age. However, once the peak had been reached the Down's syndrome infants then stayed at that level for much longer than the normal infants, who very quickly discovered other aspects of the world and altered their pattern of looking at mother to more frequent and shorter exchanges. With respect to the late onset and initial inability to maintain eye contact for any length of time, Berger and Cunningham present two possible explanations, one related to the maturity of the visual system, the other concerned with hypotonia in the eye muscles but do not commit themselves to one or other. Data on this aspect of social interaction in older Down's syndrome children is lacking but it is of interest to note that Sinson and Wetherick (1981) felt that one reason why the Down's syndrome toddlers they studied failed to integrate into a normal nursery was that the conventions associated with maintaining mutual gaze were not observed.

The suggestion that Down's syndrome children are generally more passive and less inclined to move than normal children gains considerable support from a study by Francis (1971) of the patterns of play behaviour in home-reared and institutionalised children. Four groups of children were involved, Down's syndrome children brought up at home and in an institution, and normal children similarly reared. All of the observed behaviours involved movement, ranging from diffuse undirected movements of the limbs to more sophisticated skilled movements involving object manipulation and locomotion. The results can be summarised in two parts. First there were differences between the Down's syndrome and normal children regardless of whether they were institutionalised or not. At all developmental levels, the normal children were more alert and active than those with Down's syndrome. This showed up in the early stages as more frequent movement of the limbs, later in more active exploration of objects, and finally in more locomotion. The second important conclusion Francis reached was that the

Down's child was *more* affected by institutional rearing than the normal child. For both normal and Down's children, the institutions provided fewer toys, more physical restraint, and less social contact, but these seemed to affect the Down's children more than their normal peers. In addition to the findings concerning objects in the surroundings, Francis also reports that the Down's children seemed less aware of the observer than the normal infants.

Taken together, these findings support the view that a form of self-perpetuating "sensory motor deprivation" contributes to the deviant trajectory of motor development in the young Down's syndrome child. Paucity of movement seems to be a major component of it.

Finally, it is essential to mention speech problems as one of many difficulties that Down's syndrome children may have in learning to communicate with others. Lack of clear and fluent speech is a common addition to language problems of other kinds. In a survey of speech production problems in Down's syndrome adults Schlanger and Gottslaben (1957) noted that 95% of their subjects had articulation problems, 72% voice production abnormalities and 45% were stutterers. Though these proportions are likely to have changed due to various improvements in the management of Down's syndrome, the fact that substantial numbers of Down's syndrome children do still exhibit speech production problems is indisputable (see Gunn, 1985 for a review).

To some extent unclear speech can be attributed to anatomical and physiological factors. The child with Down's syndrome often displays a reduced buccal cavity, distorted dentition, an enlarged and protruding tongue, poor salivation control, palate anomalies as well as sometimes having hearing problems. Added to this there may be frequent respiratory infections and of course the speech musculature is not exempt from hypotonia.

Although these factors must inevitably influence the child's ability to produce an already planned sequence of sounds, by themselves they do not seem to provide a complete explanation of the observed articulatory disorders. In fact, Lennenberg, Nichols and Rosenberger (1962) went so far as to discount defective articulators as being a major factor since they could find no significant relationship between the outstanding abnormalities and clarity of articulation. One reason for this is that the articulatory defects are often not entirely straightforward. For example, Down's syndrome children not only make more errors than normal children but also their errors are less consistent (Smith, 1975). When asked to imitate words they make fewer mistakes than when they say the same words spontaneously (Smith, 1975) and when asked to remember words then recall them verbally they make more errors than normal (Dodd, 1975). On the basis of these and other studies Dodd (1975) hypothesised a higher order motor planning defect as well as peripheral problems to account for these findings. However, a complete account of this issue is not relevant to this discussion. What is of more concern is the contribution these defects might make to the difficulty of Down's children to communicate with those around them. Numberous studies exist which describe similarities and differences between how Down's children and normal children communicate with their caretakers but few address the contribution of speech problems directly.

We have now considered a selection of studies which illustrate the ways in which the "motor" problems of the Down's syndrome child manifest themselves in"real-life" situations. Admittedly, there are instances where the case for assigning a major role to a "motor" deficit is stronger than others. For example, Cunningham's study of reaching documents not only the difficulties in successfully achieving a goal but also describes deviations from normal in the execution of the movements comprising the action. Thus, we have incontrovertible evidence of a problem of visuo-motor co-ordination affecting the outcome of an action. In contrast, Francis (1971) reports only a failure to perform certain kinds of movement. Proponents of other positions might argue that the paucity of movement is caused by a general lack of motivation or exploratory drive. However, this kind of problem only arises if one adopts a rather narrow view of "motor" problems which focuses on the quality of movement as opposed to the action systems of which the movements are but elements. In order to explain how deficits in the neuromotor machinery actually have their effect it is necessary to appeal to a much broader conceptual framework.

With respect to the various findings reported in this part of the paper it seems necessary to consider two different levels of explanation alongside each other. First, there is the possibility mentioned earlier, that is concerned with the control of movement per se. That is, that it takes much longer for the spatial representation of the world to become "mapped onto" the neuromotor system in the Down's syndrome child. Indeed, it might be argued that the level of refinement achieved by the normal individual is never reached by the Down's syndrome person. Hence, the lack of finesse which characterises their movement even in adulthood. At the same time, its seems essential to invoke a more abstract level of explanation which is not "motor" in the simple sense but which has to do with action. Using movement as a means of gaining access to the world seems to be deficient in the Down's syndrome child. Not only do they seem passive in the presence of objects and people but more than that they seem to lack the understanding of how to use movement to satisfy their needs and communicate with others.

CONCLUDING REMARKS

The preceding discussion has centred on the question of whether the development of motor control in Down's syndrome children follows a pattern which is unique to this particular group of genetic abberrations. Unfortunately, the existing evidence which can be called forth to support the conjectured relationship between the genetic anomaly and behaviour in the motor domain, is too fragmented to provide a clear answer to the question. Though data is accumulating, at least two major problems remain.

The first is well know, worth mentioning only because it is ubiquitous in the study of atypical groups of children. It concerns the absence of longitudinal studies and studies which focus on learning as opposed to performance. Most of the investigations that have been dealt with in this paper provide no more than a "momentary snapshot" of performance. Thus questions relating to how skills develop, how failure is compensated for, which environmental factors are conducive to learning and which are not etc. remain unanswered.

The second problem is much more difficult. How are we to bridge the gap between the different levels at which we have located attempts to analyse the deficit? It is easy to weigh a cerebellum and find that it weighs less than normal. It is also easy to observe that a child cannot catch a ball or stand on one leg, but linking these two factors will take some time.

References

Airaksinen, E.M. (1974). Tryptophan treatment of infants with Down's Syndrome. *Annals of Clinical Research, 6,* 33-39.
Ahlman, H., Grillner, S. & Udo, M. (1971). The Effect of 5-Hydroxytryptoph on the static fusimotor activity and the tonic stretch reflex of an extensor motor. *Brain, 27,* 393-396.
Anwar, F. (1983). The role of sensory modality for the reproduction of shape by the severely retarded. *British Journal of Developmental Psychology, 1,* 317-327.
Aslin, R.N. (1981). Development of smooth pursuit in human infants. In D.F. Fisher, R.A. Monty and J.W. Senders (Eds.), *Eye movements: Cognition and Visual Perception.* Hillsdale, N.J.: Lawrence Erlbaum Associates.
Aslin, R.N. & Salapatek, P. (1975). Saccadic localisation of visual targets by the very young human infant. *Perception and Psychophysics, 17,* 293-302.
Ball, M.J. & Nuttall, K. (1980). Neurofibrillary tangles, granulovacuolar degeneration, and neuron loss in Down Syndrome: Quantitative comparison with Alzheimer Dementia. *Annals of Neurology, 7,* 462-465.
Bayley, N. (1969). *Manual for the Bayley Scales of Infant Development.* New York: Psychological Corporation.
Bazelon, M., Paine, R., Cowie, V., Hunt, P., Houck, J. & Mahanand, D. (1967). Reversal of hypotonia in infants with Down's Syndrome by administration of 5-Hydroxytryptophan. *The Lancet, 1,* 1130.
Belmont, J.M. (1971). Medical-Behavioural Research in Retardation. In N.R. Ellis (Ed.), *International Review of Research in Mental Retardation.* New York: Academic Press.
Berger, J. & Cunningham, C.C. (1981). The development of eye contact between mothers and normal versus Down's Syndrome infants. *Developmental Psychology, 17,* 678-689.
Berkson, G. (1960a). An analysis of reaction time in normal and mentally deficient young men: Duration threshold experiment. *Journal of Mental Deficiency Research, 4,* 51-58.
Berkson, G. (1960b). An analysis of reaction time in normal and mentally deficient young men: Variation of complexity in reaction time tasks. *Journal of Mental Deficiency Research, 4,* 59-67.
Berkson, G. (1960c). An analysis of reaction time in normal and mentally deficient young men: Variation of complexity in reaction time tasks. *Journal of Mental Deficiency Research, 4,* 69-77.
Blanchard, I. (1964). Speech pattern and etiology in mental retardation. *American Journal of Mental Deficiency, 68,* 612-617.
Butterworth, G. & Cicchetti, D. (1978). Visual calibration of posture in normal and motor retarded Down's Syndrome infants. *Perception, 7,* 513-525.
Carr, J. (1970). Mental and motor development in young mongol children. *Journal of Mental Deficiency Research, 14,* 205-220.
Carr, J. (1975). *Young children with Down's Syndrome.* London: Butterworth.
Cicchetti, D. & Srouffe, L.A. (1976). The relationship between affective and cognitive development in Down's Syndrome infants. *Child Development, 47,* 920-929.
Coleman, M. (1975). The use of 5-Hydroxytryptophan in patients with Down's Syndrome. In R. Koch and F.F. de la Cruz (Eds.), *Down's Syndrome (Mongolism). Research, Prevention and Management.* New York: Brunner-Mazel.

Coltheart, M., Patterson, K. & Marshall, J.C. (Eds.) (1980). *Deep Dyslexia.* London: Routledge and Kegan Paul.
Connolly, K. (1973). Factors influencing the learning of manual skills in young children. In R.A. Hinde and J. Stevenson-Hinde (Eds.), *Constraints on Learning.* London: Academic Press.
Connolly, K.J. & Prechtl, H.F.R. (Eds.) (1981). *Maturation and Development. Biological and Psychological Perspectives. Clinics in Developmental Medicine, No. 77/78.* London: S.I.M.P. with Heinemann; Philadelphia: Lippincott.
Cowie, V.A. (1970). *A Study of the Early development of mongols.* Oxford: Pergamon.
Crome, I., Cowie, V. & Slater, E. (1966). Statistical note on cerebellar and brain stem weight in mongolism. *Journal of Mental Deficiency Research, 10,* 69-72.
Cunningham, C.C. (1979). Aspects of early development in Down's Syndrome infants. Ph.d thesis. University of Manchester.
Cunningham, C.C. (1982). *Down's Syndrome: An Introduction for Parents.* London: Souvenir Press (Educational & Academic Ltd.).
Cunningham, C.C. & Mittler, P.J. (1981). Maturation, Development and Mental Handicap. In K.J. Connolly and H.F.R. Prechtl (Eds.), *Maturation and Development: Biological and Psychological Perspectives. Clinics in Developmental Medicine, No. 77/78.* London: S.I.M.P. and Heinemann; Philadelphia: Lippincott.
Davidson, P.W., Pine, R., Wiles-Kettenmann, M. & Appelle, S. (1980). Haptic-visual shape matching by mentally retarded children: Exploratory activity and complexity effects. *American Journal of Mental Deficiency, 84,* 526-533.
Davis, W.E. & Kelso, J.A.S. (1982). Analysis of "invariant characteristics" in motor control of Down's Syndrome and normal subjects. *Journal of Motor Behavior, 14,* 194-212.
Davis, W.E. & Sinning, W.E. (1985). The effects of strength training on the muscle - joint system mechanical properties of Down's Syndrome and other mentally handicapped subjects. Unpublished manuscript.
Davis, W.E., Ward, T. & Sparrow, W.A. (1984). Fractionated reaction times in Down's Syndrome and other mentally handicapped adults. *American Journal of Mental Deficiency Research* (in press).
Dodd, B.J. (1975). Recognition and reproduction of words by Down's Syndrome and non-Down's Syndrome retarded children. *American Journal of Mental Deficiency, 80,* 306-311.
Dicks-Mireaux, M.J. (1972). Mental development of infants with Down's Syndrome. *American Journal of Mental Deficiency, 77,* 26-32.
Dubowitz, V. (1980). *The Floppy Infant. 2nd. Edition. Clinics in Developmental Medicine, No. 76.* London: S.I.M.P. with Heinemann. Philadelphia: Lippincott.
Dunn, J. (1981). Maturation and Early Social Development. In K.J. Connolly and H.F.R. Prechtl (Eds.), *Maturation and Development: Biological and Psychological Perspectives. Clinics in Developmental Medicine No. 77/78.* London: S.I.M.P. and Heinemann. Philadelphia: Lippincott.
Emde, R., Katz, E. & Thorpe, J. (1978). Emotional expression in infancy: II. Early deviations in Down's Syndrome. In M. Lewis and L. Rosenblum (Eds.), *The Development of Affect.* New York: Plenum Press.
Evarts, E.V., Teravainen, H. & Calne, D.B. (1981). Reaction times in Parkinson's Disease. *Brain, 104,* 167-168.
Fishler, K., Share, J. & Koch, R. (1964). Adaptation of Gesell developmental scales for evaluation of development in children with Down's Syndrome. *American Journal of Mental Deficiency, 68,* 642-646.

Fraiberg, S. (1977). *Insights from the Blind.* New York: Basic Books.
Francis, S.H. (1971). The effects of own-home and institution rearing on the behavioural development of normal and mongol children. *Journal of Child Psychology and Psychiatry, 12,* 173-190.
Frith, V. & Frith, C.D. (1974). Specific motor disabilities in Down's Syndrome *Journal of Child Psychology and Psychiatry, 15,* 293-301.
Gaussen, T. (1984). Developmental milestones or conceptual millstones? Some practical and theoretical limitations in infant assessment procedures. *Child Care, Health and Development, 10,* 99-115.
Gesell, A. & Armatruda, C.S. (1941). *Developmental Diagnosis.* New York: Harper.
Gibson, D. (1978). *Down's Syndrome: The psychology of mongolism.* Cambridge: Cambridge University Press.
Griffiths, R. (1954). *The abilities of babies.* London: University of London Press.
Gunn, P. (1985). Speech and Language. In D. Lane and B. Stratford (Eds.), *Current Approaches to Down's Syndrome.* London: Holt, Rinehart and Winston.
Gustafson, G.E. (1984). Effects of the ability to locomote on infants' social and exploratory behaviours: An experimental study. *Developmental Psychology, 20,* 397-405.
Henderson, S.E. (1985). Motor Skill Development. In D. Lane and B. Stratford (Eds.), *Current Approaches to Downs' Syndrome.* London: Holt Rinehart and Winston.
Henderson, S.E., Morris, J. & Frith, U. (1981). The Motor deficit in Down's Syndrome children: A problem of timing? *Journal of Child Psychology and Psychiatry, 22,* 233-245.
Hofsten, C. von. (1978). Development of visually guided reaching: the approach phase. *Journal of Human Movement Studies, 5,* 160-178.
Hofsten, C. von. (1980). Predictive reaching for moving objects by human infants. *Journal of Experimental Child Psychology, 30,* 369-382.
Hofsten, C. von. (1982). Eye-hand co-ordination in newborns. *Developmental Psychology, 18,* 450-461.
Hofsten, C. von. (1983). Foundations for perceptual development. In L.P. Lippsitt and C.K. Rovee-Collier (Eds.), *Advances in Infancy Research Vol. 2.* Norwood: Ablex Publishing Co.
Hogg, J. & Moss, S.C. (1983). Prehensile development in Down's Syndrome and non-handicapped pre-school children. *British Journal of Developmental Psychology, 1,* 189-204.
Kirman, B.H. (1951). Epilepsy in Mongolism. *Archives of Diseases of Childhood, 26,* 501.
Kopp, C.B. & Shaperman, J. (1973). Cognitive development in the absence of object manipulation during infancy. *Developmental Psychology, 9,* 430.
Laveck, B. & Laveck, G.D. (1977). Sex differences in development among children with Down's Syndrome. *Journal of Pediatrics, 91,* 767-769.
Lee, D.N. & Aronson, G. (1974). Visual proprioceptive control of standing in human infants. *Perception and Psychophysics, 15,* 529-532.
Lee, D.N. & Lishman, J.R. (1975). Visual proprioceptive control of stance. *Journal of Human Movement Studies, 1,* 87-95.
Lennenberg, E.H., Nichols, I.A. & Rosenberger, E.F. (1962). Primitive stages of language development in mongolism. *Proceedings, Association for Research in Nervous and Mental Disease, 42,* 119-137.
Lewis, V.A. & Bryant, P.E. (1982). Touch and vision in normal and Down's Syndrome babies. *Perception, 11,* 691-701.
Loesch-Mdzewska, D. (1968). Some aspects of the neurology of Down's Syndrome. *Journal of Mental Deficiency Research, 12,* 237-246.

McIntire, M.S. & Dutch, S.J. (1964). Mongolism and generalised hypotonia. *American Journal of Mental Deficiency, 68,* 669-670.
Molnar, G.E. (1978). Analysis of motor disorder in retarded infants and young children. *American Journal of Mental Deficiency, 83,* 213-222.
Morris, A.F., Vaughan, S.E. & Vaccaro, P. (1981). Measurement of neuromuscular tone and strength in Down's Syndrome children. *Journal of Mental Deficiency Research, 26,* 41-46.
Nashner, L.M. & Woollacott, M. (1979). The organisation of rapid postural adjustments of standing humans: An Experimental - conceptual model. In R.E. Talbot and D.R. Humphreys (Eds.), *Posture and movement.* New York: Raven Press.
Nashner, L.M. & McCollum, G. (1986). The Organisation of human postural movements: A formal basis and experimental synthesis. *The Behavioural and Brain Sciences, 8,* 135-172.
Nashner, L.M., Shumway-Cook, A. & Marin, O. (1983). Stance posture control in selected groups of children with cerebral palsy: Deficits in sensory integration and muscular co-ordination. *Experimental Brain Research, 49,* 393-409.
Price, D.L., Whitehouse, P.J., Struble, R.G., Cycle, J.T., Clark, A.W., Delong, M.R., Cork, L.C. & Hedreen, J.C. (1983). Alzheimer's Disease and Down's Syndrome. *Annals of the New York Academy of Science, 396,* 145-164.
Roy, E. (Ed.) (1985). *Neuropsychological Studies of Apraxia and related disorders.* Amsterdam: North-Holland.
Sameroff, A.J. & Chandler, M.J. (1975). Reproductive risk and the continuum of caretaking casualty. In F.D. Horowitz, M. Hetherington, S. Scarr-Salapatek and G. Siegel (Eds.), *Review of child development research (Vol. 4).* Chicago: University of Chicago Press.
Saqi, S.M. (1981). Reaction times and movement times of Down's Syndrome children. Unpublished M.Sc.Thesis. Institute of Education, University of London.
Schlanger, B. & Gottsleben, R.H. (1957). Analysis of speech defects amongst the institutionalised mentally retarded. *Journal of Speech and Hearing Disorders, 22,* 98-103.
Seyfort, B. & Spreen, O. (1979). Two-plated tapping performance by Down's Syndrome and non-Down's Syndrome retardates. *Journal of Child Psychology and Psychiatry, 20,* 351-355.
Shumway-Cook, A. & Woollacott, M.H. (1985). *Dynamics of Postural Control in the child with Down's Syndrome.* (in press).
Sinson, J.C. & Wetherick, N.E. (1981). The behaviour of children with Down's Syndrome in normal playgroups. *Journal of Mental Deficiency Research, 25,* 113-120.
Smith, N.V. (1975). Universal tendencies in the child's acquisition of phonology. In N. O'Connor (Ed.), *Language, cognitive deficits and retardation.* London: Butterworth.
Thelen, E. & Fisher, D.M. (1983). From spontaneous to Instrumental behaviour: Kinematic analysis of movement changes during very early learning. *Child Development, 54,* 129-140.
Thelen, E. & Fisher, D.M. (1983). The organisation of spontaneous leg movements in newborn infants. *Journal of Motor Behavior, 15,* 353-377.
Trevarthen, C. (1984). Biodynamic structures, cognitive correlates of motive sets and the development of motives in infants. In W. Prinz and A.F. Sanders (Eds.), *Cognition and Motor Processes.* Berlin: Springer Verlag.
Wing, A.M. (1984). Disorders of movement. In M.M. Smyth and A.M. Wing (Eds.), *The Psychology of Human Movement.* London: Academic Press.

Yang, R.K. (1979). Early infant assessment: An Overview. In J.D. Osofsky (Ed.), *Handbook of Infant Development*. New York: Wiley.

THE TRAINABILITY OF MOTOR PROCESSING STRATEGIES WITH DEVELOPMENTALLY DELAYED PERFORMERS

G. Reid

INTRODUCTION

Few scientists today would argue against the notion that cognition is a factor in motor control. However, the extent of cognitive involvement is a crucial issue, separating present day schools of information processing in which cognition rules supreme from the ecological approach to action in which cognition is minimised (Turvey & Carello, 1981; Newell, in press). The present essay, given the title, is more clearly grounded in the cognitive camp. But, as the issues regarding the direct intervention of strategic cognitive-motor processing are addressed, some questions and problems raised by ecological advocates will be highlighted.

A strategy may be defined generally as a method for approaching a task or achieving a goal (Kirby, 1984). While a strategy might be considered an annoying individual difference, the tact here is to view strategy as an important construct worthy of study in its own right. There appear to be four conceptual approaches to the term although they may not be mutually exclusive. First, strategy can refer to the production of a specific pattern of coordination, for example a backhand tennis stroke with one or two hands. Secondly, strategy may denote a pattern of behaviour across a series of trials. Such an approach was recently adopted by Brewer and Smith (1984) to explain the slow and more variable reaction times of the mentally retarded. A third use of the term is as a synonym for method or approach. A coach or teacher may choose a particular teaching strategy or game plan. Fourthly, strategy can be conceptualised as a means to remember, learn or problem solve (Brown, Bransford, Ferrara & Campione, 1983). This orientation, the focus of the present paper, emanates from an information processing perspective and is often associated with attempts to train developmentally delayed learners to be more strategic.

INFORMATION PROCESSING AND DEVELOPMENTALLY DELAYED LEARNERS

The information processing perspective of skilled performance was particularly attractive to researchers dealing with special populations for theoretical and practical reasons (e.g. Hagen, Barclay & Schewthelm, 1982; Hall, 1980; Stanovich, 1978). First, models of information processing were seen as vehicles to define and categorise learning problems. For example, Atkinson and Shiffrin's (1968) analysis of memory, included both structural and control components. Structural components (short-term sensory store, short-term store and long-term store) were viewed as permanent, unchanging and unmodifiable features. In contrast, the control processes were posited to modulate the flow of information through the structures and were regarded as transient, optional and used at the discretion of the individual. In the area of mental retardation, the notion of structure seemed logically related to intelligence and thus could be an important construct in defining retardation (Fisher & Zeaman, 1973). Definitional problems abound in special education (Torgesen & Kail, 1980) and the issue of labeling is always present. Thus a functional analysis of child's processing proficiencies and deficiencies was viewed as a way to deemphasising labels while categorising performance (Hagen et al, 1982).

The second benefit of processing models in special population research had a distinct remedial flavour. An implicit assumption was that subjects could be shown to have both strengths and weaknesses in information processing. Then, teaching would proceed by working directly with the deficit or via the strengths depending upon the bias of the instructor (Torgesen & Kail, 1980). In fact, some special educators have bemoaned the almost exclusive use of behaviour modification techniques in teaching academic, vocational, social and personal skills and have argued that neglecting cognitive training may be denying the ideology upon which special education is built (Sabatino, Miller & Schmidt, 1981).

The information processing perspective is not without its difficulties in relation to special populations. First, the structure/control process distinction while heuristically valuable is sometimes difficult to dicotomise (Winograd, 1975) and developmentalists now acknowledge that both structure and process will change, the former less slowly than the latter (Anwar, 1983; Butterfield, 1981; Campione & Brown, 1978; Newell, 1984). Thus implications for definition become cloudy. Also, at least in the area of mental retardation and physical performance, virtually all stages of information processing have been shown to be faulty (Henderson, 1985; Nettelbeck & Brewer, 1981; Newell, 1985), including attentiveness (Kirby, Nettelbeck & Thomas, 1979); perceptual processing (Nettelbeck & Lally, 1979); decision making (Brewer, 1978); response capacity and organisation (Sugden & Gray, 1981; Wade, Newell & Wallace, 1978); coincident timing (Wade, Newell & Hoover, 1982); temporal anticipation (Newell, Wade & Kelly, 1979); and short-term motor memory (Reid, 1980a). Thus information processing has been criticised as simply another description of the motor performance of retarded persons since it has not lead to a demonstration of proficiencies and deficiencies (Newell, 1985).

Current work under the information processing umbrella is best associated with control processes rather than structural features (e.g. Brown et al, 1983) although the search for specific structural deficits continues (Ellis, Deacon & Woolridge, 1985). Developmentally delayed individuals are now being characterised as passive, non-strategic learners whose difficulties may be modifiable (Brown et al, 1983). This shift in emphasis is apparent in mental retardation, learning disabilities (Hagen et al, 1982) and physical awkwardness (Wall, McClements, Bouffard, Findlay & Taylor, 1985). The remainder of the paper will focus on the salient points in training developmentally delayed learners to be strategic in their motor performance.

DEVELOPMENT OF STRATEGIC BEHAVIOURS

Identifying strategic behaviour in information processing was initiated in developmental memory (e.g. Flavell, 1970) and was soon explored with mentally retarded persons (e.g. Belmont & Butterfield, 1969; Brown, 1974;

Ellis, 1970). Flavell, Beach and Chinsky (1966) demonstrated developmental differences among 5-, 7- and 10-year old children on a task of recalling previously presented objects. Observed lip movements were used as measures of spontaneous verbal activity. This began a series of investigations by Flavell (1970), Hagen (Hagen & Stanovich, 1977) and their associates on the acquisition of strategic behaviour and its relationship to performance. It was postulated that mediated memory was seldom seen before 6 years of age and that developmental differences in memory performance were attributed to the growth of strategic behaviour. A corollary was offered by Brown (1974) who stated that tasks which did not require deliberate strategies would not likely be developmentally sensitive. Strategic behaviours identified were rehearsal, organisation, elaboration, intentional forgetting, chunking, labelling and imagery.

Two hypotheses were put forward to explain the poor memory performance of the developmentally young; meditational or production deficiencies. A mediational deficiency was one in which a strategic technique was used but failed to influence performance. In contrast, a production deficiency was presumed when potential mediators were not used and therefore could not affect performance. Differentiating between the two usually entails training subjects to be strategic, unless a direct measure of the strategy is available. If a subject is taught to be strategic and improves at the given task, then the original problem is assumed to have been one of production while a failure of the training to influence behaviour is interpreted as a mediational deficiency or poor training. While there is considerable evidence that retarded, learning disabled and nonhandicapped children do not spontaneously employ strategies there is almost as equally an abundant literature that they can be trained to do so, suggesting the original difficulty was primarily a production deficiency (Bauer, 1977, 1979; Belmont & Butterfield, 1977; Brown, 1978; Campione & Brown, 1977; Butterfield, Wambold & Belmont, 1973; Ellis, 1970; Torgesen, 1977).

Since 1970 there has been a growing body of empirical evidence with verbal tasks to support the following conclusions regarding development and training of strategic behaviour (Brown et al, 1983; Campione, Brown & Ferrara, 1982; Torgesen & Kail, 1980).

1) Preschool aged children may be strategic when the goal of the activity is clear, meaningful and the setting familiar.

2) Strategies are not a question of presence or absence. Rather, there is a gradual emergence of competency in their use. Both Brown et al (1983) and Hagen et al (1982) have specified developmental sequences.

3) In the early developmental years strategies tend to be task dependent or "welded" (Brown et al, 1983) to a domain. With maturity they evolve into more flexible and sometimes generaliseable skills.

4) While improvement in strategic behaviour with instruction by retarded and learning disabled persons is documented and there is some evidence of durability, the data supporting generalisability of acquired strategies is controversial (Borkowski & Cavanaugh, 1979; Campione & Brown, 1978).

5) Strategies can become so dominant that with experience they may resemble automatic, unconscious processing (Naus & Ornstein, 1983).

6. Strategies do not covary perfectly with age. Experience and knowledge in a domain are important (Chi, 1978, 1983; Naus & Ornstein, 1983).

7) A partially adequate strategy may be maintained and may impede progress toward more efficient strategies.

8) A strategy may be in the behavioural repertoire of a person but not accessed under appropriate circumstances.

9) The motivational perspective of the learner will affect the strategy chosen (Biggs, 1984).

There is a paucity of information regarding the development of strategies with movement related tasks. Thomas, Thomas, Lee, Testerman and Ashy (1983) showed that 9-year old children remembered both distance and location information of a jogging task more effectively than 4-year olds and that the older children were more able to articulate a specific means to remember. In a second experiment these authors instructed 5-, 9- and 12-year olds to employ a "step counting strategy" to facilitate reproduction of the criterion distance jogged. The strategy had no significant influence on the older children who appeared to spontaneously adopt a mnemonic device but the two younger groups were superior to control comparison groups who did not receive strategy training. In a subsequent study by Gallagher and Thomas (1984) a mature strategy including active rehearsal of eight movements in groupings which highlighted their inherent organisation was demonstrated to be superior to a child-like strategy of remaining at the end of each movement for 8 sec. Also the 5-year olds performed like the 7- and 11-year olds when taught to use the mature strategy. These findings are in concert with other movement data (Winther & Thomas, 1981) and the verbal literature in which manipulation of strategic behaviour can produce results suggesting the child is functioning like a more mature performer.

Deficiencies in short-term motor memory have been identified with mentally retarded subjects (Horgan, 1983a; Sugden, 1978; Reid, 1980a). To determine the trainability of these problems Reid (1980b; 1984) instructed mentally retarded subjects to focus their attention on the "feel" of the criterion movement on a linear positioning apparatus (1980b) and a ball rolling task (1984). Attention to the end position of the hand relative to another body part was also put forth as an effective strategy. The strategy instructed groups were able to recall their movements with greater facility than non-instructed groups. Horgan (1983b) has also shown that retarded subjects can improve their performance on a linear positioning task, in fact to levels attained by the nonretarded, when they are instructed to employ a recall strategy. Thus the developmental and special population research supports the notion that young and less intelligent youngsters are not spontaneously strategic with motor tasks. However the mnemonic techniques thus far identified appear quite susceptible to instruction.

While the lions share of research attention in developmental memory has focused on strategic behaviour as an explanation of age related variance, the role of the developing knowledge base must not be overlooked. Clearly a child's knowledge increases with age. Chi (1978, 1981) has argued that strategy changes cannot be adopted as solely responsible for memory development because (1) adults are usually still superior to children even if the latter are taught an adult strategy (see Gallagher & Thomas, 1984 for support of this statement in the motor domain), (2) differences between adults and children remain if both are taught a strategy, (3) if adults are prevented from being strategic, their performance typically remains superior to that of children.

Chi's (1978) oft cited study of expert chess players championed the importance of the knowledge base. When the experts were children and the novices were adults, the experts still outperformed the novices on immediate recall of chess positions (9.3 versus 5.9) despite the fact that on a digit span task the children-experts were inferior although not significantly to the adult-novices (6.1 versus 7.8). A recent model of motor development has been constructed on the assumed importance of knowledge in learning and performance (Wall et al, 1985).

Current knowledge and strategic behaviour are thus important explanatory factors in understanding memory performance and learning. Chi (1978, 1981) argued that the knowledge base is the most critical factor and that strategies should be viewed as general knowledge of heuristic rules that emerge from an increasingly rich and specific procedural and declarative knowledge base. Brown et al (1983) however suggested that the evidence regarding strategies proposed by Chi is only indirect and thus appeared to favour a position of concurrent development of strategies and knowledge and their mutual importance in influencing learning and remembering.

Strategic behaviour and the knowledge base must be investigated jointly in order to tease out the vagaries of their relationship (Naus & Ornstein, 1983). In fact Hagen et al (1982) have categorised environmental demands and person status in terms of strategies and knowledge in order to predict performance based on their interaction. Chi (1981) has added age to a similar endeavor. There is recent evidence that knowledge and processing strategies interact (Chi, 1981; Naus & Ornstein, 1983). A training implication from this evidence is that adult strategies may not be appropriate to teach youngsters in situations where the contextual knowledge is novel and unfamiliar. The challenge for motor behaviour specialists is to determine the movement related knowledge base and investigate its relationship with strategic techniques - no small task, since there may be knowledge-specific strategies (Chi, 1978) to the movement domain which heretofore have not been identified and some movement knowledge is no doubt tacit (Newell & Barclay, 1982).

Metamemory and the more generally metacognition have become domains related to the training of strategies in developmentally delayed youngsters. "Metacognition refers to one's knowledge and control of the domain cognition" (Brown et al, 1983). Two dimensions of metacognition are therefore apparent, knowledge and control (Lawson, 1984). It has been described as a fuzzy concept defying exact definition; for while there is good agreement on central instances of the concept there is considerable debate about other instances (Wellman, 1983). Arguably, it is metacognitive knowledge by which a person ascertains if a task is difficult enough to require strategic activity. Thus the production deficiencies previously noted with the developmentally immature may be influenced by their lack of metacognitive knowledge (Campione & Brown, 1977).

Flavell and Wellman (1977) have outlined two major domains of metamemory knowledge: 1) knowing whether or not a task requires planful memory strategies and 2) knowing that performance is influenced by a) memory characteristics (strengths and weakness) of the person, b) memory characteristics of the task, i.e. some tasks are more difficult than others, and c) potential strategies for the task and their relative potencies. Taking stock of available strategies is essentially what others have referred to as "executive control" of cognition (Belmont & Butterfield, 1977) and appears to be what Brown et al (1983) refer to as the regulation of cognition. These latter categories of metacognition refer to the planning, monitoring and checking of ongoing cognition in general and strategies in particular.

There is evidence that metamemory is a developmental phenomena influenced by age and experience (Flavell & Wellman, 1977; Kreutzer, Leonard & Flavell, 1975; Lawson, 1984) and that the developmentally delayed, at least the mentally retarded, are not adept at metacognitive skills such predicting the difficulty of a given task or selecting appropriate strategies (Campione & Brown, 1977). Further, some types of knowledge about memory or cognition would seem to figure strongly in effecting performance but the exact articulation of the metacognitive-cognitive response relationship is not yet available (Flavell & Wellman, 1977; Lawson, 1984; Wellman, 1983).

Metacognitive knowledge about movement is a virtually untapped research avenue although anecdotal examples exist (see Newell & Barclay, 1982). Markman (1973 as cited by Newell & Barclay, 1982) found children were almost as accurate as adults in predicting performance on the long jump. This may have resulted because the children had sufficient practice in this physical skill but they might not have fared so well on novel tasks. The need to clarify the relationships between experience, knowledge and metacognition seems obvious.

In sum, specifying the role of strategic behaviour in the motor domain from a developmental and special populations perspective while still in its infancy should adopt an interaction perspective (Brown et al, 1983) with metacognition and the motor knowledge base as critical factors. Four immediate issues in assessing the trainability of motor processing strategies are addressed in the next section.

MOVEMENT PROCESSING STRATEGIES

Task Selected: Determining the trainability of processing strategies will be influenced by the task selected. It is assumed that the ultimate goal is to enhance the acquisition of patterns of coordination. In the motor development and special population studies previously cited (e.g. Gallagher & Thomas, 1984; Horgan, 1983b; Reid, 1980b; Thomas et al, 1983) as well as the research on strategic motor learning with adults (e.g. Shea, 1977; Singer & Cauraugh, 1985) the tasks selected have been primarily cognitive in nature. Linear positioning and pursuit rotor apparatus are generally categorised as rather simple tasks or more formally as ones which place minimal demands of reducing redundant degrees of freedom (Bernstein, 1967). Even the jogging activities used by Thomas and colleagues are essentially cognitive in nature since the goal is to remember the distance or location jogged, not a pattern of coordination. Thus the "motor" work conducted thus far with the developmentally young might be argued to be simply repetitions of previous work in the cognitive domain; the motor tasks not really being very motor. This might explain why the strategic intervention data with motor tasks auger so well with the cognitive literature.

The early investigations of strategic behaviour were tied closely to specific models of information processing, for example the Atkinson and Shiffrin (1968) model. Tasks, often simple and quite meaningless were designed in order to test the model. The information processing framework thus created the task. In more recent work on strategic development and intervention, ecologically valid tasks such as studying and writing expositions (Brown et al, 1983) are selected and then investigated within relevant theoretical constructs. Strategies are still regarded as important, interacting with the developing knowledge base and metacognition. The research is nonetheless theoretical, but it is not concerned if the strategies are associated with a hypothetical stage of processing. But upon what performance criteria could the effectiveness of strategic training be based?

Ecological theorists have distinguished among coordination, control and skill (Kugler, Kelso & Turvey, 1980, 1982) and Newell (in press) has argued that coordination within this context may be operationalised as a set of relative motions. Indeed, most strategic motor learning research to date has been concerned, at best, with control or the scaling of the set of relative motions. Thus, if strategic intervention could be shown to effect the acquisition of a set of relative motions that defined a task important in the lifestyle of the disabled performer, a stingent test of motor processing strategy training would be apparent. It aided coordination! Further removed theoretically from the coordination, control and skill distinction, but possibly viable in strategic training research are the recent qualitative descriptions of developmental motor patterns which yield performance scores (Mosher & Schutz, 1983; Ulrich, 1985). Thus while more complex and real motor tasks are difficult to quantify and are seldom novel to the subjects (thus presenting research design obstacles) the full assessment of the trainability of movement processing strategies requires work with such patterns of coordination.

Identification of Strategies to Instruct: Determining the appropriate strategy to teach may be the most difficult problem in the training enterprise. Ecological psychologists have admonished the cognitive orientation for a preoccupation with the "how" of information processing to the detriment of questions pertaining to "what". In the present context Gibson's followers would demand that we be specific regarding "what" the subjects are being strategic about. What cues in the movement-environment synergy are attended to? What mnemonics are functioning? Labelling, rehearsal, elaboration organisation and chunking have a basis in fact with verbal or comprehension performance but the assumption that these strategies are operable with movement tasks is based more in faith than fact. Fleshing out the motor processing strategies may be complicated because (1) the existing empirical knowledge regarding the organisation and representation of movement is meagre, (2) the strategies may be largely tacit particularly with experienced performers and (3) training strategies may be problematic once identified since people may be strategic but have difficulty executing the task.

With these concerns in mind a task analysis may be a useful starting point. Singer and Cauraugh (1985) have proposed a task analysis framework to guide instruction of strategies for motor tasks. The procedure will likely highlight task-specific strategies, most certainly different strategies for categories of motor tasks. Their information processing task analysis includes three stages (1) information analysis which assesses information receipt and sensory-perceptual processing such as anticipation and attention to specific cues (2) response generation and organisation which pertains to sequencing and phasing and (3) response-produced feedback which purports to identify such factors as the relevant feedback cues.

Task analysis is sometimes accompanied by asking performers to make post task reports (Belmont & Butterfield, 1977). Indeed asking experts how they accomplish the task is quite common and those interested in motor processing strategies may consider interviewing expert performers, or successful coaches and teachers. Some insight into effective strategies may be gained from introspection of precocious child performers or by adopting a microgenetic analysis (Karmiloff-Smith, 1979) which follows a child or small group of children as they proceed through the learning phases of a task. Age and experience must be considered in strategy selection since strategies for the developmentally young should be compatible with cognitive competency of the child (Brown, 1978) and experience may rule out some strategies and point to others (Wade, 1976). While verbal reports have problems (Brown et al, 1983) there now exist guidelines to minimise their difficulties (Ericsson & Simon, 1980) and they may be invaluable as an initial step in identifying relevant strategies in a movement context.

Direct measures of strategic devices are also important (Belmont & Butterfield, 1977) to determine if a strategy is spontaneously used and the effects of an instructional program. Verbal reports are not direct and it is possible people will verbally report what they believe they are doing but which does not coincide with reality. Simple product outcome measures are not likely to be sensitive enough. It is possible that a trial-to-trial analysis of kinetic or kinematic variables may be helpful (see Brewer & Smith, 1984, for an example). Some of the suggestions may prove effective in identifying strategies used by learners. However, whatever method is used, their effectiveness must be assessed by a training protocol.

Demonstrating Strategic Training Efficacy: Empirical vertification of strategic training efficiency is required to verify the task analysis. Since the assumption is that developmentally delayed learners are not spontaneously strategic, a test-train-test protocol (Campione, Brown & Ferrara, 1982) is suggested. The logic of the training study follows. The initial test confirms that they have problems with the motor task. From the task analysis, interviews with experts etc., it is hypothesised that successful performance on the task is dependent upon components A, B, and C and that the developmentally delayed youngsters do poorly because of A. To test this hypothesis, subjects are trained to do A and retested on the criterion task. If performance improves the task analysis is reinforced as well as the hypothesis about the subjects' difficulties. If A were not important or if the subjects were already efficient with A, performance should not improve. As Campione et al (1982) argue, the test-train-test design is an iterative one as new hypotheses and task analyses are generated on the basis of the findings.

Multiple assessment will reinforce the role of strategic involvement in motor performance (Campione et al, 1982). The demonstration of strategic trainability with the developmentally delayed and their initial ineptitude supports the link from strategy to performance. Also, showing that non-delayed persons are strategically involved in their learning but suffer when prevented from exercising their mediating techniques would garner evidence for the proposed link. Convergent measures of strategy are thus desired.

Research endeavors in the early 1970's indicated that cognitive processing strategies were ameneable to training. However, the effectiveness of a training regime must be evaluated against three criteria (1) initial effects, (2) durability or maintenance and (3) generalisability. To date only two published studies in motor learning have addressed the generalisability issue (Brown, Singer, Cauraugh & Lucariello, 1985; Singer & Cauraugh, 1984) and both used adult nonhandicapped subjects. Campione and Brown (1977) suggested maintenance of strategy training with retarded persons could be realised but that the evidence was weak regarding generalisation. Borkowski and Cavanaugh (1979), in contrast, interpret the evidence to support generalisation if the training is adequate. Their suggestions to promote maintenance and generalisation which seem applicable to physical skills follow.

Maintenance and generalisation may represent an assessment of metacognition (Belmont & Butterfield, 1977). If a strategy is used at a latter point on the same task or is invoked when a new task is introduced then the subject has elected to employ the strategy in light of tasks demands, an execution function. Maintenance of a strategy may be facilitated by (1) sufficient training experiences, (2) variation in strategy training such as changing or fading instructors during training, (3) identifying the most effective strategies, (4) explaining to subjects via feedback that the use of strategies are related to outcome measures (Borkowski & Cavanaugh, 1979).

Strategy maintenance is likely a necessary condition for generalisation but not a sufficient one. Thus generalisation should be advanced by the maintenance procedures as well as some suggestions from the cognitive behaviour modification literature. The latter include (1) ensuring that strategies are maintained in the new environment by natural consequences, (2) using multiple exemplars in training, that is, two or three tasks, (3) reinforce generalisation, (4) train the strategy on a task in a context similar to that of the generalisation task.

Subject Selection: Definitional problems of developmentally delayed children which confront special educators have particular relevance for the researcher interested in cognitive processing. The category learning disabilities is a particular case in point. These youngsters are often classified differently in various regions within a country, across countries and among different researchers. This makes comparisons of reports and generating conclusions difficult to impossible (Torgesen & Kail, 1980). Also the definitions are very broad, indeed, they are often linked to poor readings scores, the causes of which are enormous. Researchers are thus faced with extreme heterogeneity on the dependent variable.

In the present context it would be expected to find learning disabled children who are proficient strategically and others who are rather passive in exercising their control processes. If this broad range of disabled youngsters were used in a study it would not be surprising to find that the training of strategies was minimally effective if at all. Ignoring the variance issue of statistical significance for a movement, it is conceivable that the instructed strategies were already spontaneously functioning in a large segment of the sample and thus the training had no influence on them. What is needed are ways to classify children with learning problems (Torgesen & Kail, 1980). At the least, the strategy training researcher should pretest subjects to identify those who do and do not demonstrate strategic behaviours.

Subject selection also involves the decision to use nondisabled or developmentally disabled persons. An acknowledged model for investigating developmental phenomena is to select children deficient in the hypothesised process, observe them on a range of tasks related to the process and use instruction to ameliorate the problem (Hagen et al, 1982). This model has guided Brown, Campione and students who have used mentally retarded persons to determine the relationship between strategic behaviour, metacognition and intelligence (Campione et al, 1982). They point out that handicapped subjects are not necessary if one views intelligence as the ability to perform adequately on academic tasks. In this case, work with poor performers is not necessary, although possibly helpful, because the theory relates to normal functioning. If, however, intelligence is viewed as an individual difference construct then the theory must explain how people differ from each other. In this instance, as Campione et al (1982) cogently put forth, comparative research is not only nice but necessary.

In a developmental physical skills context what would be an appropriate comparison group for strategy research? Physically awkward children should be considered since they represent a manifestation of individual differences in skilled movement (Wall, 1982). Also despite some difficulties of identification (Keogh, Sugden, Reynard & Calkins, 1979) there is converging evidence of subclassifications (Dare & Gordon, 1970; Henderson & Hall, 1982) the necessity of which was noted. Separating physically awkward children into groups with and without concomitant learning problems in the classroom would be desirable to assess the efficacy of strategic intervention.

CONCLUSION

Research findings of information processing in a movement context have not enjoyed wide application possibly because researchers have confined themselves to simple tasks, and in laboratory settings and/or because educators have been unable or unwilling to see instructional possibilities. The discussion of the trainability of strategies under the headings task selection, identification, demonstrating efficacy and subject selection attempted to provide ways to enhance the applicability of the findings. It is assumed the real impact of strategy research will not be apparent until it is translated into educational practice (Torgesen & Kail, 1980).

The focus of this paper has been on control processes, strategies, but it should not be inferred that some structural limits do not contain the performance of handicapped persons. Although structural deficits with the mentally retarded have not been identified (although Ellis et al, 1985 take issue with this) it does not mean they do not exist. Some (e.g. Belmont & Butterfield, 1977) argue as if structural deficits do not exist and training may eliminate retardation. However, not to accept some motion of structural deficits begs the question of why mentally retarded persons are retarded (Ellis et al, 1985). Similarly, if a strategies research program aids the physical skills of clumsy children one must ask (1) if they are "at par" or simply improved and (2) why were they awkward and nonstrategic in the first place.

The present essay has stressed the trainability of strategies. Others have argued that they are not really ameneable to intervention, they are not importantly related to education phenomena and that they can only be learned incidently as part of a task (Brown et al, 1983). Also, the followers of the ecological perspective would cringe at the continual reference to cognitive strategies, and in particular executive functioning. However, while many questions remain with regard to engineering strategic techniques in a movement context, to deny their existance is to imply too passive a posture to the intelligent human condition.

References

Anwar, F. (1983). Vision and kinaesthesis in motor movements. In J. Hogg and P.J. Mittler (Eds.), *Advances in mental handicap research (Vol. 1)*. New York: Wiley & Sons.

Atkinson, R.E. & Shiffrin, R.M. (1968). Human memory: A proposed system and its control process. In K.W. Spence and J.T. Spence (Eds.), *The psychology of learning and motivation (Vol. 2)*. New York: Academic Press.

Bauer, R. (1977). Short term memory in learning disabled and nondisabled children. *Bulletin of the Psychonomic Society, 10*, 128-130.

Bauer, R. (1979). Memory, acquisition, and category clustering in learning disabled children. *Journal of Experimental Child Psychology, 27*, 365-383.

Belmont, J.M. & Butterfield, E.C. (1969). The relations of short-term memory to development and intelligence. In L.C. Lipsett and H.W. Reese (Eds.), *Advances in child development and behavior (Vol. 4)*. New York: Academic Press.

Belmont, J.M. & Butterfield, E.C. (1977). The instructional approach to developmental cognitive research. In R.V. Kail Jr. and J.W. Hagen (Eds.), *Perspectives on the development of memory and cognition*. Hillsdale, N.J.: Lawrence Erlbaum.

Bernstein, N. (1967). *The coordination and regulation of movement*. New York: Pergamon Press.

Biggs, J.B. (1984). Learning strategies, student motivation patterns, and subjectively perceived success. In J.R. Kirby (Ed.), *Cognitive strategies and educational performance*. New York: Academic Press.

Borkowski, J.G. & Cavanaugh, J.C. (1979). Maintenance and generalisation of skills and strategies by the retarded. In N.R. Ellis (Ed.), *Handbook of Mental Deficiency (2nd. Ed.)*. Hillsdale, N.J.: Lawrence Erlbaum.

Brewer, N. (1978). Motor components in the choice reaction time of mildly retarded adults. *American Journal of Mental Deficiency, 82*, 565-572.

Brewer, N. & Smith, G.A. (1984). How normal and retarded individuals monitor and regulate speed and accuracy of responding in serial choice tasks. *Journal of Experimental Psychology: General, 113*, 71-93.

Brown, A.L. (1974). The role of strategic behavior in retardate memory. In R.N. Ellis (Ed.), *International review of research in mental retardation (Vol. 7)*. New York: Academic Press.

Brown, A.L. (1978). Knowing when, where, and how to remember: A problem of metacognition. In R. Glaser (Ed.), *Advances in instructional psychology (Vol. 1)*. Hillsdale, N.J.: Lawrence Erlbaum.

Brown, A.L., Bransford, J.D., Ferrara, R.A. & Campione, J.C. (1983). Learning, remembering and understanding. In P.H. Mussen (Ed.), *Handbook of child psychology (4th. Ed., Vol. 4)*. New York: Wiley & Sons.

Brown, H.J., Singer, R.N., Cauraugh, J.H. & Lucariello, G. (1985). Cognitive style and learner strategy interaction in the performance of primary and related maze tasks. *Research Quarterly for Exercise and Sport, 56*, 10-14.

Butterfield, E.C. (1981). Testing process theories of intelligence. In M.P. Friedman, J.P. Das, N. O'Connor (Eds.), *Intelligence and learning*. New York: Plenum Press.

Butterfield, E.C., Wambold, C. & Belmont, J.M. (1973). On the theory and practice of improving short-term memory. *American Journal of Mental Deficiency, 77*, 654-669.

Campione, J.C. & Brown, A.L. (1977). Memory and metamemory development in educable retarded children. In R.V. Kail Jr. and J.W. Hagen (Eds.), *Perspectives on the development of memory and cognition*. Hillsdale, N.J.: Lawrence Erlbaum.

Campione, J.C. & Brown, A.L. (1978). Toward a theory of intelligence: Contributions from research with retarded children. *Intelligence, 2,* 279-304.

Campione, J.C., Brown, A.L. & Ferrara, R.A. (1982). Mental retardation and intelligence. In R.J. Sternberg (Ed.), *Handbook of human intelligence.* New York: Cambridge University Press.

Chi, M.T.H. (1978). Knowledge structures and memory development. In R. Siegler (Ed.), *Children's thinking. What develops?* Hillsdale, N.J.: Lawrence Erlbaum.

Chi, M.T.H. (1981). Knowledge development and memory performance. In M.P. Friedman, J.P. Das and N. O'Connor (Eds.), *Intelligence and learning.* New York: Plenum.

Chi, M.T.H. (Ed.) (1983). *Trends in memory development.* New York: Karger.

Dare, M.T. & Gordon, N. (1970). Clumsy children: A disorder of perception and motor organisation. *Developmental Medicine and Child Neurology, 12,* 178-185.

Ellis, N.R. (1970). Memory processes in retardates and normals. In N.R. Ellis (Ed.), *International review of research in mental retardation (Vol. 4).* New York: Academic Press.

Ellis, N.R., Deacon, J.R. & Woolridge, P.W. (1985). Structural memory deficits of mentally retarded persons. *American Journal of Mental Deficiency, 89,* 393-403.

Ericsson, K.A. & Simon, H.A. (1980). Verbal reports as data. *Psychological Review, 87,* 215-251.

Fisher, M.A. & Zeaman, D. (1973). An attention-retention theory of retardates' discrimination learning. In N.R. Ellis (Ed.), *International review of research in mental retardation (Vol. 6).* New York: Academic Press.

Flavell, J.H. (1970). Developmental studies of mediated memory. In H.W. Reese and L.P. Lipsitt (Eds.), *Advances in child development and behavior (Vol. 5).* New York: Academic Press.

Flavell, J.H., Beach, D.H. & Chinsky, J.M. (1966). Spontaneous verbal rehearsal in a memory task as a function of age. *Child Development, 37,* 283-299.

Flavell, J.H. & Wellman, H.M. (1977). Metamemory. In R.V. Kail Jr. and J.W. Hagen (Eds.), *Perspectives on the development of memory and cognition.* Hillsdale, N.J.: Lawrence Erlbaum.

Gallagher, J.D. & Thomas, J.R. (1984). Rehearsal strategy effects on developmental differences for recall of a movement series. *Research Quarterly for Exercise and Sport, 55,* 123-128.

Hagen, J.W., Barclay, C.R. & Schewthelm, B. (1982). Cognitive development of the learning disabled child. In N.R. Ellis (Ed.), *International review of research in mental retardation (Vol. 11).* New York: Academic Press.

Hagen, J.W. & Stanovich, K.E. (1977). Memory: Strategies of acquisition. In R.V. Kail Jr. and J.W. Hagen (Eds.), *Perspectives on the development of memory and cognition.* Hillsdale, N.J.: Lawrence Erlbaum.

Hall, R.J. (1980). An information-processing approach to the study of exceptional children. In B.K. Keogh (Ed.), *Advances in Special Education (Vol. 2).* Greenwich, C.T.: JAI Press.

Henderson, S.E. (1985). Motor skill development. In D. Lane and B. Stratford (Eds.), *Current approaches to Down's Syndrome.* London: Holt, Rinehart & Winston.

Henderson, S.E. & Hall, D. (1982). Concomitants of clumsiness in young school children. *Developmental Medicine and Child Neurology, 24,* 448-460.

Horgan, J.S. (1983a). Measurement bias in memory for movement by mentally retarded and nonretarded children. *Perceptual and Motor Skills, 56,* 663-670.

Horgan, J.S. (1983b). Mnemonic strategy instruction in coding, processing and recall of movement related cues by mentally retarded children. *Perceptual and Motor Skills, 57,* 547-557.

Karmiloff-Smith, A. (1979). Micro- and macro-developmental changes in language acquisition and other representational systems. *Cognitive Science, 3,* 91-118.

Keogh, J.F., Sugden, D.A., Reynard, C.L. & Calkins, J.A. (1979). Identification of clumsy children: Comparisons and comments. *Journal of Human Movement Studies, 5,* 32-41.

Kirby, N.H. (Ed.) (1984). *Cognitive strategies and educational performance.* New York: Academic Press.

Kirby, N.H., Nettelbeck, T. & Thomas, P. (1979). Vigilance performance of mildly mentally retarded children. *American Journal of Mental Deficiency, 84,* 184-187.

Kreutzer, M.A., Leonard, S.C. & Flavell, J.H. (1975). An interview of children's knowledge about memory. *Monographs of the Society for Research in Child Development, 40,* (1, Serial No. 159).

Kugler, P.H., Kelso, J.A.S. & Turvey, M.T. (1980). On the concept of co-ordinative structures as dissipative structures: 1. Theoretical lines of convergence. In G.E. Stelmach and J. Requin (Eds.), *Tutorials in Motor Behavior.* Amsterdam: North-Holland.

Kugler, P.H., Kelso, J.A.S. & Turvey, M.T. (1982). On the control and coordination of naturally developing systems. In J.A.S. Kelso and J.E. Clark (Eds.), *The development of movement control and coordination.* New York: Wiley & Sons.

Lawson, M.J. (1984). Being executive about metacognition. In J.R. Kirby (Ed.), *Cognitive strategies and educational performance.* New York: Academic Press.

Mosher, R. & Schutz, R. (1983). The development of a test of overarm throwing: An application of generalizability theory. *Canadian Journal of Applied Sport Sciences, 8,* 1-8.

Naus, M.T. & Ornstein, P.A. (1983). Development of memory strategies: Analysis, questions and issues. In M.T.H. Chi (Ed.), *Trends in memory research.* New York: Karger.

Nettelbeck, T. & Lally, M. (1979). Age, intelligence and inspection time. *American Journal of Mental Deficiency, 83,* 398-401.

Nettelbeck, T. & Brewer, N. (1981). Studies of mild mental retardation and timed performance. In N.R. Ellis (Ed.), *International review of research in mental retardation (Vol. 10).* New York: Academic Press.

Newell, K.M. (1984). Physical constraints to development of motor skills. In J.R. Thomas (Ed.), *Motor development during childhood and adolescence.* Minneapolis, MN: Burgess.

Newell, K.M. (1985). Motor skill acquisition and mental retardation: Overview of traditional and current orientations. In J.E. Clark and J.H. Humphrey (Eds.), *Motor development: current selected research (Vol. 1).* Princeton, NJ: Princeton Book Company.

Newell, K.M. (in press). Coordination, control and skill. In D. Goodman, I. Franks and R. Wilberg (Eds.), *Differing perspectives in motor control.* Amsterdam: North Holland.

Newell, K.M. & Barclay, C.R. (1982). Developing knowledge about action. In J. A.S. Kelso and J.E. Clark (Eds.), *The development of movement control and coordination.* New York: Wiley & Sons.

Newell, K.M., Wade, M.G. & Kelly, T.M. (1979). Temporal anticipation of response initiation in retarded persons. *American Journal of Mental Deficiency, 84,* 289-296.

Reid, R. (1980a). Overt and covert rehearsal in short-term motor memory of mentally retarded and nonretarded persons. *American Journal of Mental Deficiency, 85,* 69-77.

Reid, G. (1980b). The effects of memory strategy instruction in the short term motor memory of the mentally retarded. *Journal of Motor Behavior, 12,* 221-227.

Reid, G. (1984, July). A kinesthetic memory strategy for mentally retarded adults: Initial effects and maintenance. Paper presented at the Olympic Scientific Congress, University of Oregon.

Sabatino, D.A., Miller, P.F. & Schmidt, C. (1981). Can intelligence be altered through cognitive training. *Journal of Special Education, 15,* 125-144.

Shea, J.B. (1977). Effects of labeling on motor short-term memory. *Journal of Experimental Psychology: Human Learning and Memory, 3,* 92-99.

Singer, R.N. & Cauraugh, J.H. (1984). Generalization of psychomotor learning strategies to related psychomotor tasks. *Human Learning, 3,* 215-225.

Singer, R.N. & Cauraugh, J.H. (1985). The generalizability effect of learning strategies for categories of psychomotor skills. *Quest, 37,* 103-119.

Stanovich, K.E. (1978). Information processing in mentally retarded individuals. In N.R. Ellis (Ed.), *International review of research in mental retardation (Vol. 9).* New York: Academic Press.

Sugden, D.A. (1978). Visual motor short term memory in educationally subnormal boys. *British Journal of Educational Psychology, 48,* 330-339.

Sugden, D.A. & Gray, S.M. (1981). Capacity and strategies of educationally subnormal boys on serial and discrete tasks involving movement speed. *British Journal of Educational Psychology, 51,* 77-82.

Thomas, J.R., Thomas, K.T., Lee, A.M., Testerman, E. & Ashy, M. (1983). Age differences in use of strategy for recall of movement in a large scale environment. *Research Quarterly for Exercise and Sport, 54,* 264-272.

Torgesen, J.K. (1977). Memorization processes in exceptional children. *Journal of Educational Psychology, 69,* 571-578.

Torgesen, J.K. & Kail, R.V. Jr. (1980). Memory processes in exceptional children. In B.K. Keogh (Ed.); *Advances in Special Education (Vol. 1).* Greenwich, CT: JAI Press.

Turvey, M.T. & Carello, C. (1981). Cognition. The view from ecological realism. *Cognition, 10,* 313-321.

Ulrich, D.A. (1985). *Test of gross motor development.* Austin, TX: Pro Ed.

Wade, M.G. (1976). Developmental motor learning. In J. Keogh and R.S. Hutton (Eds.), *Exercise and sport science reviews (Vol. 4).* Santa Barbara, CA: Journal Publishing Affiliates.

Wade, M.G., Newell, K.M. & Wallace, S.A. (1978). Decision time and movement time as a function of response complexity in the motor performance of retarded persons. *American Journal of Mental Deficiency, 83,* 135-144.

Wade, M.G., Newell, K.M. & Hoover, J.H. (1982). Coincident timing behavior in young mentally handicapped workers under varying conditions of target velocity and exposure. *American Journal of Mental Deficiency, 86,* 643-649.

Wall, A.E. (1982). Physically awkward children: A motor development perspective. In J.P. Das, R.F. Mulcahy and A.E. Wall (Eds.), *Theory and research in learning disabilities.* New York: Plenum Press.

Wall, A.E., McClements, J., Bouffard, M., Findlay, H. & Taylor, M.J. (1985). A knowledge-based approach to motor development: Implications for the physically awkward. *Adapted Physical Activity Quarterly, 2,* 21-42.
Wellman, M.H. (1983). Metamemory revisited. In M.T.H. Chi (Ed.), *Trends in Memory Development Research.* New York: Karger.
Winograd, T. (1975). Frame representations and the declarative/procedural controversy. In D.G. Bobrow and A. Collins (Eds.), *Representation and Understanding: Studies in Cognitive Science.* New York: Academic Press.
Winther, K.T. & Thomas, J.R. (1981). Developmental differences in children's labeling of movement. *Journal of Motor Behavior, 13,* 77-90.

MOTOR DYSFUNCTIONS IN CHILDREN. TOWARDS A PROCESS-ORIENTED DIAGNOSIS.

W. Hulstijn and T. Mulder

A great number of children, estimations range from five to ten percent (Huyberechts, 1984), are more or less hindered by motor dysfunctions. These children are usually described as "clumsy" or "non-optimal" (Schellekens, Kalverboer & Scholten, 1981). Their non-optimal motor behaviour expresses itself in a great variety of symptoms, such as writing and drawing problems at school, and also gross motor problems can frequently be observed. This chapter addresses the problem how to diagnose or classify this variety in motoric problems. In particular, evidence will be presented for the diagnostic power of one type of data: error data.

The experiments that will be described are concerned with the fine motor activity in drawing. After a short introduction emphasising a process-oriented approach in the diagnosis of motor dysfunctions, data from a reaction-time experiment will be presented. Next the movement times obtained in a Fitts' type task will be considered. Both of these experiments gave rise to error data which, as will be shown, proved to have considerable diagnostic power. For this reason, the last experiment reported focuses on the analysis of different types of errors made in copying figures under different conditions.

Imagine a clumsy child in the first years of the elementary school, when her or his motor problems usually become manifest in writing and gymnastics. Or think of a more seriously handicapped child, who is given daily training in a rehabilitation centre by special teachers and occupational therapists. How should their motor deficiences be analysed and characterised? There are several perspectives. In addition to research objectives, for example, in the investigation of long lasting effects of birth traumas, motor skills are also tested in neurological examinations. However, in both types of assessment the investigator is not interested in motor behaviour *per se*, but rather in using errors made in some specific test-movements - like pointing to the nose or rotating the hand - as diagnostic signs of a neurological disorder.

In addition to these procedures aimed at a medical diagnosis, there exist a number of psychomotor tests, which focus more on the behavioural aspects of the problem. These tests, such as the 'Oseretzky', the 'Ayres', the 'Frostig', the 'Benton' and the 'Bender', consist of a series of tasks (of increasing difficulty) - like standing on one leg, tying shoelaces or drawing a figure - use as criterion the number of tasks successfully passed. The child's performance is compared to his or her average age level. Since only the observable end results of the specific motor tasks are analysed, this approach can be qualified as a 'product' or 'result-oriented' approach. It may give a good impression of what a child is able to perform with respect to his peers but it does not give an answer to the question why certain activities cannot be executed. A good insight into the nature of the motoric problems, in particular into the processes responsible for the observed motor performance delays, is essential in choosing the best targets for training (see Laszlo & Bairstow, 1985, for similar arguments).

In addition to this product way of working we attempted to develop a process oriented diagnostic procedure. In this approach only a few tasks are employed. In this Chapter one of these tasks, a drawing task, will be described: subjects were required to copy figures, that were presented to them. It was assumed that by varying certain aspects of the task, i.e. complexity or accuracy, specific motor control processes would be tapped. Originally our conceptualisation of these processes was strongly influenced by the sequential stage models of Sternberg (1969) and Sanders (1980). However on the basis of acquired data (Hulstijn & Van Galen, 1983) and recent discussions in the literature (Broadbent, 1984) a strict stage-approach was discarded in favour of a more parallel processing model.

If a child is asked to copy a figure, for example the character 8, a number of processes will occur. These can roughly be grouped into input, decision and output processes. Before the character 8 can be drawn, the figure has to be perceived and identified correctly. Next this perceived image of the stimulus figure has to be 'transformed' into a series of adequately timed motor impulses addressed to the relevant muscles. This translation process, from image to act, is termed 'programming'. Programming in our view (see also Hulstijn & Van Galen, 1983; Hulstijn, in preparation; Van Galen, 1980; Van Galen & Teulings, 1983) must fulfil at least three requirements: the movement sequence must be planned, correctly parameterised and finally be coordinated with other movements like those for maintaining posture.

The planning of a well learned movement starts with the retrieval of an abstract motor plan from long term motor memory. This plan contains the number of separate control units of which the total movement consists. The content of this plan depends largely on the novelty of the actual motor problem. For experienced writers, letters or, in the case of a signature, even a combination of letters may be the units. Hence, in the example of writing the character 8 the movement can be planned as one unit. However in children the situation may be different. In young children the 8 might be planned as two circles on top of each other.

Another aspect of the planning process is the determination of the starting point of the movement and the endpoint. For example, most Dutch writers have learned to start their 8 in the middle, at the top of the lowest circle, while most English writers start on top of the upper circle.

It is not proposed that a programme runs off without the evaluation of feedback. On the contrary, part of the planning has to do with feedforward control. This is not only done to check whether the intended response requirements are being met, but also to monitor the progress of the movement against the planned sequence. The more common situation in motor behaviour is that two activities are performed together, for example, writing and the conceptualising and formulating of the contents of the to be written text.

Therefore part of the planning of a movement sequence in units allows the termination of an unit to be signalled to a higher control level. In terms of the writing example, this would mean that planning of the motor sequence is a requirement for the thinking, formulating and writing organism to know where the pen is, or how far behind the pen is, in relation to his or her thoughts (see also Hulstijn, in preparation).

As argued, a motor plan is conceived of as an abstract representation specifying the sequence of different types of sub-movements. Hence the plan for the character 8 does not specify its size, nor its position on the paper and therefore not the muscles that have to be used. This means that after constructing or retrieving the movement plan, this plan must be supplied with proper parameters like size, spatial position, speed, and required accuracy. By this parameterising the abstract plan turns into a more concrete programme fitted to the actual requirements of the task. Finally this programme has to be translated into muscle commands and linked or coordinated with other movements and with postural control.

This conceptualisation of motor programming is very much in line with ideas formulated in slightly different versions by Schmidt (1975), Keele (1981), and in our laboratory by Van Galen (1980, see also Sheridan, 1984 and Van Galen & Wing, 1984). The main controversies between these authors are concerned with the nature of the abstract plan or programme. In a very recent study carried out in the Nijmegen handwriting laboratory Teulings, Thomassen and Van Galen (in press) investigated which movement aspect in the repeated writing of the same letter is most invariant: force, time or the spatial structure. They very convincingly demonstrated that variations in forces are higher than variations in timing, but that both are larger than variations in the spatial characteristics. The most invariant characteristic is the most likely candidate for the type of information that is stored in motor memory. Therefore their study suggests that it is something which comes very close to spatial information which is contained in stored motor programmes. This is in accordance with Bernstein's notion of a topological representation of movements (see Whiting, 1984). Hence, here, we have an example of a tight relation between perception and action.

Thus far we described motor control in terms of a few processes. How this approach can be applied to the diagnosis of motor dysfunctions, will be explained in the next section.

EXPERIMENT 1

The first process of which the diagnostic relevance will be investigated is the planning process. From the experimental literature it is known that longer movement sequences require more advance programming, or, in other words, require a longer planning period, which is reflected in an increased reaction time (Henry & Rogers, 1960; Klapp, 1977). In slightly modified form, this original idea still has a great deal of support today (Henry, 1980; Klapp, 1980; Fischman, 1984; Hulstijn, in preparation). The increase in reaction time with sequence length therefore may be taken as a measure of programming load. Therefore it is predicted that in subjects with planning problems this reaction time increase must be higher than in normal subjects.

In general, the employed strategy starts from a well documented experimental effect, such as the effect of sequence length or, as in Experiment 2, the influence of target width in a Fitts' type task. The experimental task measuring this effect is adapted to children and presented to normal control children as well as to children with minor motor difficulties. The obvious hypothesis being that, at least for a subgroup of the children with motoric problems, larger effects of the task variables will be found.

METHODS

Four groups of subjects were used. The control group (N) consisted of normal children, recruited from an ordinary elementary school. There were three age groups - 6 years, 8 years and 10 years - with 10 subjects in each of these groups. Children with minor motor difficulties (MMD), educated at a special school for children with learning and educational problems, formed the second group. There were 15 of these children, their mean age was 8.4 years. These were children, according to their teacher, with a very poor handwriting or a low sporting ability. The third group consisted of 12 cerebral palsy children (CP), with a mean age of 8.7 years. This is a mixed group of pupils of an elementary school for external patients at a local rehabilitation centre. Most of these children were diagnosed in a neurological examination as suffering from an infantile or post-traumatic encephalitis. The occupational therapists only selected children with a 'normal' intelligence and attentional capacity. These children could, therefore, easily understand the instructions and could concentrate on the experiment for the required 30 minutes. In fact they were used to these types of procedures. Finally a group of 10 adult student subjects (A) was run for reasons that will be explained later.

The apparatus used for presenting the stimuli and the recording of the pen movements consisted of an Apple II microcomputer and Apple Graphics tablet or digitiser. With this (very portable) apparatus the position of the pen was recorded with a precision of 0.1 mm and a frequency of 100 Hz.

Six different stimuli were presented six times each in a random order. Five of the stimulus patterns are pictured below the X-axis in Figure 1. The stimuli numbered 1, 2, and 3 in Figure 1 had the same initial stroke, but differed in the number of strokes which, as has been stated earlier, was assumed to influence the duration of the programming process and thereby the reaction time. The same holds more or less for the difference between stimuli 4 and 5, although these stimuli differed also in degree of familiarity and were selected for other reasons. The sixth stimulus was, like stimulus 1, a simple upward stroke, not in the upper right direction however, but to the upper left. A stroke in this latter direction was not allowed to be made with a simple turning of the hand around the wrist, but required the coordinate movements of a number of finger and thumb joints. The results of the comparison between these latter two stimuli will be reported elsewhere.

RESULTS

Before presenting the reaction time results as a function of sequence length, the group averages for reaction time (RT) and movement time (MT) will be described. The reaction time, measured from the stimulus onset to the start of the drawing movement on the paper surface, decreased with age, from 1020 msec for the 6 year old children to 770 msec for the 10 year olds and 580 msec for the adult group. The normal group on the average had a very much lower mean RT (940 msec) than the two groups with motoric problems (1290 msec for the MMD group and 1300 msec for the CP group).

Like the reaction times, the movement times (i.e. the total time taken to draw a figure), significantly decreased with age (from 1255 msec for the 6 year old children to 950 msec for the 10 year olds and 530 msec in the adult group). However, quite contrary to the expectations, children having motor problems had the same movement times as their normal controls (1200 msec for the MMD children and 1150 for the CP group). This holds even for the more complex patterns, i.e. the numbers 3 and 5 in Figure 1.

The error data presented in Table 1 show that achieving this equal movement was at the expense of an enormous increase in errors. Four types of errors are given in Table 1. Absolute errors were errors in which the stimulus figure was hardly discernable. They could mostly be characterised as very serious form errors in which half or more of the pattern was distorted. Form errors were scored when one element was lacking, added or disturbed. Errors in the orientation of the drawing were scored in those instances in which the relationship between the figure elements was more or less correct, but in which the whole pattern was tilted more than 45 degrees to the right or the left. Errors in size were counted if the drawn figure was larger than three times the required size.

Table 1. Percentage of trials with errors of different types, averaged over subgroups.

Error type	Normals 6 yr.	8 yr.	10 yr.	MMD	CP
Absolute	2.8	2.1	1.2	10.3	12.4
Form	8.7	1.9	1.8	17.2	19.3
Orientation	12.3	10.3	6.5	24.6	24.3
Size	1.6	0.4	0.9	14.6	37.0

Errors generally and significantly decreased with age. It is clearly evident in Table 1 that the groups with minor motor difficulties and the cerebral palsy group had much higher percentages of errors.

The effects of age and the differences between the groups in mean RT and MT having been characterised, the data testing the main hypothesis can be evaluated. As stated earlier, a longer sequence length should manifest itself in a longer reaction time, which effect should be larger for the groups with motoric problems.

The effect of sequence length is best tested with the patterns 1 through 3 in Figure 1, since stimuli 4 and 5 also differed in familiarity. In contrast to the main assumption, the increase in the number of stimulus-strokes does

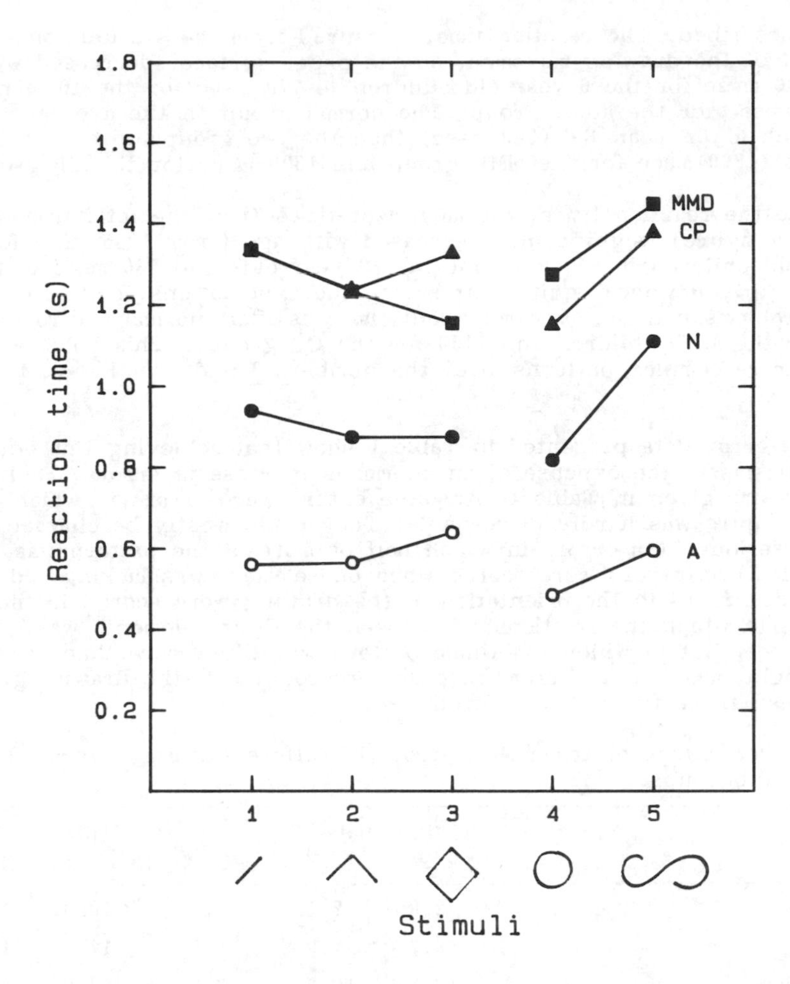

Fig. 1. Reaction times to draw the five stimuli, averaged per group (A= Adult, N= Normal, CP= Cerebral Palsy, MMD= Minor Motor Dysfunction).

not lead to an increase in reaction time. This holds for the normal children as well as for the MMD and CP children. These negative results explain why later an extra group of adult subjects was incorporated in the experiment. Most of the earlier positive results gathered in our laboratory were obtained from the usual laboratory subjects, i.e. students. As is quite clear in Figure 1, these normal student results were replicated in this experiment, even with only six trials per stimulus. Although the rise in RT is a few milliseconds from stimulus 1 to 2, there is a significant increase from the two-stroke pattern to the four-stroke figure.

DISCUSSION

It must be concluded that the question whether children with motoric problems are having planning difficulties cannot be answered since the main assumption was not satisfied, at least for children. One reason for the difference in effect of sequence length between children and adults may be found in what should be called 'preparatory movements' (Hulstijn & Mulder, 1985). Children, unlike adults, perform a lot of movements with the pen above the paper before they actually start the writing movement. In normal children these preparatory movements occur during about 150 msec before the actual writing movement. In children with motor problems these movements last about 350 msec, while in adults they are observed quite rarely, taking a 25 msec on the average. Mostly the function of these movements is to place the pen and the hand in a proper starting position, in order to start the first stroke ballisticly. A negative by-product of this time-consuming initial positioning may have been the masking of any positive sequence effect.

The second reason for the failure to find an increasing RT with more complex figures may be sought in strategy differences. Adults probably plan the total sequence, while children or subjects having difficulty with planning may only plan one stroke at a time.

EXPERIMENT 2

In the second experiment a Fitts' type task was used. In this task the subjects had to draw simple straight lines to targets (circles) differing in width, in distance and in direction. Since each line could be planned as one element, it was assumed that the planning was equal for all these lines. They only differed in the parameters that had to be supplied. The variables target width and distance are assumed to influence movement time (Fitts, 1954; Fitts & Peterson, 1964; see Schmidt, 1982). The direction of the line effects the number of muscles that have to be coordinated. The hypotheses were more or less similar to those in Experiment 1. If pointing to a small target takes more time than reaching a larger target, then the resulting increase in movement time should be most prominent for children with particular problems in pointing.

METHOD

On a sheet of paper eight little men were pictured each holding a stick with a set of three balloons. One balloon of each set was not connected properly to the stick and the child was asked to draw the connecting line. There were eight sheets, each having eight missing lines. In half of the sheets the missing lines were partly drawn as straight dotted lines. In this condition (the accuracy condition) the child had to trace the dotted line as accurately as possible, without much time pressure. On the other four sheets the trajectory was not indicated. The child was instructed to draw the missing lines as quickly as possible after a 'go' signal, without paying to much attention to accuracy (the velocity condition).

Within a sheet, the required eight lines differed in length (i.e. 1 or 2 cm), in direction (i.e. upward left and upward right), and in target size (i.e. the balloon having an outer diameter of 2 or 5 mm).

The same three groups of children as in the first experiment were used.

RESULTS

The main independent variable, i.e. target width, had diverse effects on movement time (MT), which is taken here as the time to draw a connecting stroke between the stick and the balloon. In the velocity condition the MT to the smaller target was slightly higher. Although this effect was in the assumed direction, it was not as large as expected. Moreover, this effect was about equal for all groups. In the accuracy condition the reverse held; the MT to the smaller target was larger. Group differences were small and insignificant.

Figure 2b gives the movement times averaged over target size, target distance and movement direction. The inter-response time (IT), which was the period between the drawing of two successive lines, i.e. the period in which the pen was positioned above the paper surface to start the next line, is presented in Figure 2a. There was a significant group effect in inter-response time, which was largely due to the much higher values of the cerebral palsy children.

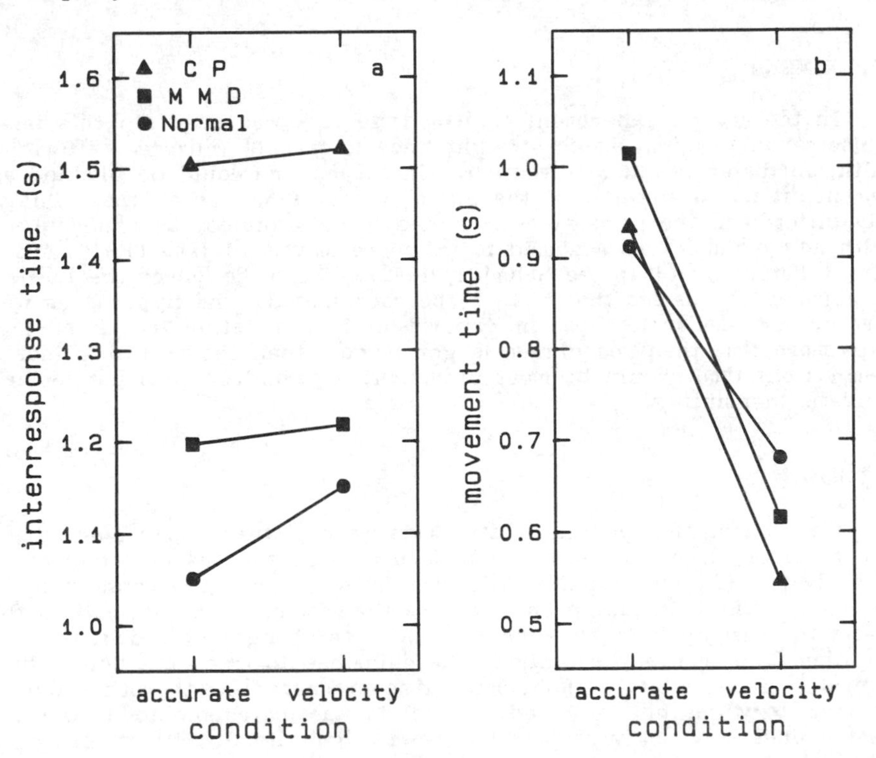

Fig. 2. Inter-response time (panel a) and movement time (panel b) in two drawing conditions, averaged for three groups.

With respect to movement time: no main group effect was found. There was a marginal significant interaction between groups and condition, meaning that the extra time taken in the accurate condition, compared to the time in the fast condition, is slightly longer for the non-optimal children. But, none of the effects of the other parameters - target size, distance and direction - interacted with group differences.

In Figure 3, two error measures are presented. In Figure 3a the absolute distance between the end of the line drawn and the circumference of the target circle is given, and in Figure 3b the average length of the drawn line is displayed. This last measure gives an impression of the size of the deviation from a straight line. As is quite clear in Figure 3, there were large, and highly significant group differences in both error measures.

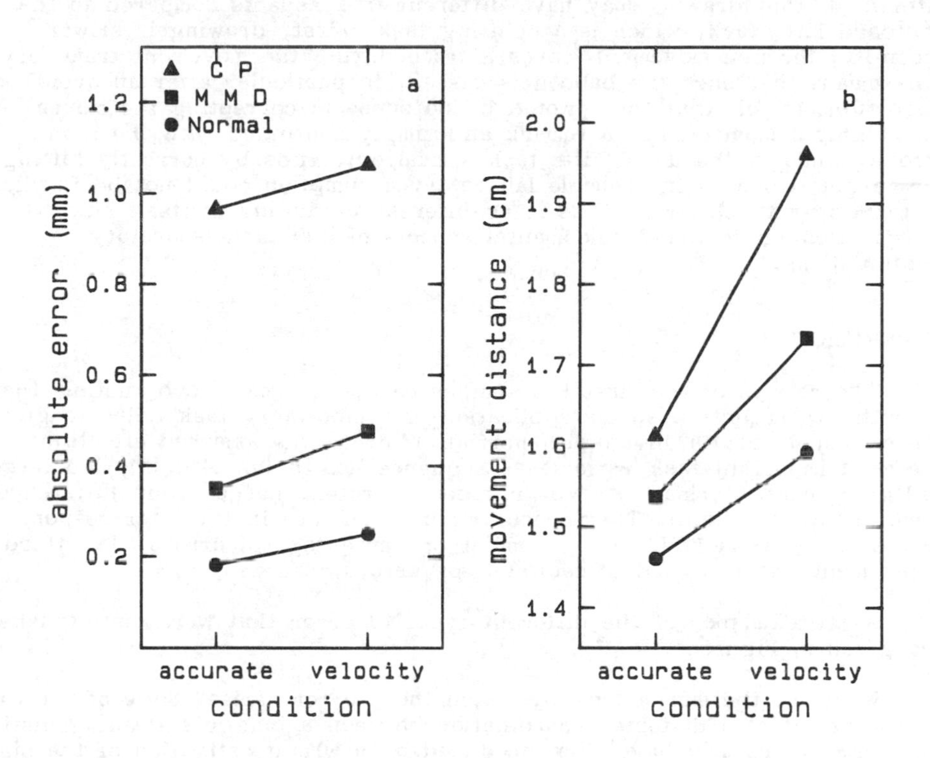

Fig. 3. Absolute error (panel a) and movement distance (panel b) in two drawing conditions, averaged for three groups.

Age effects in both time measures (MT and IT) and both error measures were very small, none of them being statistically significant.

DISCUSSION

The correspondence in results between Experiment 1 and Experiment 2 is striking. In both studies there were no group differences in movement time, however, interesting differences in the time to prepare the movement (RT and IT) were found and very large differences in error scores were counted. Moreover, size was the only error measure in Experiment 1 differentiating between the two groups with motor problems. This finding is quite compatible with the differences between group MMD and CP in the error measures in this second task.

Although the hypothesis, that moving to a smaller target requires more time, sounded reasonable at the start of the experiment, it was realised afterwards that drawing may have different task aspects compared to the standard Fitts task, which is a pointing task. First, drawing is slower, secondly, the pen movement leaves a trace during the movement trajectory. This means that once the balloon is missed, in particular after an overshoot, most subjects felt that there would be no sense in correcting the movement. The children mostly made a remark and simply continued with the next stroke, while in the usual Fitts task a trial only ends by correctly hitting the target. Once again a simple laboratory assumption could not be fulfilled in working with children. This is an interesting finding in itself since it draws attention to the developmental aspects of standard laboratory manipulations.

EXPERIMENT 3

The results of the first two studies can be summarised by noting that in both experiments a simple application of a laboratory task failed to give the expected results. Even with normal children, the assumed effects of the most important task variables - sequence length for planning and target width for parameterisation - was not demonstrated. Large group differences were, however, found. These occurred in mean RT, in the inter-response time and, most marked, in the number or percentage of errors. The third experiment was designed to capitalise on errors.

A few examples of the different types of error that were distinguished are given in Figure 4.

What are the mechanisms by which these errors arise? Some of them may be the result of a distorted coordination between agonistic and antagonistic muscles. Others may have been produced by a wrong estimation of the size or force parameter resulting in strokes that are too short or in the wrong direction, and which are successively being corrected. Reversals may be caused by perceptual errors. But, how should the first example in the category of form errors be explained? It is even difficult to describe what actually was drawn. Is it characterised by an improper extra upstroke at the end? Is the second "valley" a repetition of the first C-shaped element, or is the subject unable to reverse the counter-clockwise rotation of the first part in a clockwise rotation needed for the second part of the correct pattern? Is this error produced by improper perception of the stimulus? Is the movement wrongly planned in successive perseverative C's, or did the subject have insufficient muscle control resulting in a failure to change the rotation direction?

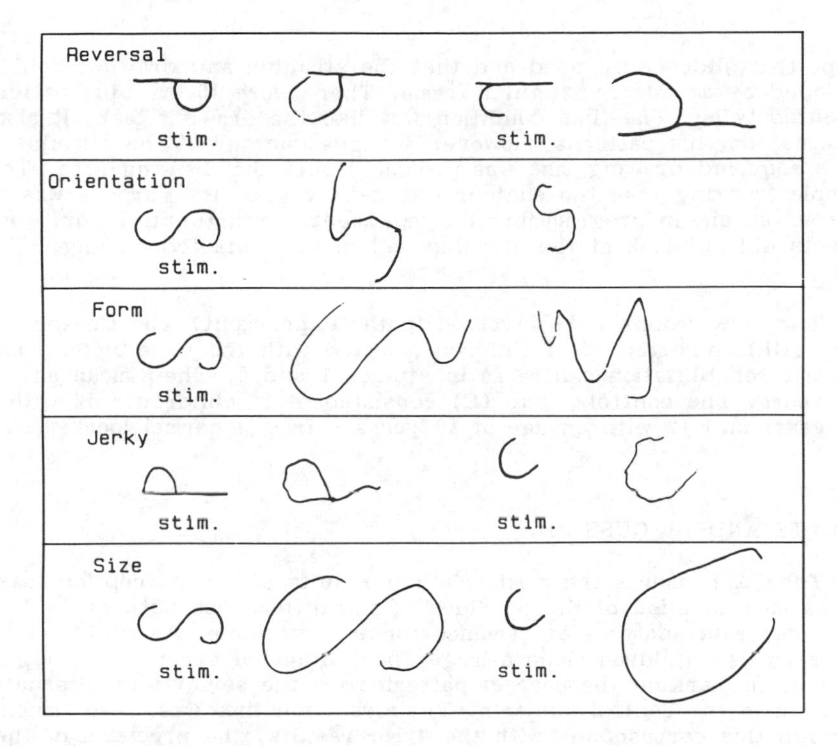

Fig. 4. Typical examples of five categories of drawing errors. The correct patterns are indicated by the term 'stim'.

These are not three exclusive and exhaustive hypotheses. They are only put forward to transmit the idea that a simple categorising and counting of errors cannot give much insight into the specific motor processes that are disturbed. Instead, what should be done is to change the conditions in these drawing tasks and explore the effects such changes have on the frequency with which different types of errors are made. Secondly, correlations or combinations between different types of error should be calculated to investigate whether ambiguous errors can be related to errors with a more clearcut cause.

The final experiment was an attempt to meet these objectives.

METHOD

There were three conditions. In the first, a perception task, the stimulus figure had to be recognised from a set of four alternatives, that were presented in a row below the stimulus figure. The stimuli were not presented on the monitor, as was done in the first two studies, but by means of a slide-projector projecting on a mirror positioned at 45 degrees above the X-Y tablet. The stimulus patterns were projected directly onto the writing paper on the upper half of the tablet. The subject had to mark the right alternative by drawing a small line in the correct rectangle, with the pen of the tablet.

The second condition was similar to the drawing task of Experiment 1, except that slides were used and that the stimulus and drawing field were enveloped by a wide rectangular frame. There were 15 stimulus patterns, presented twice. The final condition was like the drawing task, it also used the same stimulus patterns, however a vague contour of the stimulus pattern at the required drawing size was projected onto the drawing area. To avoid a simple tracking task the contour was kept vague. Its purpose was to serve as an aid in programming the movement. Unfortunately, quite a lot of subjects did not look at the stimulus and directly started tracing.

Two new groups were involved in the experiment. The Cerebral Palsy group (CP) consisted of 14 children selected with the same criteria and from the same rehabilitation centre as in studies 1 and 2. Their mean age was 10.6 years. The control group (C) consisted of 24 children - 12 with an age of 8 years and 12 with an age of 10 years - from a normal local elementary school.

RESULTS AND DISCUSSION

Table 2 presents the most relevant results of the perception task, as well as an indication of the p-values of the differences between both groups in the separate analyses of variance for each variable. As might be expected, cerebral palsy children made a larger percentage of errors or wrong decisions in marking the correct pattern from the set of four alternatives, compared to the control subjects. Their reaction time was, also, much slower. Although this corresponds with the error results, the precision of the pointing movements of this task may have required extra time. The other data in Table 2 give some impression of the quality of the simple line that was drawn to mark the right alternative. A few of the cerebral palsy children made that stroke very slowly and with a low velocity.

Table 2. The results of the perception task.

subjects	Control	Cerebral Palsy	p
Percentage of errors	5.3%	13.1%	$< .001$
Reaction Time	2.383 sec	3.017 sec	$< .001$
Movement time	.215 sec	.276 sec	$< .01$
Maximum velocity	34.9 cm/sec	24.3 cm/sec	$< .05$

In particular from the error data it may be concluded that the incidence of perceptual problems in the brain-damaged group is larger. This, of course, is not a new finding. In fact the conclusion should be reversed. The perception task that was used was sensitive enough to produce large differences between cerebral palsy children and controls.

The results of the other two conditions are presented in Table 3. This table does not give the data of the control subjects. These control children made very few errors and their reaction times, as well as their movement times were shorter. Therefore the differences between both groups were very much like those in the perception task.

Table 3. The results of the drawing and contourdrawing task.

Task	Drawing	Contourdrawing	p
Errors			
Reversal	0.9%	0.1%	< .05
Orientation	5.4%	4.3%	ns
Form	5.8%	5.6%	ns
Absolute	2.6%	1.8%	ns
Jerkiness	4.0%	7.6%	< .01
Size	6.1%	1.2%	< .05
Reaction Time	1.958 sec	1.777 sec	< .10
Movement Time	1.645 sec	1.523 sec	< .10
Movement Distance	4.79 cm	4.02 cm	< .05

What is the effect of adding a contour? The reaction time and the movement time are not significantly different in drawing with or without a contour. The movement distance, i.e. the length of the pen trajectory on the paper, was shorter in the contour condition. Obviously, the contour, by forcing the subjects to keep the pen within its boundaries, tends to suppress the natural tendency in these children to draw large.

The change in the frequency of errors over the two conditions gives some insight into the nature of these errors. Examples were given in Figure 4. Reversals turned out to be an infrequent type of error. As expected, they are effectively blocked in the contour condition. In contrast to this result, and more or less against the expectations, orientation errors, form errors and absolute errors - which may be seen as very serious form errors - seem to persist in the contour drawing task. This is a very interesting finding since it suggests that most of these errors are not caused by an inadequate perception, but by a lack of sufficient motor control. The last two error types are anti-polar. The smaller movement distance, to which the subjects were forced in the contour task, with the resultant reduction in size errors, had to be paid for by an increase in cramped, trembulous or jerky movements.

As was pointed out before, errors of different types and in different conditions should be combined in order to categorise different types of movement problems. Table 4 is an attempt to do this. On the left of the table the various types of errors, discussed previously are listed. In addition to error scores various 'hard' data are presented, i.e. reaction time, movement time in connection with jerkiness and movement distance as the more exact measurement of size errors. On the top row, the identification numbers of the fourteen subjects are listed. The data for each subject are given in a separate column. In the columns is indicated whether a subject is an exceptional scorer on a specific error type. In order to be able to do this, the mean and standard deviation were calculated, separately under each condition, for the frequency of each error type and of each of the other dependent variables. If the score of an individual subject was higher than one standard deviation above the mean for that condition, this subject was marked by a cross (X). If the subject was clearly above the mean, but not as high as one SD, he was marked by a small dot (.) in the table. The order of the subjects is such that a few subgroups would appear.

Table 4. Indications of error frequency in all individual subjects, (.= well above the mean; X= more than one SD above the mean) in the three tasks (P= perception, D= drawing, CD= contour drawing).

	Task	Subjects (Nr) 4	1	9	6	2	10	3	5	8	7	11	13	12	14
Reaction	P		.			X		.		.		.		X	X
Time	D							.		.		.		X	X
	CD		.							.	.	.		X	X
Errors in	P		.	X	X									.	X
Reversal	D		X			.	X				.		.	X	X
	CD				X										X
Orientation	D			X			.			.				X	
	CD		.	.			.			.			.	X	
Form	D			.			X	.						.	X
	CD			.			X	X		.				.	.
Absolute	D		.				.	X						X	X
	CD		.				.	X							X
Jerkiness	D							X	X					.	X
	CD							X	X					.	X
Movement	D					.		X	X					.	X
Time	CD					.		X	.					.	X
Size	D			.							X	X	X		
	CD									X					
Movement	D				.		.	.			X	X	X		
Distance	CD									X					

The first subject on the left, Nr *4*, has no single dot or cross. At the other side of the continuum, subjects *12* and *14* have a dot or cross in almost every row. The subjects positioned in between those extremes are the most interesting. Going from the right of the table back to the left, three or four subjects are encountered (the subjects numbered *13*, *11*, *7* and *8*), whose main characteristic is that they draw too large. It is remarkable that these subjects have no other "cross". Even the two children with most movement problems, subjects *12* and *14* do not score high in this size category.

Going more to the left, there are two subjects (subject *3* and *5*), with long movement times and many jerky movements. An interesting comparison can be made between subject *10* and subject *3*. Both had a large number of form errors and absolute errors. However, in subject *3* these might have been caused by his lack of sufficient muscle control, evidenced by his large amount of jerkiness. Subject *10* on the contrary was rather fluent, but showed a great many reversals. His perception scores were relatively good. Probably subject *10* has a planning disorder.

The block at the left of the table, subjects *1*, *9*, and *6*, may be classified as perception disturbances. The combination of perception errors and reversals, probably explain the orientation errors and the occasional form and absolute errors.

We may conclude that Table 4 gives a good impression of the great diversity of the fourteen CP subjects in this experiment. Moreover, this table shows a method of categorising these diversities. If the effects of task manipulations on different error types are combined, and if these error frequencies are supported by temporal data, then the combining of extreme error frequencies may be an avenue to classify these subjects. The task manipulations that should be chosen in the future must be those that have the least disputed relations with the programming processes referred to in the introduction. It should also be task manipulations that are relevant in therapeutic training programmes.

GENERAL DISCUSSION

The results of the first two experiments revealed an important problem, namely, the impossibility to transfer simple laboratory manipulations directly to applied research with children. The measurement of reaction time did not prove to be the right procedure in acquiring insight into the nature of the processes that may be disturbed. One reason for this may be that the movements of children, although superficially resembling those of adults, are governed by different processes or different strategies. The children's slowness, i.e. their long reaction and movement times may be caused by their inability to use overlearned stored motor programmes. They could not perform the task in a rapid, more or less ballistic way. Instead, they copied the figures, controlling their movements by making a strong use of visual feed-back. This closed loop control strategy will have interfered with the demands of a reaction time study, thereby preventing the effect of the planning variable - sequence length - to appear in the reaction time results.

However, there is an interesting alternative to the measurement of reaction time. One of the more promising procedures is the analysis of errors. This should not be taken to be the simple counting of errors, but the manipulation of specific aspects of the task, e.g. increasing complexity or accuracy, and the investigation of the effects of these manipulations on error frequency. Since errors can be distinguished in several types, they convey more information than reaction time. But this information may be misleading, as was shown by some data in the third experiment. Form errors, for instance, may be caused by disturbances in several processes. Which process is responsible can only be checked by varying, for each process, those aspects of the task which are assumed to influence that process most directly. This should be done for normal children, to test the effect of the task manipulations, and for children with motor problems, to see whether the effect of some specific task manipulation is larger for them.

In addition to an error analysis, one can analyse the invariant characteristics of the drawing and writing movements over repetitions. In the introduction the study by Teulings et al (in press) was mentioned showing that force or time parameters were not the most invariant characteristics over several repetitions of the same drawing movement, but the spatial features of the movements. Maybe this is true for experienced writers only, so it would be interesting to see whether it holds for children of different ages. Moreover, it may form the basis for a strategy in studying distorted movements of children. If a child consistently produces the same, wrong spatial characteristics, one can argue that a distortion on the level of a perception or planning process probably is the cause. If on the other hand the observed form errors vary from trial to trial, then probably force or time parameters are not properly adjusted.

The development of diagnostic procedures along these lines is not only of theoretical interest, it will have an immediate spin off to therapy. For example, if a child has great problems in writing letters, it is important to know whether form aspects should be emphasised in training or whether training exercises should focus on force or timing aspects. It is the parallel interest of diagnosis and therapy which should lead to more process-oriented diagnostic research.

References

Broadbent, D.E. (1984). The Maltese cross: A new simplistic model for memory. *The Behavioral and Brain Sciences, 7,* 55-94.

Fischman, M.G. (1984). Programming time as a function of number of movement parts and changes in movement direction. *Journal of Motor Behavior, 16,* 405-423.

Fitts, P.M. (1954). The information capacity of the human motor system in controlling the amplitude of movement. *Journal of Experimental Psychology, 47,* 381-391.

Fitts, P.M. & Peterson, J.R. (1964). Information capacity of discrete motor responses. *Journal of Experimental Psychology, 67,* 103-112.

Henry, F.M. (1980). Use of simple reaction time in motor programming studies: A reply to Klapp, Wyatt and Lingo. *Journal of Motor Behavior, 12,* 163-168.

Henry, F.M. & Rogers, D.E. (1960). Increased response latency for complicated movements and a "memory drum" theory of neuromotor reaction. *Research Quarterly, 31,* 448-458.

Hulstijn, W. (in preparation). Programming of verbal and non-verbal motor behaviour. In H.F.M. Peters and W. Hulstijn (Eds.), *Speech motor dynamics in stuttering.*

Hulstijn, W. & Mulder, Th. (1985). Stoornissen in de fijne motoriek. Een poging tot diagnostiek. In A.J.W.M. Thomassen, G.P. van Galen and L.F.W. de Klerk (Eds.), *Studies over de schrijfmotoriek: Theorie en toepassing in onderwijs.* Lisse: Swets & Zeitlinger.

Hulstijn, W. & Galen, G.P. van (1983). Programming in handwriting: reaction time and movement time as a function of sequence length. *Acta Psychologica, 54,* 23-49.

Huyberechts, B. (1984). Fysiotherapeutische evaluatie van perceptueel motorische dysfunkties bij het jonge kind. *Nederlands Tijdschrift voor Fysiotherapie, 94,* 90-85.

Laszlo, J.I. & Bairstow, P.J. (1985). *Perceptual Motor Behavior. Developmental assessment and therapy.* London: Holt, Rinehart and Winston.

Keele, S.W. (1981). Behavioral analysis of movement. In V.B. Brooks (Ed.), *Handbook of physiology, sectionI: the nervous system. Volume II, Motor Control, Part 2.* Baltimore: American Physiological Society.

Klapp, S.T. (1977). Reaction time analysis of programmed control. In H.R. Hutton (Ed.), *Exercise and sports science reviews.* Santa Barbara, Ca.: Journal Publishing Affiliates.

Klapp, S.T. (1980). The memory drum theory after twenty years: Comments on Henry's note. *Journal of Motor Behavior, 12,* 169-171.

Sanders, A.F. (1980). Stage analysis of reaction processes. In G.E. Stelmach and J. Requin (Eds.), *Tutorials in motor behavior.* Amsterdam: North Holland.

Schellekens, J.M.H., Kalverboer, A.F. & Scholten, C.A. (1981). Analyse van hand en armbewegingen bij kinderen met lichte neurologische dysfunkties (M.B.D.). *Heymans Bulletin.* Psychologische Instituten Rijksuniversiteit Groningen: nr. HB-81-553-EX.

Schmidt, R.A. (1975). A schema theory of discrete motor skill learning. *Psychological Review, 82,* 225-260.

Schmidt, R.A. (1982). *Motor control and learning. A behavioral emphasis.* Champaign: Human Kinetics Publishers.

Sheridan, M.R. (1984). Planning and controlling simple movements. In M.M. Smyth and A.M. Wing (Eds.), *The psychology of human movement.* London: Academic Press.

Sternberg, S. (1969). The discovery of processing stages: Extensions of Donders' method. *Acta Psychologica, 30,* 276-315.
Teulings, H.L., Thomassen, A.J.W.M. & Galen, G.P. van (in press). Invariants in handwriting: The information contained in a motor program. In H.S.R. Kao, G.P. van Galen and R. Hoosain (Eds.), *Graphonomics: Contempary research in handwriting.* Amsterdam: North-Holland.
Van Galen, G.P. (1980). Storage and retrieval of handwriting patterns: A two-stage model of complex motor behavior. In G.E. Stelmach and J. Requin (Eds.), *Tutorials in motor behavior.* Amsterdam: North Holland.
Van Galen, G.P. & Teulings, H.L. (1983). The independent monitoring of form and scale factors in handwriting. *Acta Psychologica, 54,* 9-22.
Van Galen, G.P. & Wing, A.M. (1984). The sequencing of movements. In M.M. Smyth and A.M. Wing (Eds.), *The psychology of human movement.* London: Academic Press.
Whiting, H.T.A. (Ed.) (1984). *Human motor actions - Bernstein reassessed.* Amsterdam: North-Holland.

INFORMATION PROCESSING AND MOTIVATION AS DETERMINANTS OF PERFORMANCE IN CHILDREN WITH LEARNING DISABILITIES

J.P. Das

Children with learning difficulties in reading and in arithmetic are more frequently clumsy than their class mates who have no such problem in school work. Neither their scholastic handicap nor their deviation from the norm in motor performance can be easily explained. Are they deficient in information processing even if they have normal intelligence? Is the motor deficiency parsimoniously explained by the same construct which can account for their problems with school work? This chapter starts out with a discussion of the relation between cognitive information processing and motor behaviour to show that the two are intimately related. Description of a model of cognitive processes is provided next. The model is recommended for use in interpreting motor performance of the kind which requires prior planning and deliberation. This is the first part of the paper, which ends with the consideration of clumsy children specially in terms of their learning difficulties. The second part of the paper reports a study on the interactions between motivational and information processing factors in the context of reading performance of children who are normal or poor in reading. The main finding of the study is that whereas both factors jointly predict the reading performance of normal readers, only one of the factors does so for poor readers. A threshold of reading competence must be reached above which motivational factors seem to influence reading.

Information Processing is a framework within which various accounts of how the mind works can be accommodated. Computer analogy of mental processes is only one such account. Artificial intelligence is closely related to the description of mental processes in computer terms. Objections have been raised to such an approach to understanding mental processes, mainly because of the fact that the human being is not a computer. Computers do not make scientific discoveries or engage in creative thinking. Artificial intelligence calls for an artificial organism (Skinner, 1985).

An alternative to the computer analogy is offered by neuropsychological models of mental or cognitive functions. Clinical evidence of disorders in processing information are obtained and integrated to suggest a coherent model of how the mind works. One of these models divides cognitive functions into three categories which are arousal, simultaneous and successive coding, and planning (Luria, 1966; Das, Kirby & Jarman, 1975). This model of information-integration is presented in a subsequent section of the chapter. Motor performance is viewed within this model; it is closely related to planning, and to the output component of information integration. The other components are input and central processing. Children with learning disabilities but of average or above average IQ are described in the context of the model as those who may have a deficit in simultaneous and successive coding of information or in the utilisation of the coded information. Strategies for utilisation of information are included in planning function. A failure to plan affects output adversely. In this chapter, the nature of planning has been discussed in some detail because it provides a link for relating motor skills to cognitive processes.

PART I

COGNITION AND MOTOR ACTIVITY: ARE THESE SEPARATE IN PLANFUL BEHAVIOUR?

Theoreticians among motor skills insist that the image or the plan of the activity is of the greatest importance in guiding motor activity. Let us review some of the contemporary cognitive theories in this regard.

The first to be reviewed is Whiting's image of the Act (Whiting, 1982). He believes that movement and cognition may not be separable. The mental or cognitive realm is intrinsically motoric like all the nervous system (cited by Whiting from Weimer). Chase and Chi are also cited in support: there is not in fact, much theoretical justification for differentiating perceptual-motor and cognitive skills. Whiting also draws heavily from the writings of the Soviet psychologist, Bernstein, who believes that we have an objective representation of the external world by monitoring the feedback from our own motor activity. Bernstein's statement, it seems to me, is almost an echo of Piaget's notion that the representation of reality becomes possible by operating on it. Images of Act are a specification of the essential form of the movements necessary to tackle a particular motor problem. Whiting proposes a *central motor controller* whose structural base is in the central motor cortex.

Keogh uses movement consistency and 'movement constancy' - clever homophones - as the key concepts in his process interpreation of motor skills. Acquisition of refined and reliable movement skills are to be used in day to day living. A *flexible* use of these movement skills is named movement constancy. The production of movement is represented as the rsult of processing information within a personal-social surrounding. Sensory input is gathered from internal or external sources, perceptual cognitive systems interpret the information and formulate plans for action. Neuro-motor systems then produce movement. All of these including performance must take into account the personal and social environment (Keogh, 1982).

Roy (1978) divides movement into three kinds based on research evidence from apraxia. Apraxia seems to be a cognitive disturbance in as much as *planning* apraxia shows up in an inability to plan motor behaviour. Executive apraxia is seen in the inability to *execute* planned behaviour.

The two kinds of apraxia are isomorphic to generation of plans and execution of selected plan. Roy does not include an inbetween stage which is the *selection* of an appropriate plan for execution. Perhaps a selection difficulty is seen in planning for motor responses.

Wall (1982) tries to explain the process of moving from an intention to specific action. There is one type of process for automated or well-learned, should we say, habitual action, and another for new or nonentrenched action patterns. It is obviously the latter that presents a complex problem and involves the use of complex psychological processing. Therefore, it is also subject to attentional and motivational influences. Wall draws his theory from many contemporary sources including the research on planning by Shallice (Norman & Shallice, 1980; Shallice & Evans, 1978). While making meta-theoretical points about action, Wall refers to Ann Brown's writings on knowledge. He suggests that acquired knowledge relating to action should be divided into procedural, declarative and affective knowledge. Higher mental processes such as attentional control which essentially indicates the voluntary control an individual can exercise over his or her own cognitive processes (metacognition) are important for performing complex tasks skilfully. Conscious control of action is the keyword here, and it is offered as the reason why average children are superior to awkward children. The awkward children lack procedural knowledge and metacognitive skills.

All of the above theories carry at least two messages for me: (1) *that planning and decision making are essential for competence in motor performance and* (2) *therefore 'motor' and 'mental' domains are not separate.*

We know from brain physiology that the motor cortex is a controller for motor response, especially its initiation involves the cells in the motor cortex.

The structural base of planning, the frontal lobes, have close connections with the motor cortex which is housed in the frontal lobes. And at the same time, the frontal lobes, especially the prefrontal area where 'planning' seems to be concentrated, is closely related (has many bands of connecting neurons) to the lower subcortical areas such as the limbic systems, and the brain-stem in general.

PLANNING: WHAT DOES PLANNING MEAN CONCEPTUALLY?

First consider the frontal lobe functions, and the reference to motor activity. The structural base for planning, broadly defined, is the frontal lobes (cf. Luria, 1966). The frontal lobes "regulate the 'active state' of the organism, control the essential elements of the subject's intentions, programme complex forms of activity and constantly monitor all aspects of activity" (Hecaen & Albert, 1979, p. 376). Luria (1969) had observed that injury to the frontal lobes disturbs impulse control, regulation of voluntary action, and perception as in visual search. It has an adverse effect on memory that requires the adoption of strategies. Above all, symbolic functions are badly affected, because it leads to incorrect choice of programs and results in an inability to restrain premature operations.

There seems to be good neurophysiological reason to justify the important role which the frontal lobes play in planning. As Luria wrote:

> The frontal lobes of the brain are the last acquisition of the evolutionary process and occupy nearly one third of the human hemispheres...They are intimately related to the reticular formation of the brain stem, being densely supplied with ascending and descending fibres...They have intimate connections with the motor cortex and with the structures of the second block...their structures become mature only during the 4th to 5th year of life, and their development makes a rapid leap during the period which is of decisive

significance for the first forms of conscious control of behaviour (Sapir & Nitzburg, 1973, p. 118).

The neuropsychological conceptualisation can be easily related to an information processing model of planning. Miller, Galanter and Pribram's (1960) classic book "Plans and the Structure of Behavior" provides the link. The publication of the book 25 years ago has been the most influential event in the growth of cognitive psychology as a discipline. A major distinction in the book has been made between images and plans.

IMAGE AND PLAN

Image. The Image is all the accumulated, organised knowledge that the organism has about itself and its world. The Image consists of a great deal more than imagery. What we have in mind when we use this term is essentially the same kind of private representation that other cognitive theorists have demanded. It includes everything the individual has learned - values as well as facts which have been organised by the concepts, images, or relations which have been acquired.

Plan. Any complete description of behaviour should be adequate to serve as a set of instructions, that is, it should have the characteristics of a plan that can guide the action described. Plan refers to a *hierarchy* of instructions. *A Plan is any hierarchical process in the organism that can control the order in which a sequence of operations is to be performed.*

PREDICTION AND SEARCH: THE TWO KINDS OF COGNITIVE PROCESSES THAT MAKE UP PLANFUL ACTIVITY

According to Miller et al searching provides a model for all processes which are involved in problem solving. Searching involves discrimination or discernment, and selection. Searching also includes exploring alternatives. But can all problem solvings be modelled after search? The authors distinguish between *problems to find* and *problems to prove*. The problem to prove is concerned with testing the truth of a statement. It seems to me that *problem to prove* may not fit a search model.

In summary, Millet et al suggest that the two ways for representing information processing that goes on during planful behaviour are prediction and search. Both are assumed in the general model of searching. However, prediction is concerned more with image, whereas searching for a target from a large number of alternatives is closely related to plans.

CONSCIOUSNESS, AND THE VERBAL REGULATION OF MOTOR BEHAVIOUR

How are plans and consciousness related in the neuropsychological writings of Luria? Consciousness, is the ability to assess sensory information, to respond to it with critical thought and actions, and to retain memory traces in order that such traces or actions may be used in the future. While fulfilling all of these functions, consciousness is closely related to speech. It is on the basis of speech that complex processes of regulation of man's own actions are formed. This complex form of brain activity which is consciousness entails the analysis of incoming information, the evaluation and selection of its significant elements, the use of memory traces, control over the course of goal activity, and finally, the evaluation of the consequences of its own activity. It is easy to see the parallel between Miller, Galanter and Pribram's *image* and *plan* which formed the core of cognitive activity, and the definition of consciousness given by Luria. Luria emphasises the *role of speech* in the formation of conscious activity. By means of speech, a person can analyse a situation, distinguish its important components and formulate programs of action. In forming images and plans, speech too has an extremely important role.

Luria lists three characteristics of goal directed activity: (1) recoding of information; (2) the formation of action programs with selection of approrpiate responses and inhibition of interfering ones; and (3) a comparison of the effect of action with the original intention. These three are the characteristic features of conscious activity. To reiterate, conscious activities are carried out with the intimate participation of speech processes. I think the recognition of the role of internal speech in planning motor activity is the salient link we have been looking for between cognition and action.

WHERE DOES PLANNING BELONG IN A SYSTEM OF COGNITIVE FUNCTIONS?

I have been working on a model of information integration. The initial impetus for this model came from Luria's research on the functional organisation of the brain. Briefly, the model can be described as follows; detailed description and evaluation of the model are given in a book (Das, Kirby & Jarman, 1979).

Simultaneous integration refers to the synthesis of separate elements into groups, these groups often taking on spatial overtones. The essential nature of this sort of processing is that any portion of the result is at once surveyable without dependence upon its position in the whole.

Successive information processing refers to processing of information in a serial order. The important distinction between this type of information processing and simultaneous processing is that in successive processing the system is not totally surveyable at any point in time. Rather, a system of cues consecutively activates the components.

The central processing unit has three major components: that which processes separate information into simultaneous groups, that which processes discrete information into temporally organised successive series, and the decision-making and planning components which uses the information so integrated by the other components. The model assumes that the two modes of processing information are equally available to the individual. The selection of either or both depends on two conditions: (1) the individual's habitual mode of processing information as determined by social-cultural and genetic factors; and (2) the demands of the task. The third component, planning, uses coded information and determines the best possible plan for action.

Now turning to the output aspect of the model, both simultaneous and successive processing can be involved in all forms of responding. This is the case irrespective of the method of input presentation. The output unit determines and organises performance in accordance with the requirements of the task. Take the example of memory tasks; a subject may be required to recall *serially* or recall the items in *categories;* thus, appropriate output organisation is necessary.

An example of motor planning in a simultaneous processing task will further clarify the functions of the output unit as well as the information processing nature of motor activity. The task is copying the figure of a cube. The figure is exposed for 5 seconds after which it is removed. The child is then asked to draw a likeness of the figure, which comprises the construction of the figure's image from memory. A schema of the figure must be formed in the mind; this requires simultaneous processing. Then the figure is constructed which involves a set of successive movements, while the figure's representation is held in the mind. We may record the time taken to construct, as well as the accuracy of construction. The time score should reflect output efficiency much more than the accuracy score which should be a measure of encoding and processing.

Any performance is determined not only by the two coding processes, simultaneous and successive, and the planning functions, but also by arousal and attention. Since it is rather difficult to separate arousal from attention as they influence performance in a meaningful task, let us consider the two together. They are the basic prerequisites for efficient coding and planning. Without adequate attention to the relevant cues in a task, processing is likely to be improverished. In Luria's neuropsychological model, arousal-attention are functions of the limbic system; the reticular formation is an important structure for this function. We can regard motivation to have its neural basis mainly in the interaction between the frontal lobe and the limbic and other structures in the brain-stem. We can also suggest that motor activity is planned and structured through the direct involvement of coding, planning and the arousal-attention functions. Motivation has its neural basis predominantly in those structures that mediate planful behaviour and attentional responses. It is also important to recognise the role of knowledge-base for all of our cognitive and motor functions. Both the processing of input and the organisation of output functions must depend on the cumulative store of knowledge that an individual has.

THE LEARNING DISABLED AND THE CLUMSY CHILDREN: ARE THEY OVERLAPPING SETS?

In the final section of the first part of the chapter, I wish to consider the above question. Taylor's study carried out under the supervision of Professor Wall on the Learning (Reading) Disabled and Physically Awkward Children tries to answer this (Taylor, 1982).

Jane Taylor asked a very interesting question in her dissertation: "Are the reading disabled children physically awkward?" She tried to answer this by giving a battery of motor tasks such as throw and catch, target throw, stork balance, etc, to normal readers and reading disabled children. Her results showed a significantly poor performance by the reading disabled children on 11 out of 15 of these common games that children of their age would normally play. Looking at Taylor's results more closely, she labelled a group of the children as physically awkward if they were below the 20th percentile in a large number of the tests in the motor performance battery. Then she counted the number of physically awkward children among the reading disabled and among the non-disabled or normal readers. Some 13%

of the normal readers were 'awkward' whereas nearly 28% of the disabled readers were awkward. There is a predominance of 'awkward' children among the reading disabled; but only the reading disabled were not physically awkward by any means. It seems to me that the reading disabled children have, relatively speaking, poor motor performance in game situations, but they are not, as a group, generally clumsy. Rather than assigning the reading disabled children another label, of clumsiness, subtle difficulties noticed in their strategies or plans for motor activity should be identified, and if possible, remedied. An analysis of their errors during motor performance revealed the following:

1. Lack of motor control;
2. Inability to follow a pattern;
3. Inability to recognise errors;
4. Deficiencies in specific skills, and
5. Inability to use advice on what strategies are to be followed.

Let us attempt to identify the deficit in information processing underlying these errors. I suggest that 1. can be related to planning, specially, to difficulties in motor programming. 2. is an instance of coding failure involving both simultaneous and successive processing. 3. indicates a planning dysfunction, which is characterised by deficit in evaluating feedback. On the other hand, 4. does not point to processing deficits at all; it implies that there is an inadequate knowledge-base. Lastly, 5. refers to an inability to use feedback even if evaluating feedbacks can still occur; this is a planning dysfunction.

PART II

COGNITIVE PERFORMANCE AND INTRINSIC-EXTRINSIC ORIENTATION IN BACKWARD AND AVERAGE READERS*

Backward readers appear to have a deficit in processing sequential or successive information. This has been noticed in the classroom as well as in empirical studies (Torgeson, 1978; Jorm, 1983). In a previous study in which good and poor readers were compared on memory span type tasks as well as on non-span tasks, it was observed that if reading disability is *severe*, amounting to at least two years delay in reading, then the backward readers are found to be inferior in *both* span and non-span tasks when compared to average readers (Das, 1984). However, if the children are not so severely disabled, and are still retained in regular classrooms with occasional help by a special teacher, they are found to be particularly poor in the span tasks. Such children who are slightly backward may still demonstrate some amount of deficiency in non-span tasks. The non-span tasks included tests such as Figure Copying, Memory for Design, Visual Search and Trail-making (Das, Snart & Mulcahy, 1982). These tasks were given to Grade 4 children who were divided into backward, average and superior readers in a study by Das, Bisanz and Mancini (1984). The span tasks showed an increment in performance across the reading groups, but the non-span tasks did not show a consistent trend. We investigated further into the relationship between span and reading disability by examining the role of phonemic encoding, since children with reading disability appear to be relatively poor in this. Rhyming (BCDGPTV) and nonrhyming (HKRQLSW) letter series were used to test memory span. Superior average and backward readers were compared

* Assistance of Dr. Murphy in running this study is appreciated.

(Das, Bisanz & Mancini, 1984). Although superior readers were better than the other two groups in recall, the backward compared to the average readers did not show poor phonemic encoding. Thus it appears that a poor memory span may be the characteristic deficit of most, but not all reading disabled children.

The cognitive processes which contribute to a poor memory span have not been identified. Nevertheless, memory span has been implicated as an explanation for competence in reading (Baddeley & Lewis, 1981). Hence, poor performance in span task and in reading should be positively related. Research on reading relating to span have used the concepts of automaticity and working memory capacity (cf. Baddeley, 1981; Lesgold & Perfetti, 1978). One may reasonably conclude from these that the backward readers' poor performance in sequential tasks, such as memory span, and consequently in decoding, may be primarily due to their slow endocing time for letters and words. But is their slowness in encoding specific to verbal stimuli or not? No definitive answer is available; but one suspects that it is a general characteristic of severely backward readers who perform poorly not only in tasks that relate to reading, but in many other congitive tasks (Das, Leong & Williams, 1978). A general slowness in encoding may be inferred from this. The present study has for one of its objectives the comparison of average readers and backward readers in mainly span and nonspan tasks, but it uses midly backward readers as subjects.

The second objective of the study is a simple one. It is to determine if developmental trends in grades three to six could be obtained for both the average and the backward readers. The cognitive tasks in the present study, which have been used previously to measure simultaneous and successive coding and planning processes, have been shown to be sensitive to chronological age (Das, Bisanz & Mancini, 1984). Therefore it is fully expected to find a similar increment in performance on instances of tasks measuring the three processes with age for both average and backward readers. However, there may be a reason to suppose that the backward readers have atypical cognitive development. Such a view would be derived from assuming that the backward readers have not only a developmental lag, but a defect. In a previous study we considered the defect vs. developmental lag view (Das, Bisanz & Mancini, 1984); our data supported the latter. even if the critical difference between the two groups of readers would lie in a general speed of encoding, there would be no reason to suspect a qualitative difference in encoding speed.

The third, and final, objective of the present investigation is to determine the interaction between cognitive and motivational factors as they relate to reading competence. Obviously, cognitive tests measuring various kinds of processing would correlate with reading performance, especially decoding or word recognition skills. However, reading disabled children have been suspected of poor classroom motivation. They are thought to be more extrinsically oriented, typically lacking curiosity, a desire for mastery and a sense of challenge in their school work. Susan Harter (1981) has recently published a scale for measuring extrinsic and intrinsic orientation in the classroom; we have used this scale in a previous study in which we compared average and backward readers in grades three to six (Das & Murphy, Note 1)*. It was heartening to find that the backward readers were quite

---

* Das, J.P. & Murphy, D. *The development of intrinsic and extrinsic motivational orientation in normal and disabled readers.* An unpublished paper submitted to the Alberta Mental Health Advisory Council.

comparable with average readers in their intrinsic orientation until grade five. Only in grades five and six were they relatively more extrinsic in some of the subscales of the Harter scale. Our objective in the present report is to determine whether or not the motivational and the cognitive variables, together, predict reading performance in each of the two groups. Since the Harter scale is new, there are no studies which address the question of determining the variance contributed by the subscales of the Harter scale and cognitive process measures to reading. However, locus of control scales such as Crandall, Kratkovsky and Crandall's (1965) scale of Intellectual Achievement Responsibility comes closest, conceptually, to the Harter scale. Another one that has often been used to measure locus of control is the Nowicki-Strickland locus of control scale for children (Nowicki & Strickland, 1973). Using Crandall's locus of control scale in predicting reading and arithmetic achievement, Das, Manos and Kanungo (1975) obtained a significant contribution from locus of control to these achievement measures along with such other noncognitive variables as parental aspirations for children's academic achievement and socio-economic status. Similarly, Swanson (1981) has obtained a significant correlation between the other locus of control scale and reading and arithmetic measures in learning disabled children. In fact, there is no dearth of studies which demonstrate that motivational factors such as locus of control have a weak to moderate level of correlation with academic achievement (see the review by Uguroglu & Walberg, 1979). What is lacking, however, is the examination of the joint contribution of tests of intellectual functions and locus of control type motivational variables to a basic scholastic achievement such as reading. Additionally, it has not been clear whether or not the relative influence of intellectual and internal/external motivation to reading remains the same for children with reading disability.

We hypothesise that the backward readers in comparison with the average, will perform poorly in cognitive tasks which measure short-term memory span. In nonspan tasks they may or may not be different. Further, both groups of readers will improve in their cognitive processing measured across grades three through six. Their patterns of development will be similar even when a developmental lag is found for some of the tasks. In regard to the joint contribution of cognitive and motivational factors, we have no strong basis for a hypothesis; both should significantly contribute to the variance in reading performance.

METHOD

Subjects

The subjects were children in grades three to six who were attending The Edmonton Separate School System. Two groups of children were involved in this study.

The first was a group of average readers, and consisted of those children whose IQ was above 80 and whose reading skills were at or above the 50th percentile on the Canadian Test of Basic skills. All the average readers came from nine schools, three at each SES level, low, middle and high. Teachers in these schools were asked to confirm the appropriateness of each subject's inclusion in the average reading group. Those subjects on whom there was disagreement were eliminated from the study. For the remaining children, parental permission was obtained. This process resulted in 42 subjects from each of the grades three to six, who were finally selected to participate in this study.

The second group consisted of backward readers. These subjects were initially identified using the school system's "Computer Assisted Screening of Children with Learning Disabilities", which is based on the Bond and Tinker (1967) Years in School Formula. This computer program examines the children's IQ scores (in grade three, the Primary Mental Abilities Test, and in grades four to six, the Lorge-Thorndike) and Reading Achievement Scores (in grade three, the Gates-MacGinitie, and in grades four to six, the Canadian Test of Basic Skills). Children who obtain scores of below one-third of their reading expectancy are assigned a Read Score Value of 0.00. For the present study, children whose Read Score Value was -.5 and below were selected for grades three, four, and five. This cut-off was raised to -.3 for grade six children, in order to obtain a sufficient number of subjects. The Resource Room teacher was asked to confirm the appropriateness of each subject's inclusion in the backward reading group. Subjects about whom there was disagreement, or who had emotional, behavioural or sensory problems, as well as those for whom English was a second language, were further eliminated. Of the remaining children, only those having the most difficulty with reading were finally selected for inclusion. Parental consent was then sought for these subjects. This process resulted in 50 subjects from each of the grades three to six who finally participated.

Tests

A. *Measures of Cognitive Processes*

Five tests were used to measure cognitive processes. Three were measures of successive processing (Visual Digit Span, Auditory Serial Recall and Sentence Repetition), one measured simultaneous processing (Figure Copying) and one measured planning (Trail-making). These tests will now be described briefly.

Visual Digit Span:

This test is based on the Digit Span subtest of the WISC-R (1974). The subject is presented with a series of digits of increasing length. Each digit in the series is displayed on an index card. The subject is required to verbally recall each series. The score is the maximum list length correctly recalled.

Auditory Serial Recall:

This test consists of 16 lists of words. The lists vary in length from four to seven words. The lists of words are read to the subject, one list at a time, at the rate of one word per second. The subject then is required to verbally recall the word in its correct position. The number of words recalled in the correct serial order is recorded, for a maximum score of 96.

Sentence Repetition:

This test consists of a list of 20 sentences of increasing length, which are read by the tester. The subject is required to recall the sentences verbatim. A score of one is given for each sentence correctly recalled.

Figure Copying:

This test is adapted from one used by Ilg and Ames (1964). It consists of a 15 page booklet containing a geometric figure on one half of each page. The figures are of increasing complexity. The subject is required to reproduce the figures, which are scored two, one or zero, according to accuracy.

Trail-making:

This test was originally developed by Armitage (1946) to measure planning ability. The subject is required to join a sequence of numbers which are distributed randomly over a page. Two pages are presented and the times for each are recorded separately and then totalled.

B. *Measure of Motivation*

The measure of motivation used in this study was the Intrinsic-Extrinsic Motivation Scale developed by Harter (1981). Her original scale was used in spite of the unreliability of some of its items.

C. *Measures of Reading Achievement*

The Schonell Graded Word Reading Test:

This test of reading words was developed by Schonell (1955). It consists of 100 words of increasing difficulty which the subject is required to read aloud. The total number of words correctly read is converted into a reading age score.

The Gates-MacGinitie Reading Tests

This is a norm referenced group administered test which provides a measure of reading attainment in vocabulary and comprehension. The Canadian Edition (1979) of this test was used. In the present study, raw scores were converted into grade equivalents.

Canadian Test of Basic Skills

This is a norm referenced, group administered test which examines attainment in the areas of reading, language, work-study skills and mathematics. In the present study, both vocabulary and comprehension were of interest. Here, raw scores were converted into grade equivalents.

Test Administration

With the exception of the Gates-MacGinitie and the Canadian Test of Basic Skills, which were administered by the School Board, the other tests were administered by several testers, all of whom had elementary school experience. The tests were presented in random order.

Because backward readers were also of interest in this study, it was thought advisable to modify the standard administration of the motivation scale. In this study, the tester, rather than the subject, read the items to avoid the confounding effects of poor reading skill. The other tests were administered in the standard manner.

All children were administered the Schonell word reading test.

RESULTS AND DISCUSSION

Performance of average and backward readers on the five motivation and cognitive tasks as well as on Schonell has been summarised in Table 1. Multivariate analysis of variance was carried out on the five cognitive tests (Figure Copying, Trail-making, Auditory Serial Recall, Digit Span and Sentence Repetition) with 2(group) X 4(grades) on a total number of 357 subjects. Both F-ratios for groups and grades were highly significant ($p < .01$). Their values were 19.87 and 11.39 respectively.

Table 1. Mean scores on motivation subscales and cognitive tasks of average (N= 170) and backward (N= 187) readers.

	Extrinsic-Intrinsic Motivation Scales				
Readers	Challenge	Curiosity	Mastery	Judgement	Criteria
Average	3.03	3.03	2.91	2.12	2.51
Backward	2.90	2.95	2.68	1.88	2.08

	Cognitive Tasks					
	Figure Copying	Trail-making (seconds)	Serial Recall	Digit Span	Sentence Repetition	Schonell
Average	16.92	58.39	37.51	5.05	12.15	10.31
Backward	13.68	68.06	27.90	4.56	11.80	8.76

The df= 5 and 345 for the groups, and df= 15 and 952 for grades. The interaction term was also significant: $F(15,952)= 2.82$, $p < .01$. These overall results show that there is a general advantage for the average over backward readers when all cognitive tasks are taken together, and a developmental increment in performance is observed across grades three through six. The interaction term is not very informative in the context of the hypothesis of this study. In fact, the overall difference between the groups is not very informative either, because it does not show how each test behaved in distinguishing between the groups at each grade. Therefore, follow-up analyses of variance were carried out for each test for grades three to six separately. In grade 3, all tests except Sentence Repetition discriminated between average and backward readers: F-ratios were significant beyond .01 level. These results were to be expected from examining the means. In grade 4, only Figure Copying and Trail-making had significant F-ratios ($p < .01$). In view of the fact that the grade four average readers compared to backward readers were less than a year above in Schonell word reading, even these differences were unexpected. Continuing with test by test analysis, in grade 5, F-ratios for Trail-making ($p= .02$), Serial Recall and Digit Span ($p < .01$) were significant. For grade six, significant F-ratios were obtained for Figure Copying, Serial Recall ($p< .01$), and for Sentence Repetition ($p = .01$). Taking into consideration these test by test comparisons between average and backward readers, one does not see that the latter group shows a consistent disadvantage in span or successive tasks. An overall disadvantage exists for them when all tests are combined, across all grades.

These results show that both average and backward readers improve over grades 3 to 6, and their pattern of development is indistinguishable. But, the backward readers did not have a reading disability which was severe; hence significant retardation in every cognitive test in each grade was not observed. Incidentally, Sentence Repetition does not appear to be a strong test, as given in the present study, in order to detect either developmental or group differences.

Multiple Regression Analyses were carried out next in order to determine the relative contribution of cognitive processes and motivational variables to reading competence. The predicted variable in the first set of analyses was Schonell Word Reading. Stepwise multiple regression on data from the backward readers showed that Figure Copying contributed 20% of the variance followed by Auditory Serial Recall which increased the value to 28.9% and Sentence Repetition (32%). $\underline{F}$ for each of these was significant beyond the .001 level. For backward readers, none of the motivational measures contributed to the prediction of reading, but they did in the case of the sample of average readers. In order of importance, Auditory Serial Recall (25.6%), Judgment (36.7%), Trail-making (42.9%), Figure Copying (46%), and Challenge (47.7%) contributed significantly to predicting reading - for all $\underline{F}$ ratios, $p < .01$).

The Schonell word reading measures only one component of reading competence, namely word encoding. The other components, vocabulary and comprehension as indicated by Gates-MacGinitie and Canadian Test of Basic Skills (CTBS) were also examined by carrying out separate multiple-regression analyses. As mentioned in the Method section, Gates-MacGinitie Vocabulary and Comprehension tasks were given to grade 3, and CTBS Vocabulary and Comprehension tasks to Grades 4, 5, and 6. The structure of the two tests were comparable and the scores for vocabulary as well as for comprehension, given in grade equivalents - for both tests. Hence, we treated these scores as equivalent, and entered them in the regression analysis which is described below. Since the vocabulary and comprehension scores were obtained from school records, these may be less reliable than Schonell which was administered by us. In spite of this, the results were consistent with those obtained in predicting Schonell word reading.

Vocabulary and comprehension scores of the backward readers were predicted by Auditory Serial Recall (R^2= 17.8%, and 18.5%) which was increased to R^2 of 28.8% and 31.9% by the addition of Figure Copying. No other cognitive tests made a statistically significant contribution. However, as before, the reading scores of average readers were predicted by both cognitive and motivational variables. Cumulative percentage of variance are reported below for vocabulary: Auditory Serial Recall (32.6%), Judgment (40.0%), Trail-making (43.8%), Figure Copying (47.5%), Criteria (50.6%), and Curiosity (51.0%). Values for Gates-MacGinitie comprehension performance were 30.8% for Auditory Serial Recall; it increased to 36.7% for Criteria, 39.0% for Trail-making, 42.6% for Judgment and 44.8% when Figure Copying was added. All value increments were significant ($p < .01$).

Some of the motivational measures, then, influence the reading competence of children who are average or better in reading; motivation does not contribute to the reading competence of backward readers. One interpretation of the average and backward readers' performance considered together may be as follows: Basic cognitive processes are of primary importance to reading competence; only when a *threshold of competence* has been crossed can noncognitive processes such as motivational traits influence reading. For backward readers, one would then assume that their level of reading is below this threshold because they are still acquiring the rudiments of word-attack skill. Those who have mastered these skills will be above this threshold. For instance, Swanson (1981) observed that locus of control influenced the scholastic achievement of older learning disabled children. Thus the notion of a threshold is a plausible one. It can be thought of as a minimum level of competence in decoding printed material which in turn would imply an adequate encoding speed. The latter increases with age in the early school years; like many cognitive skills, its growth is sensitive to both maturation and instruction in school. Backward readers reach the threshold later than average readers, and after they have crossed the threshold, their reading competence is subject to motivational influence as that of the average readers in grades three to six. A subsequent study to test this suggestion on beginning average readers and relatively proficient backward readers seems to be worthwhile.

In conclusion, both groups of children generally improve in their performance on the span and nonspan tasks from grades three to six; however, their performance in adjacent grades are not always significantly apart. Examining the superiority of the average over backward readers, a general trend is noticed, but the discriminant power of each of the five tests for distinguishing between the groups is not uniform. Even the span-type successive tests do not discriminate between the average and backward reader in grade four. Had we taken backward readers who were substantially more than two years behind in reading, their performance on cognitive tasks would have been significantly poorer. As their mean Schonell scores show, in grade four, the difference was even less than one year!
The most notable finding of this study is in the multiple regressions. A threshold seems to be operating, allowing one to conclude that motivational factors begin to determine reading competence only after children have acquired an adequate level of initial reading skills. Is this threshold largely determined by encoding speed? Existing research would suggest that it is. The nature of encoding, then, should be understood. Are the backward readers slower in encoding the spatial and temporal characteristics of the stimulus as well as its semantic attributes? These problem ought to be included in subsequent research in reading disability.

ACKNOWLEDGEMENTS

The research in Part II of the chapter was supported by a grant from Alberta Mental Health to J.P. Das and a grant from IBM to Drs. A.E. Wall, R. Mulcahy and J.P. Das. We are grateful to the Separate School Board and the staff and students of the Separate School System, Edmonton, for making this research possible. Thanks are due to Drs. Judy Lupart, Ann Price, Robert Mulcahy and A.E. Wall for help in selecting subjects and standardised test scores.

References

Armitage, S.G. (1946). An analysis of certain psychological tests used for the evaluation of brain damage. *Psychological Monographs, 60,* Whole No. 277.

Baddeley, A.D. (1981). Cognitive psychology and psychometric theory. In M.P. Friedman, J.P. Das and N. O'Connor (Eds.), *Intelligence and learning.* New York: Plenum Press.

Baddeley, A.D. & Lewis, L. (1981). Inner active processes in reading: The inner voice, the inner ear, and the inner eye. In A.M. Lesgold and C.A. Perfetti (Eds.), *Interactive processes in reading.* Hillsdale, N.J.: Lawrence Erlbaum.

Bond, G. & Tinker, M. (1967). *Reading difficulties: Their diagnosis and correction.* 2nd Edition. New York: Appleton-Century Crofts.

Crandall, V.C., Kratkovsky, W. & Crandall, V.J. (1965). Children's beliefs in their own control of reinforcements in intellectual academic achievement situations. *Child Development, 36,* 91-109.

Das, J.P. (1984). Simultaneous and successive processing in children with reading disability. *Topics in Language Disorders, 4,* 34-47.

Das, J.P., Bisanz, G.L. & Mancini, G. (1984). Performance of good and poor readers on cognitive tasks: Changes due to development and reading competence. *Journal of Learning Disabilities, 17,* 549-555.

Das, J.P., Kirby, J. & Jarman, R. F. (1975). Simultaneous and successive syntheses: An alternative model for Cognitive Abilities. *Psychological Bulletin, 82,* 87-103.

Das, J.P., Kirby, J. & Jarman, R. (1979). *Simultaneous and successive cognitive processes.* New York: Academic Press.

Das, J.P., Leong, C.K. & Williams, N.H. (1978). The relationship between learning disability and simultaneous-successive processing. *Journal of Learning Disabilities, 11,* 16-23.

Das, J.P., Manos, J. & Kanungo, R.N. (1975). Performance of Canadian native, black and white children on some cognitive and personality tests. *The Alberta Journal of Educational Research, 21,* 183-195.

Das, J.P., Snart, F. & Mulcahy, R. (1982). Reading disability and its relation to information-integration. In J.P. Das, R.F. Mulcahy and A.E. Wall (Eds.), *Theory and research in learning disabilities.* New York: Plenum Press.

Harter, S. (1981). A new self-report scale of intrinsic versus extrinsic orientation in the classroom: Motivational and information components. *Developmental Psychology, 7,* 300-312.

Hecaen, H. & Albert, M. (1979). *Human neuropsychology.* New York: Wiley.

Ilg, F.L. & Ames, L.B. (1964). *School readiness: Behavior tests used at the Gesell Institution.* New York: Harper & Row.

Keogh, J. (1982). The study of movement learning disabilities. In J.P. Das, R.F. Mulcahy and A.E. Wall (Eds.), *Theory and research in learning disabilities.* New York: Plenum Press.

Jorm, A.F. (1983). Specific reading retardation and working memory: A review. *British Journal of Psychology, 74,* 311-342.

Lesgold, A. & Perfetti, C. (1978). Interactive processes in reading comprehension. *Discourse Processes, 1,* 323-336.

Luria, A.R. (1966). *Human brain and psychological processes.* New York: Harper and Row.

Luria, A.R. (1969). *The Origin and Cerebral Organization of Man's Conscious Action.* A lecture given to the XIX International Congress of Psychology, London.

Miller, G.A., Galanter, E. & Pribram, K.H. (1960). *Plans and the Structure of Behavior*. Holt, Rinehart and Winston, Inc.
Norman, D.A. & Shallice, T. (1980). *Attention to action: Willed and automatic control of behavior*. (Techn. Rep.). San Diego: University of California, Center for Human Information and Processing.
Nowicki, S. & Strickland, B. (1973). A locus of control scale for children. *Journal of Consulting and Clinical Psychology, 14,* 148-154.
Roy, E.A. (1978). Apraxia: A new look at an old syndrome. *Journal of Human Movement Studies, 4,* 191-210.
Sapir, T. & Nitzburg, A.C. (1973). *Children with learning problems*. New York: Brunner/Mazel.
Schonell, F.J. (1955). *Schonell graded word reading test*. Scotland: Oliver & Boyd.
Shallice, T. & Evans, M.E. (1978). The involvement of the frontal lobes in cognitive estimation. *Cortex, 14,* 294-303.
Skinner, B.F. (1985). Cognitive science and behaviorism. *British Journal of Psychology, 76,* 291-301.
Swanson, L. (1981). Locus of control and academic achievement in learning disabled children. *The Journal of Social Psychology, 113,* 141-142.
Taylor, K.J. (1982). Physical awkwardness of reading Disability: a Descriptive study. M.Sc. Dissertation, University of Alberta, Canada.
Torgesen, J.K. (1978). Performance of reading disabled children in serial learning tasks: A review. *Reading Research Quarterly, 19,* 57-87.
Uguroglu, M.E. & Walberg, H.J. (1979). Motivation and achievement: A quantitative synthesis. *American Educational Research Journal, 16,* 375-389.
Wall, A.E. (1982). Physically awkward children: A motor development perspective. In J.P. Das, R.F. Mulcahy and A.E. Wall (Eds.), *Theory and research in learning disabilities*. New York: Plenum Press.
Whiting, H.T.A. (1982). Image of the Act. In J.P. Das, R.F. Mulcahy and A.E. Wall (Eds.), *Theory and research in learning disabilities*. New York: Plenum Press.

DEVELOPMENT OF COORDINATION AND CONTROL IN THE MENTALLY HANDICAPPED

W.E. Davis

From the relatively few studies of motor development with persons labeled as mentally handicapped, it is abundantly clear that motor deficiency is concomitant with a deficiency in cognitive development. There are, of course, wide variations within this population. However, virtually all studies comparing mentally handicapped subjects to non-handicapped subjects find a definite and often marked performance difference on a variety of motor development measures. Most of these measures provide only global descriptions, offering little insight into the underlying problems of motor coordination and control in mentally handicapped populations (see Henderson, 1985; Newell, 1985 for reviews). There have been few "explanations" of the motor deficiency of mentally handicapped subjects and these have not been that useful.

Some researchers have suggested that motor performance deficiencies in mentally handicapped persons represent only a delay in development rather than a deviation from the normal course (e.g., Francis & Rarick, 1959) and some supporting evidence of this claim exists with such tasks as throwing (Roberton & DiRocco, 1981) and prehension (Moss & Hogg, 1981). Others contend that specific underlying deficiencies account for performance lags, or at least certain performance decrements. For example, perceptual and attentional deficits have been cited as reasons for low performance on aiming and on discrimination tasks (Anwar, 1981, 1983; Zeaman & House, 1963). From an information processing approach (see Hoover & Wade, 1985 for a review), it has been suggested that central processing capacity shortage affects memory and cognition necessary in motor skills (Wade, Hoover & Newell, 1983). The difficulty with this latter notion is that deficiencies have been found at every point along the processing chain (cf. Nettelbeck & Brewer, 1981; Wade, Newell & Wallace, 1978). In a review of this literature, Newell (1985) concluded that this approach has turned out to be only another level of description, contributing little to our understanding of coordination and control in the mentally handicapped. The most often implicated motor deficiency in Down syndrome subjects* is hypotonia, a decrease or absence of muscle tone. None of these claims, however, are fully substantiated. The implication here is that one essential element lacking in mentally handicapped research has been a viable theoretical framework from which to address this problem of motor deficiency. This "deficiency in research", if you will, has been made explicit by Henderson (1985) and Newell (1985).

---
* see over.

THEORY AND POSTULATE

One theoretical approach offering insight into motor deficiency in mentally handicapped subjects views coordination and control as arising from a mutually constrained actor-environment system (Fowler & Turvey, 1978). The one aspect of this approach, that is important for this paper, is the distinction made between coordination and control. Such distinction is not made in most of the motor control and motor development literature. According to Kugler, Kelso and Turvey (1980), coordination is seen as the process that constrains the system's free variables into a behavioural unit and control is the process by which the values are assigned to that behavioural unit. An example by Saltzman and Kelso (1985) is most relevant. They offer that the arm will act as a reaching device if organised as a damped mass-spring. This process of organising or constraining the muscle-joint system to behave as a damped mass-spring, is equated with coordination. The fact that such organisation may occur across all reaching situations is referred to as the "organisational invariant" (Fowler & Turvey, 1978; Saltzman & Kelso, 1985). In a self-organising system, values are assigned to the various dynamic variables, such as the stiffness and damping co-efficients. During each separate reaching performance, different values may need to be assigned to these variables in order to allow for different trajectories. This process of assigning values to the parameters of the system is equated with control.

It is suggested that the parameterising is achieved by constraints specified by perceptual information specific to the immediate actor-environment context, as for example, the "time to contact variable" in the execution of the long jump (Lee, Lishman & Thomson, 1982) and in baseball striking (Fitch & Turvey, 1977; Hubbard & Seng, 1960). In goal directed behaviour (for example, aiming at a target), if the appropriate parameters of the system are specified, the moving limb will stop at a new equilibrium point corresponding to the specific target to be reached. Thus, the movement goal will be accomplished. Consistent optimal specification of the parameters is referred to as "skill" (Newell, 1985).

Before proceeding it may be well to pause and review some of the basic ideas of the mass-spring system model even though more elaborate discussions are well known in the motor control literature (e.g. Feldman & Latash, 1982; Kelso & Holt, 1980). A simple mass-spring system is described by the equation $F= -K\ (1-1_o)$, where F is an external force, -K is stiffness, 1 is the current length of the spring, and 1_o is the length of the spring when no forces are acting on it. The movement characteristics (displacement, velocity, acceleration, *etc.)* are determined by the parameters of force.

---

* Down syndrome subjects represent the most significant subgroup in the mentally handicapped population. They have been a well-delineated group of individuals being visually recognisable because of their distinct appearance and the fact that they are prevalent in all societies of the world (Smith, 1981). Both similarities and differences are found between Down syndrome and other non-distinguished mentally handicapped subjects and thus the two groups of subjects are distinguished here. It has not always been the case that researchers have even made this distinction in describing their population. Data, to support a simple postulate, are presented here on both Down syndrome and mentally handicapped subjects. In this case, the important aspects of the data do not differ between Down syndrome and other mentally handicapped subjects, and thus the postulate would hold for both.

stiffness, and zero length. The latter are called dynamic parameters and the former are kinematic parameters.

In a mechanical mass-spring system the parameters of stiffness and zero length are fixed and thus changes in movement (actual length of the spring) are determined solely by an external force. To make the system controllable is to be able to alter the stiffness and zero length parameters. For example, as illustrated in Figure 1A, systematically adding weight to a mechanical spring changes the length of that spring systematically. The systematic change is plotted as a length by force (weight) function (Figure 1). If the zero length of the spring were changed (Figure 1B) and the same weights systematically added, a parallel and non-intersecting curve would be generated. Change the stiffness of the spring but hold the zero length constant and again systematically add weight and a new curve (Figure 1C) will be generated which intersects at the zero point but with a different slope. By alternating stiffness and zero length separately or together, sets of curves could be generated which would cross every point in two-dimensional space. Transpose such a system to a limb and all types of movements are possible by simply altering the force, stiffness, and zero length parameters. To reiterate, organising the system's variables to behave as a mass-spring system is equated with coordination; altering the values of these variables is equated with controlling the system.

Given this perspective, a tentative postulation can be derived from the results of the few studies of motor coordination and control with mentally handicapped subjects. It is suggested that motor deficiency in mentally handicapped populations, including Down syndrome, lies not in the fundamental organisation of the actor-environment system, i.e., in motor coordination but in the parameterisation of the functional unit, i.e., in motor control. It must be noted here that the evidence supporting this claim is limited and thus the tentative nature of this postulate is underscored. It is also to be noted that the postulate being offered here does not provide immediate insights into understanding motor deficiency in mentally handicapped subjects. Rather, it is offered as a basis, grounded in theory, for directing future research. As pointed out recently by Newell (1985), the nature of the variables of coordination "is one of the fundamental unknowns in the theory of action" (p. 12). Nevertheless, it may be stated that if a group of muscles, constrained to act as a functional unit behaving as a mass-spring system, is an organisational invariant; then, evidence exists that such organisation characterises both non-handicapped and mentally handicapped individuals. On coordination, the two groups do not differ. They do differ, however, on the assigning of values, the parameterising of this functional unit. They display a deficiency in control.

EMPIRICAL EVIDENCE

The initial evidence comes from a study by Davis and Kelso (1982) who followed the now classic experiment of Asatryan and Feldman (1965). Using a step unloading technique, plots of the static moment versus joint angle of the human muscle-joint system were obtained. Plots were obtained from seven Down syndrome and six non-handicapped subjects. The task required subjects to move to an established initial joint angle and to maintain that angle against an external load (torque). Torque was systematically changed via partial unloading in order to obtain torque by length (joint angle) functions at three separate initial joint angles. Instructions required subjects

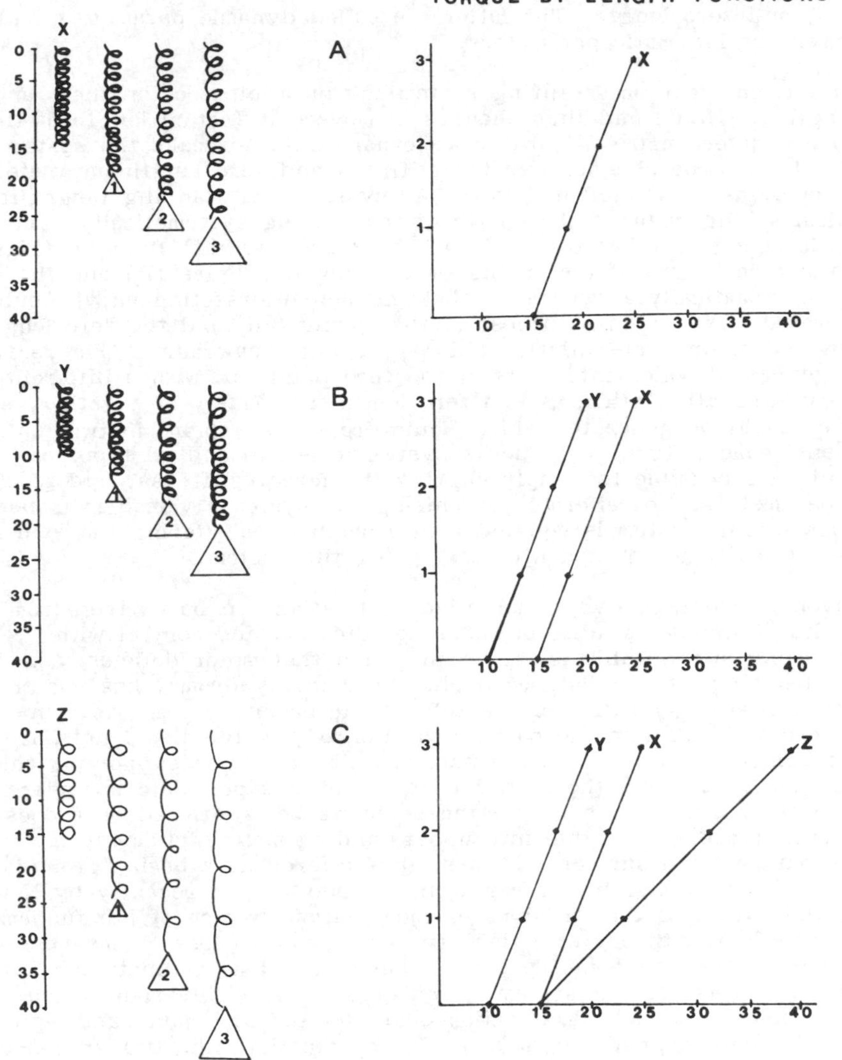

Fig. 1. Characteristics of a simple mechanical mass-spring system. Changes in the length as a function of changes in force (added weight). A) The force/length function of spring "X". B) Comparison of the same function in springs X and Y. Their stiffness is the same but their zero length differs. C) Comparison of the same function in springs X and Z. Their zero length is the same but their stiffness differs.

"not to intervene" when unloading occurred. Figure 2 shows identical parallel and non-intersecting curves for both Down syndrome and non-handicapped subjects, a finding consistent with previous studies of non-handicapped adults (Asatryan & Feldman, 1965; Feldman, 1966a, 1966b). This finding is particularly important in light of the recent evidence that

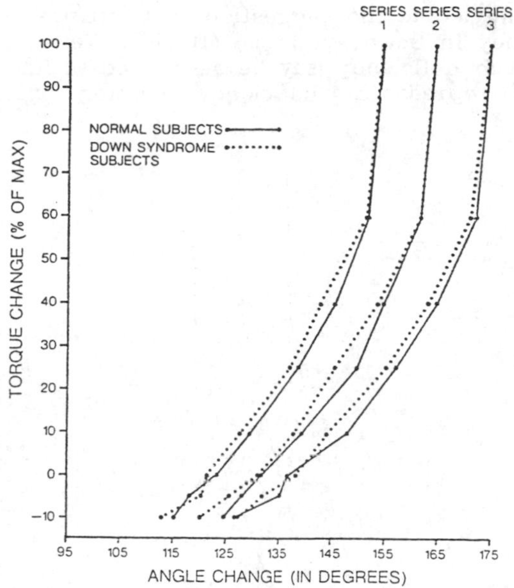

Fig. 2. Angle change as a function of torque change under the instructions "do not intervene". The large dots represent the mean angle change for the group on each of the seven unloadings. (Reproduced with permission from Davis & Kelso, 1982).

a means of controlling the muscle-joint system is by shifts along the invariant characteristics (e.g. Feldman, 1982a, 1982b; Feldman & Latash, 1982).

The identical slopes of these curves suggest that background muscle activity (muscle stiffness) of Down syndrome subjects during the statis posture, is similar to non-handicapped populations (Figure 2). This finding regarding muscle stiffness is supported by Shumway-Cook and Woollacott (1985) but does raise questions about the popularly held opinion that muscle hypotonia is responsible for motor deficiency in Down syndrome. It is worthy to note here that also being seriously challenged is the long held belief that muscle hypertonia (the opposite of hypotonia) accounts for motor deficiency in cerebral palsy and other motor disorders (Barlow & Abbs, 1984; Dietz & Berger, 1983).

In the Davis and Kelso (1982) study, it was also demonstrated that Down syndrome subjects could, upon request, increase the stiffness level of the muscle-joint system. The experimental procedure was the same as in Experiment 1, except that subjects were asked to tense (co-contract) their muscles in an effort to maintain a constant joint angle against the perturbation. Each subject was given some practice prior to the experiment proper to ensure that the instructions were understood. In the experimental trials, upon reaching the target angle, subjects were asked to "stiffen their muscles" to maintain the joint angle. As shown by the slope of the torque by angle function in Figure 3 (compare Figure 2), Down syndrome subjects were able to voluntarily change the stiffness parameter. However, the level of increase in stiffness was significantly below that of the non-handicapped subjects

(Figure 3). This finding led to the suggestion that stiffness was a sensitive index of motor deficiency in Down syndrome (Davis & Kelso, 1982). It is suggested here that such deficiency may be associated with the parameterising of the system and thus represents a deficiency in motor control.

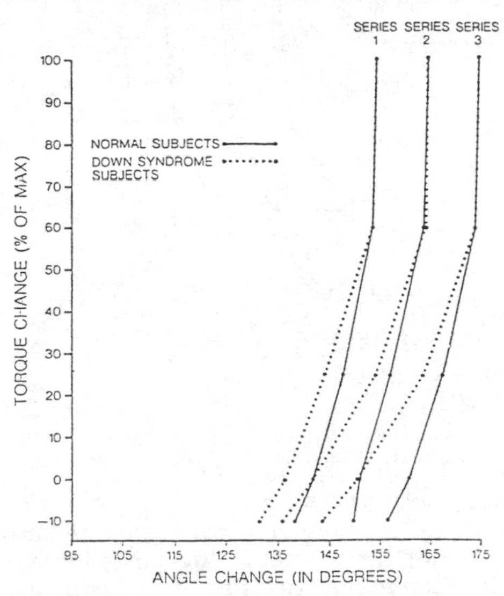

Fig. 3. Angle change as a function of torque change under the instructions "stiffen your muscles". The large dots represent the mean angle change for the group on each of the four unloadings. (Reproduced with permission from Davis & Kelso, 1982).

In a more recent study (Davis & Sinning, 1985) similar results were found for both Down syndrome and other mentally handicapped subjects on torque by IEMG (integrated electromyogram) magnitude functions. In this study, subjects were asked to maintain a constant elbow joint angle during a step loading procedure. IEMG magnitude measures of the flexor muscles were obtained and plotted against the torque measures. In Figure 4, means of the IEMG magnitudes for each of the three groups are plotted against the mean torque values. These means are expressed as percentage of maximum in order to control for possible measurement differences (Bigland-Ritchie, 1982). Plots of the actual values of IEMG and torque magnitudes for an individual subject from each group are shown in Figure 5. The slopes of these curves were taken as an index of flexor stiffness (e.g., Bigland & Lippold, 1954; Bigland-Ritchie, 1982).

The mean slopes of the IEMG/torque curves for the two groups of handicapped subjects did not differ from non-handicapped subjects. (Significant differences between groups were not found in either analysis of the means as percentage or the means as actual values). Rather, the important difference, as in the first study, was in the magnitude of torque generated. As shown in Figure 6, the non-handicapped group exhibited greater maximum voluntary contractions (MVC) than either the Down syndrome or mentally handicapped groups.

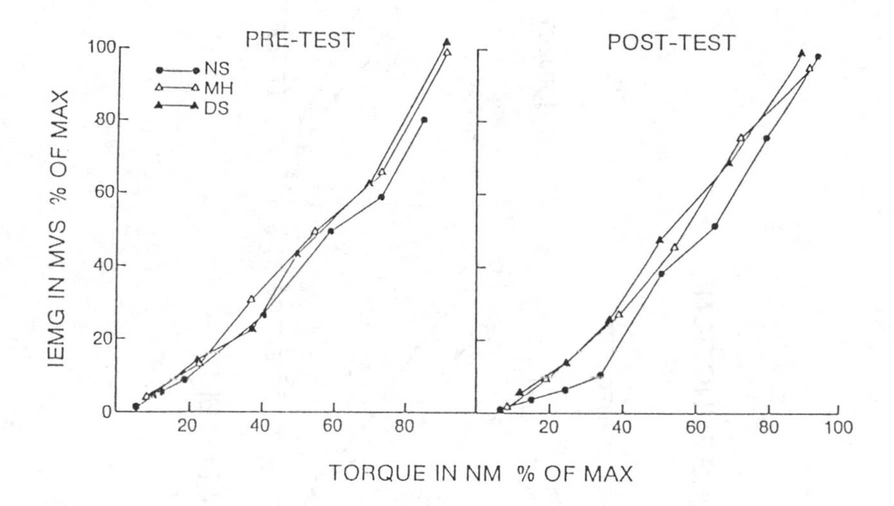

Fig. 4. Individual IEMG by torque functions taken, during a step loading procedure, from the elbow flexor muscles contracted isometrically. (Reproduced with permission from Davis & Sinning, 1985).

In addition, it was found that mentally handicapped subjects produced a significantly lower magnitude of force per unit of muscle tissue than the non-handicapped subjects (Figure 7). In turn, Down syndrome subjects were significantly lower than the mentally handicapped subjects. However, extreme caution must be taken in regard to this finding. Measurement technique does not allow for determination of the percentage of intrafiber fat tissue. Muscle mass is determined by measuring the fat layer above the muscle. If the intramuscular fat contents were high, as might be expected in many mentally handicapped subjects, particularly Down syndrome individuals, the amount of available muscle tissue would be over estimated leading to a low force to cross-section value.

Further evidence of a deficiency in control is the relative difficulty these subjects have in maintaining a constant resistance to an external force (Davis & Sinning, 1985; Davis & Kelso, 1982). As shown by the movement tracing in Figure 8, Down syndrome subjects experienced difficulty in reaching the target angle when movement was made against a load. They were also unable to maintain the constant angle in contrast to the performance of the non-handicapped subjects. Similar difficulty, during maintenance of a steady resistance for 2 seconds under isometric conditions, was observed with both mentally handicapped and Down syndrome subjects in the Davis and Sinning (1985) study.

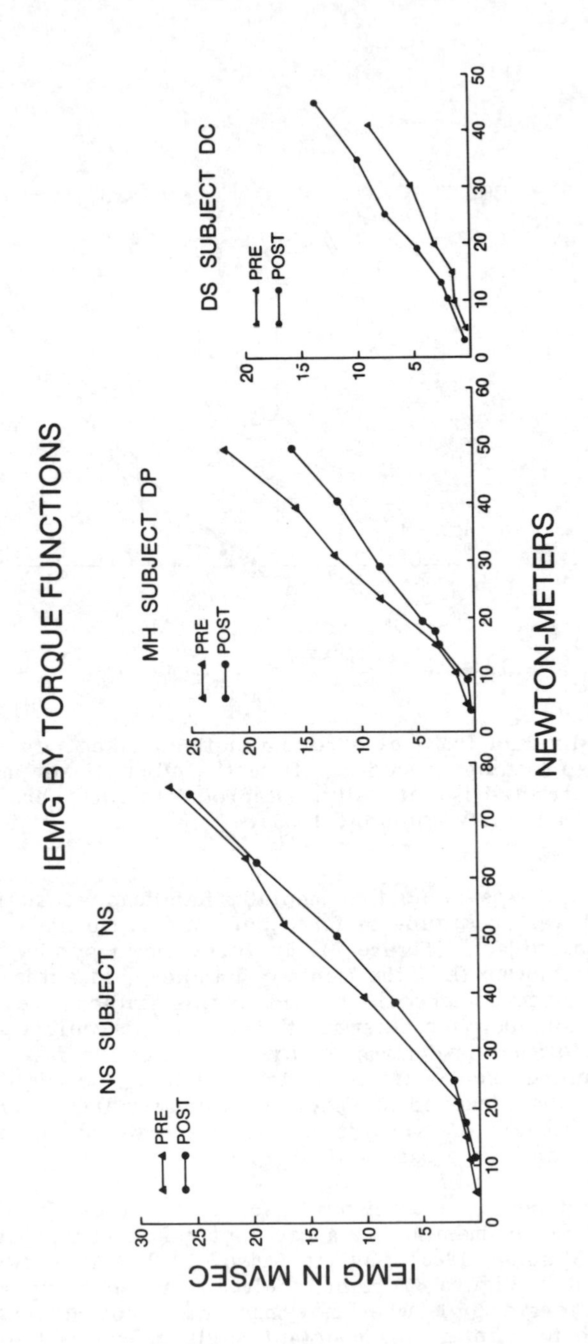

Fig. 5. Group differences in mean maximum voluntary contractions of the elbow flexor muscles. (Reproduced with permission from Davis & Sinning, 1985).

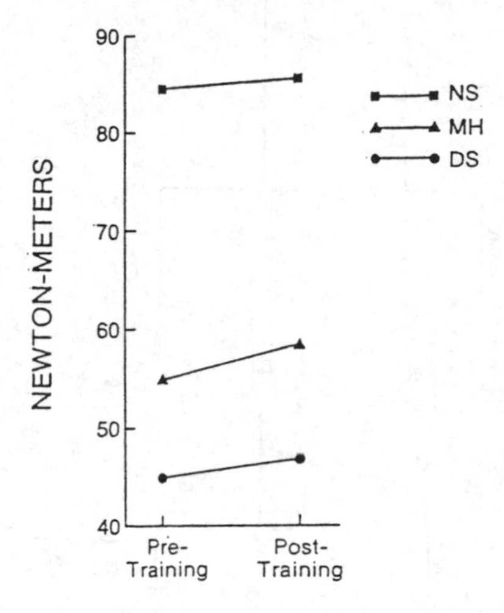

Fig. 6. Group differences in torque per volume of muscle tissue. (Reproduced with permission from Davis & Sinning, 1985).

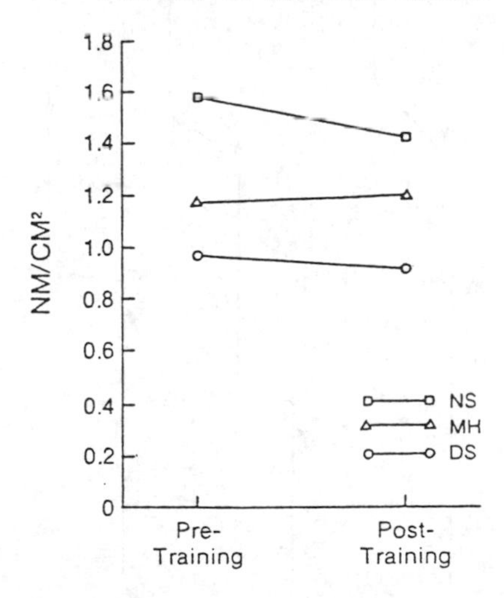

Fig. 7. Tracings of finger movements of individual subjects. Tracings for non-handicapped subjects were taken directly from the computer and tracing from Down syndrome subjects were taken from the visicorder. (Reproduced with permission from Davis & Kelso, 1982).

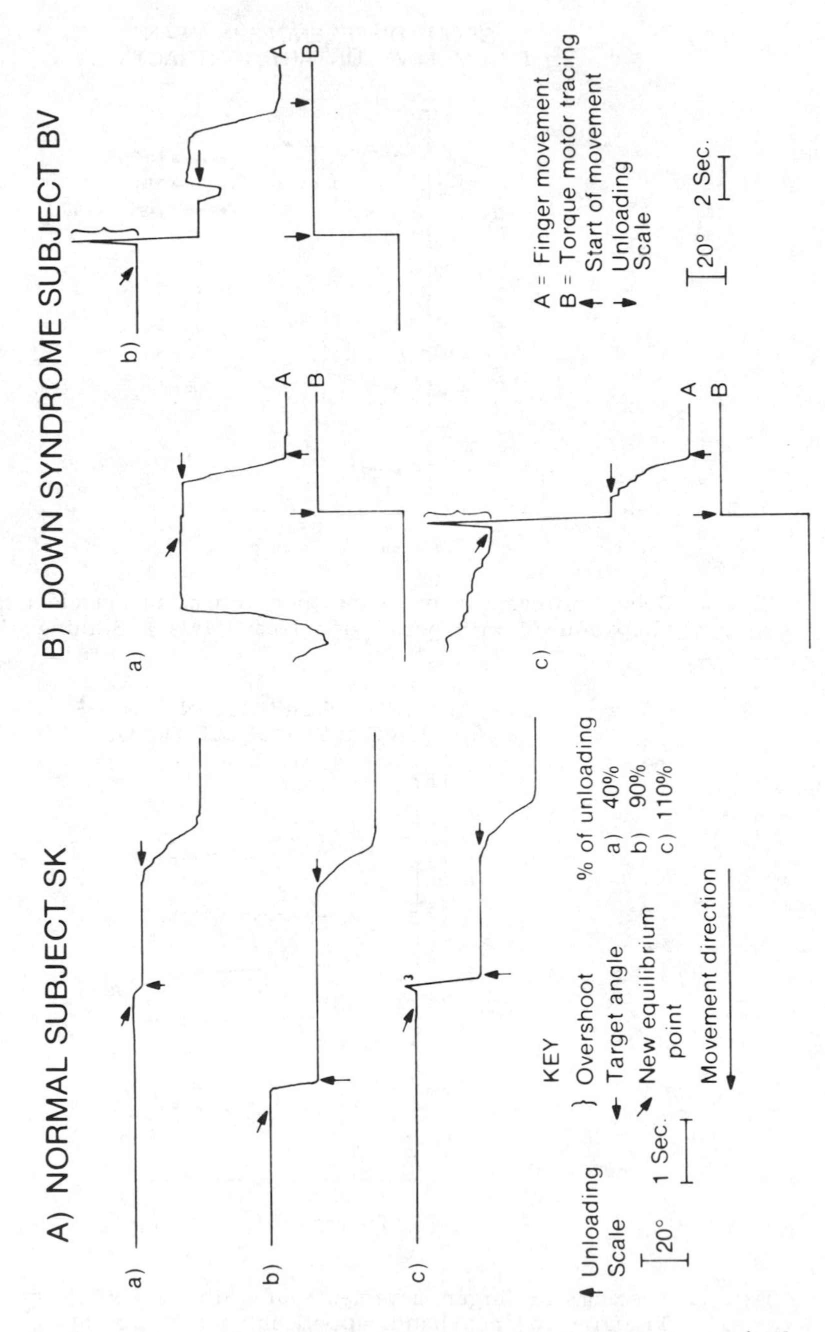

Fig. 8. Comparison of temporal delay between distal and proximal muscles in non-handicapped and Down syndrome children. (Reproduced with permission from Shumway-Cooke & Woollacott, *Physical Therapy*, 1985).

These results, along with previous findings, led to the notion that, on a physiological level, a deficiency in muscle activation describes mentally handicapped subjects (Davis & Sinning, 1985). That is, mentally handicapped subjects are unable to generate relatively high magnitude of muscle activity, and they are unable to maintain constant levels of muscle activation during movement against a resistance. This muscle activation may be associated with the parameterisation of the muscle-joint system during the maintenance of simple postures. If so, then upheld is the notion that movement deficiency of mentally handicapped individuals lies in control, at least under these limited postural conditions.

Additional support for this postulation comes from studies by Shumway-Cook and Woollacott (1985). These researchers followed previous research by Nashner (e.g., Nashner, 1977, 1981) that demonstrated remarkable consistencies in the sequence and timing of postural muscles EMG activity of non-handicapped adults during balance tasks. This muscle synergy was interpreted as evidence of an organisational invariant. Shumway-Cooke and Woollacott (1985) found that, in a similar postural situation, Down syndrome children were able to produce directionally specific postural response patterns similar to, though more variable than, non-handicapped children. As shown in Figure 9, the first muscle response to forward sway was gastrocnemius than hamstring, and to backward sway was tibialis anterior and quadriceps. All subjects showed this same response pattern. Thus, both the Down syndrome and non-handicapped children in Shumway-Cook and Woollacott's study evidenced the appearance of the same organisational invariant as the normal adults.

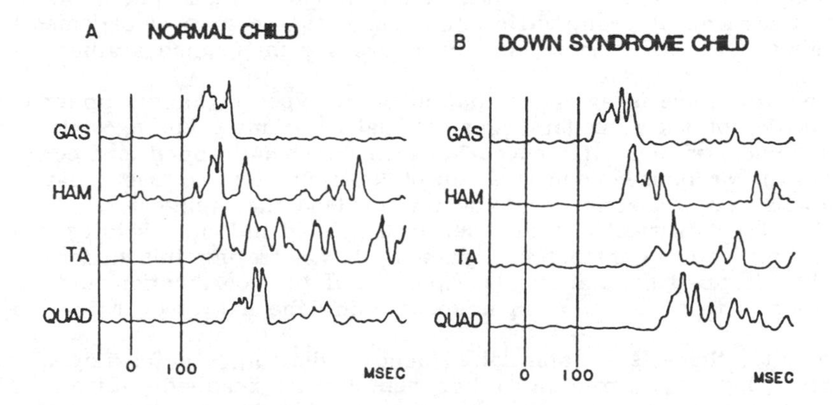

Fig. 9. Comparison of temporal delay between distal and proximal muscles in non-handicapped and Down Syndrome children (Reproduced with permission from Shumway-Cook & Woollacott, Physical Therapy, 1985).

In these same studies, important differences were also found. EMG measures were more variable and onset latencies were longer in Down syndrome subjects. Shumway-Cook and Woollacott (1985) suggested that "delayed activation of postural responses in Down syndrome children could not be attributed to reduced segmental motoneuron excitability in light of (1) normal myotatic latencies and (2) presence of low level tonic background activity in many trials, indicative of suprathreshold motoneuron excitability" (p. 14 preprint). As previously noted, these conclusions concurred with those of Davis and Kelso (1982).

This *delay* in activation of the muscle synergy is a finding consistent with a large body of literature. Slow responses are a robust finding with mentally handicapped populations, especially Down syndrome, under a variety of conditions. Much less attention has been given to the study of movement speed with this population. This paucity stands out, in particular, when contrasted to all the rapid movement studies conducted with non-handicapped subjects. However, slow movements may be a very important manifestation of this muscle activation deficiency.

SUMMARY

By way of summary, I want to make three points. First, evidence was presented which suggests that the same organisational structure exists with mentally handicapped subjects as with non-handicapped subjects. More evidence is clearly needed to substantiate the postulate that mentally handicapped subjects do not differ from non-handicapped subjects on motor coordination. Clearly, it may be the case that under more dynamic situations (i.e., movement vs posture) the organisational invariant (coordination) may not be the same in the two groups of subjects. Also, the appearance of co-ordination may be delayed in the mentally handicapped. Some evidence for this delay already exists as shown in the Shumway-Cook and Woollacott (1985) study. Questions of group differences, in both the form of organisation and the timing of its appearance, will be addressed in planned studies.

Second, there is evidence that in other types of handicapping conditions, subjects do not show similar organisational invariants. For example, Beuter (1984) found striking differences between non-handicapped and cerebral palsy subjects in her phase plane analysis of knee and hip movement data. Typical individuals have trajectories in the phase plane that suggest a self-contained second-order dynamical system. Cerebral palsied individuals have self-intersecting loops in their phase planes. Demonstrating this difference in other handicapped populations is important if the coordination and control distinction is to be of value in understanding the nature of motor deficiency.

Finally, there is substantial evidence indicating a deficiency in motor control of Down syndrome and other mentally handicapped subjects. That is, these subjects experience difficulty in parameterising the functional motor unit. If this parameterising is achieved by constraints specified by the perceptual information specific to the immediate actor-environment context, the implication for both the researcher and clinician is clear. For the researcher there is a need to identify precisely the specific information relevant to the task/mentally handicapped person system for a variety of tasks. To date, there has been little work in identifying the invariant information for non-handicapped subjects much less mentally handicapped ones. Notable exceptions are the work of Lee in vision and Kugler in haptics, but much work remains. For the clinician, assisting the mentally handicapped person in detecting the task specific information is important for a successful intervention strategy.

References

Anwar, F. (1981). Visual-motor localizations in normal and subnormal development. *British Journal of Psychology, 72,* 43-57.
Anwar, F. (1983). The role of sensory modality for the reproduction of shape by the severely retarded. *British Journal of Developmental Psychology, 1,* 317-327.
Asatryan, D.E. & Feldman, A.G. (1965). Functional tuning of nervous system with control of movement or maintenance of a steady posture-I. *Biophysics, 10,* 833-846.
Barlow, S.M. & Abbs, J.II. (1984). Orofacial fine motor control impairments in congenital spasticity: Evidence against hypertonus-related performance deficits. *Neurology, 34,* 145-150.
Beuter, A. (1984). Describing multijoint coordination: Preliminary investigation with non-handicapped, cerebral palsied, and elderly individuals. *Adapted Physical Education Quarterly, 1,* 105-111.
Bigland, B. & Lippold, O. (1954). The relation between force, velocity, and integrated electrical activity in human muscles. *Journal of Physiology,* (London), *123,* 214-224.
Bigland-Ritchie, B. (1982). EMG/Force relations and fatigue of human voluntary contractions. In D.I. Miller (Ed.), *Exercise & Sport Science Reviews (Vol. 9).* New York: MacMillan.
Davis, W.E. & Kelso, J.A.S. (1982). Analysis of "invariant characteristics" in the motor control of Down's syndrome and normal subjects. *Journal of Motor Behavior, 14,* 194-212.
Davis, W.E. & Sinning, W.E. (1985). The effects of strength training on muscle-joint system mechanical properties of Down syndrome and other mentally handicapped subjects. *Adapted Physical Activity Quarterly* (under review).
Dietz, V. & Berger, W. (1983). Normal and impaired regulation of muscle stiffness in gait: A new hypothesis about muscle hypertonia. *Experimental Neurology, 79,* 680-687.
Feldman, A.G. (1966a). Functional tuning of the nervous system with control of movement or maintenance of a steady posture II: Controllable parameters of the movement. *Biophysics, 11,* 498-508.
Feldman, A.G. (1966b). Functional tuning of the nervous system during control of movement or maintenance of a steady posture III: Mechanographic analysis of the execution by man of the simplest motor task. *Biophysics, 11,* 667-675.
Feldman, A.G. (1980a). Superposition of motor programs-I. Rhythmic forearm movements in man. *Neuroscience, 5,* 81-90.
Feldman, A.G. (1980b). Superposition of motor programs-II. Rapid forearm flexion in man. *Neuroscience, 5,* 91-95.
Feldman, A.G. & Latash, M.L. (1982). Interaction of afferent and efferent signals underlying joint position sense: Empirical and theoretical approaches. *Journal of Motor Behavior, 14,* 174-193.
Fitch, H.L. & Turvey, M.T. (1977). On the control of activity: Some remarks from an ecological point of view. In D.M. Landers and R.W. Christina (Eds.), *Psychology of Motor Behavior and Sport.* Champaign, Il: Human Kinetics.
Fowler, C. & Turvey, M.T. (1978). Skill acquisition: An event approach with special reference to searching for the optimum of a function of several variables. In G.E. Stelmach (Ed.), *Information processing in motor control and learning.* New York: Academic Press.
Francis, R.J. & Rarick, G.L. (1959). Motor characteristics of the mentally retarded. *American Journal of Mental Deficiency, 63,* 792-811.

Henderson, S.E. (1985). Motor skills development in Down's syndrome. In D. Lane and B. Stratford (Eds.), *Current approaches to Down's syndrome*. London: Rhine, Holt & Winston (in press).
Hoover, J.H. & Wade, M.G. (1985). Motor learning theory and mentally retarded persons: A historical review. *Adapted Physical Activity Quarterly* (in press).
Hubbard, A.W. & Seng, C.N. (1954). Visual movement of batters. *Research Quarterly, 25,* 42-57.
Kelso, J.A.S. & Holt, K.G. (1980). Exploring a vibratory systems account of human movement production. *Journal of Neurophysiology, 43,* 1183-1196.
Kugler, P.N., Kelso, J.A.S. & Turvey, M.T. (1980). On the concept of co-ordinative structures as dissipative structures: I. Theoretical lines of convergence. In G.E. Stelmach and J. Requin (Eds.), *Tutorials in motor behavior*. New York: North-Holland Publishers.
Lee, D.N., Lishman, J.R. & Thomson, J.A. (1982). Regulation of gait in long jumping. *Journal of Experimental Psychology, 8,* 448-459.
Moss, S.C. & Hogg, J. (1981). The development of hand function in mentally handicapped and non-handicapped preschool children. In P. Mittler (Ed.), *Frontiers of knowledge in mental retardation*. Baltimore, MD: University Park Press.
Nashner, L.M. (1977). Fixed patterns of rapid postural responses among leg muscles during stance. *Experimental Brain Research, 30,* 13-24.
Nashner, L.M. (1981). Analysis of stance posture in humans. In A.L. Towe and E.S. Luscher (Eds.), *Handbook of behavioral neurobiology (Vol. 5)*. New York: Plenum Press.
Nettelbeck, T. & Brewer, N. (1981). Studies of mild mental retardation and timed performance. *International review of research in mental retardation*. New York: Academic Press.
Newell, K.M. (1985). Motor skill acquisition and mental retardation: Overview of traditional and current theories. In J.E. Clark and J.H. Humpheries (Eds.), *Current selected research in motor development*. Vol. 1. Princeton, J.J.: Princeton Book Company.
Roberton, M.A. & DiRocco, P. (1981). Validating a motor skill sequence for mentally retarded children. *American Corrective Therapy Journal, 35,* 148-154.
Saltzman, E.L. & Kelso, J.A.S. (1985). Toward a dynamical account of motor memory and control. In R. Magill (Ed.), *Memory and control of action*. Amsterdam: North-Holland.
Shumway-Cook, A. & Woollacott, M.H. (1985). The development of postural control mechanisms in normal and Down's syndrome children. *Physical Therapy* (in press).
Smith, G.F. (1981). The history of progress in Down's syndrome. In P. Mittler (Ed.), *Frontiers of knowledge in mental retardation, Vol. II: Biomedical aspects*. Baltimore, MD: University Park Press.
Wade, M.G., Hoover, J.H. & Newell, K.M. (1983). Training and trainability in motor skills performance of mentally retarded persons. In J. Hogg and P.J. Mittler (Eds.), *Advances in mental handicap research, Vol. 2*. New York: Wiley.
Wade, M.G., Newell, K.M. & Wallace, S.A. (1978). Decision time and movement time as a function of response complexity in retarded persons. *American Journal of Mental Deficiency, 83,* 135-144.
Zeaman, D. & House, B.J. (1963). The role of attention in retardate discrimination learning. In N.R. Ellis (Ed.), *Handbook of mental deficiency*. New York: McGraw-Hill.

MANUAL LANGUAGE: ITS RELEVANCE TO COMMUNICATION ACQUISITION IN AUTISTIC CHILDREN

M.M. Konstantareas

During the 1960s, when speech training techniques were established (cf. Lovaas, Berberich, Perloff & Schaeffer, 1966), the fields of psycholinguistics, developmental psychology, and sign language research were in their infancy. This resulted in a limited view of what constitutes language acquisition in normal children, hence how language training for nonspeaking children should proceed. In this early view the prevalent working equation was: Language or Communication = Speech. The hope of the radical behaviourists was that the children treated through speech training would not only learn to talk spontaneously but would in fact come to appreciate their place in the world, hence shed off their autistic isolation. Thus spoken language development was thought to be a pivotal acquisition, paving the way for much needed personal changes. To quote from the Lovaas et al (1973) follow-up: "...in the beginning, we searched for one behaviour which, when altered, would produce a profound 'personality change'...We had once hoped, for example, that when a child was taught his name ("My name is Ricky") that his awareness of himself (or some such thing) would emerge. It did not" (p. 100).

Almost two decades after the original publication of this work, however, a considerable number of developments in a variety of cognate areas has expanded our theoretical knowledge and repertoire of techniques for assisting severely dysfunctional children to communicate. These additional developments have also made us better aware of the importance of patient characteristics, cognitive developmental theory (Piaget, 1970) as it relates to normal cognitive, social and linguistic skills development, and a rediscovery of the concept of developmental readiness. As in other fields, through the application of the original speech training technologies, we have also come to better understand the modifications required for improving these technologies. A good review of these developments has been provided by Goetz, Shuler and Sailor (1979), for example, in which issues of optimal steps to follow in early speech training and modes of improving spontaneity have been discussed at some length.

In beginning to consider these new developments, let me comment on the emergence of our broader perspective on language which encompasses much more than the original delimited view proposed by the radical behaviourists. The fact that spoken language has constituted the main medium of communication across human cultures is not fortuitous, since spoken language allows for elements of meaning to be combined and coded in a variety of ways. It provides a rapid medium for processing which does not rely on concrete sensory input. In effect, spoken languages have liberated us from the tyranny of our senses (Eccles, 1975) and have speeded up our communication and cognitive abilities dramatically. Yet they require, among other things, sequential coordinated movements of the larynx and supralaryngeal structures as well as the ability to decode spoken utterances by analysing their pitch, intensity and duration in a systematic and rule obeying fashion. Furthermore, there is a growing awareness of the fact that speech does not necessarily constitute communication and should not be equated with it. Many echolalic individuals can use extensive, well articulated, spoken utterances which are fully noncommunicative (Kanner, 1943; Fay & Schuler, 1980).Conversely, nonspoken systems of communication such as sign language, plastic symbol language, blissymbolics, etc. can allow for complex and meaningful communication to occur in non-speaking individuals. Further support for the notion that speech is not a necessary and/or sufficient condition for language or communication comes from work with nonhuman primates. Studies have demonstrated that either sign language (Gardner & Gardner, 1969, 1975) or a symbol system (Premack, 1971) can allow nonverbal primates to communicate competently, in the absence of a vocal-auditory-articulatory system suitable for speech decoding, encoding and production. Thus, despite a wired-in lack of readiness for speech processing, apes can utilise alternatives at least for expressing basic communicative intent which bypass the need to plan and execute a series of coordinated movements of the vocal chords, larynx and supralaryngeal structures as well as the need to rely on a temporal analysis of the speech sounds of others. While earlier efforts to teach nonhuman primates to communicate through spoken language proved ineffective (Hayes, 1951; Kellogg, 1968), the more recent attempts showed that medium choice was the pivotal variable for demonstrating communicative competence. As we shall see below, a parallel development is evident in existing efforts to help low functioning, autistic and other severely dysfunctional children to communicate. Furthermore, much earlier, sign language has evolved naturally by the deaf to allow for a smooth and natural medium of social exchange.

Approximately a decade ago, the early unquestionable emphasis on speech was replaced by a search for alternatives which bypass the specific processing limitations of many nonverbal children in a variety of dimensions. This review is intended to provide a summary of existing evidence on the factors relevant to the use of one such alternative system, simultaneous communication, i.e., sign language combined with speech, for overcoming some of these limitations of at least one subgroup, autistic children. It will expand upon earlier treatments of this issue by the author (Konstantareas, 1982, in press) and will attempt to address some issues not sufficiently emphasised in this field. The intended aim is to provide the reader with an up-to-date appreciation of the goodness of fit between the approach under consideration and the autistic child's special presenting characteristics. First, problems with speech training techniques will be considered. Second, the autistic child's information processing peculiarities and idiosyncracies will be reviewed. Third, the developmental delay and the concomitant motivational features of the autistic child will be considered as they relate to choice of intervention strategies relevant to the child's level. Finally, an attempt will be made to demonstrate how some properties of sign language may be successful for overcoming the autistic child's deficits and special needs.

SIMULTANEOUS COMMUNICATION: MATCHING SYSTEM CHARACTERISTICS TO POPULATION NEEDS

A. Limitations of Speech Training Techniques

The key factor for alerting therapists to the need for alternatives to speech-only training has been its many limitations, particularly when it is employed with the mute or minimally verbal autistic children. Thus, although the techniques can be successful with many autistic children, there is considerable individual variation in responsiveness to them. This is indirectly admitted to in the Lovaas, Koegel, Simmons & Long (1973) follow-up. They state: "this (operant speech training) was not necessarily the most beneficial therapeutic approach for all children. Many of them have benefited more from a program emphasising non-verbal communication" (p. 135). Even prior to this follow-up study, the U.C.L.A. group had observed and systematically investigated "overselectivity", i.e., the tendency of some autistic children to respond preferentially to one of two or more components of a stimulus complex (Lovaas & Schreibman, 1971). Yet in the early work and its follow-up evaluation we are not given more specific information as to the characteristics of children who are not responsive to speech training or the alternative techniques employed with them. In another follow-up of 51 autistic children exposed to speech training techniques over a period of up to 4 years at the Clarke Institute in Toronto an even less successful outcome in terms of communication gains was obtained (Mack, Webster & Gokcen, 1980). Although many of the children displayed decreased levels of self-stimulation and improvement in tantrums, toileting and general manageability, the vast majority did not acquire spoken language, despite their therapists' extensive and sustained efforts. Comparable lack of success was reported by Fulwiler and Fouts (1976), Creedon (1973), Bonvillian and Nelson (1978) and Konstantareas, Oxman and Webster (1977). In fact, it was this lack of success which prompted the use of simultaneous communication by these investigators in the first place. In sum, one of the most serious disadvantages of speech training techniques is their inapplicability to all autistic children. Even when successful, speech training has been criticised on additional grounds.

First, it is considered to be quite arduous and time consuming, particularly with some children. Hingtgen and Churchill (1969), for example, reported that after 6 hours per day, for five weeks, three of the four autistic children trained acquired 60, 25 and 16 words each, with the fourth child acquiring only 9 sounds. A second problem is the poor generalisation of the acquired spoken language to other settings or people (cf. Lovaas et al, 1973; Schaeffer, 1978; Schell, Stark & Giddan, 1967). A third reported limitation is in the quality of spoken language production of children exposed to speech training. Pitch, intonation and stress, i.e., the prosodic elements of spoken language relating to fine modulation of sound to reflect communicative intent, are quite poor. Thus operant trained language has been criticised as having a wooden, automatic quality which renders it inflexible, stilted and passive rather than spontaneous, generative and active (Goetz, Schuler & Sailor, 1979; Kiernan, 1983). A fourth major drawback of trained speech, mainly with the previously nonverbal children, is its lack of spontaneity (Schaeffer, 1978). These autistic children, after having been taught to verbalise, tend to use their speech only on demand, in the context of the treatment situation or in similar settings, and only with few individuals whom they have previously encountered. Such children appear to display a limited repertoire of self-generated language through which they could spontaneously request things or activities from new people in new situations. Their speech is elicited in the form of S-R chains, with the stimulus being provided primarily by the therapist or parent. Furthermore, the answers contain all the functors, i.e., prepositions, pronouns, etc. in the inflexible and correct, albeit pedantic, grammatical sequence in which they were originally trained rather than in the more flexible, conventionalised, and abbreviated form employed in everyday discourse. For example, to the question: "Would you like another piece, Timmy?", the child's answer may be "Yes, I would like another piece please" enunciated in a flat and droning manner rather than "Yes please" or "Yes, I'd like some more,thanks".

In sum, and as we shall develop in more detail later, speech training may be suited primarily to the verbal and relatively cognitively advanced subgroup of children (cf. Carr, 1979), although even then it has a number of limitations in that it is qualitatively different from the spontaneous generative language of normal children. As indicated earlier, even when speech training is the obvious method of choice as it may be true with the verbal and high functioning children, considerable modifications need to be introduced to counteract some of the limitations just mentioned (see Goetz et al, 1979). For some writers, even for the high functioning verbal autistic child, sign language superimposed on speech training may in fact be superior to speech-only training at least in the early stages of acquisition (Brown, 1977; Schaeffer, 1978), despite these children's ability to verbalise.

B. Information Processing Deficits in Autistic Children

Although early efforts at training communication could be described as unidimensional, assuming complete homogeneity of the children's presenting characteristics, we now know that, in practically all areas of development, autistic children fall along a continuum (Oxman & Konstantareas, 1981). This more recent appreciation fits in well with our increasingly improved understanding of causation in which brain damage or dysfunction are given primary consideration (cf. DeMyer, Hingtgen & Jackson, 1981; Oxman & Konstantareas, 1981). Clearly brain damage is unlikely to affect cortical structures in an all-or-none manner. It is therefore equally unlikely that there would be abrupt, saltatory discontinuities in the autistic children's observable behavioural characteristics. Yet, for purposes of simplification, we have come to dichotomise autistic children into high, mid and low functioning (DeMyer, 1976), mentally retarded and normally intelligent (Bartak & Rutter, 1976), verbal and non-verbal (Lovaas et al, 1973), etc. Clearly these are broad divisions which allow a means of systematisation and communication but do not seem to do justice to the complex permutations and combinations of strengths and deficits of individual autistic children which only a concept of a continuum in different areas of functioning can fully accommodate. Of these continua, communication and cognitive ability appear to be particularly relevant to treatment in that they are systematically related to outcome at follow-up (cf. Bartak, Rutter & Cox, 1975; Konstantareas, in press). Thus, in understanding the processing abilities of autistic children, many studies have employed dichotomies in the areas of cognition and language. Indeed in some cases arguments have been advanced suggesting that only autistic children of high cognitive ability may in fact be considered since otherwise one cannot distinguish between them and retarded children, and that research on autism should be restricted to the high functioning group (Prior, 1979). The obvious potential pitfall in this view is that studying only the high functioning subgroup will yield results specific to it. Generalising then to all autistic children will be unwarranted. Instead, studies in which children with different known presenting characteristics are included and their data are looked upon systematically as a function of their presenting relative strengths and deficits may be more promising. They can alert us to differences along these dimensions in the responsiveness of the children, and hence be used to arrive at more specific and appropriate therapeutic efforts on their behalf.

In reviewing the characteristics of the entire group, therefore, it is important to consider both overall commonalities and within group differences which may allow for subgrouping along different dimensions. In the area addressed in this section, we have evidence related to both. First, let me clarify that workers in the area of simultaneous communication training did not, as elegance would have dictated, know the information processing peculiarities of at least some autistic children before they devised alternatives to speech training. In actual fact, the practical inability to meet some of these children's needs in the classroom or clinic has compelled workers to try the alternative strategies, and, having been impressed by the effectiveness of these approaches, to look for confirmation in existing research or to devise new studies to clarify clinical hunches. This has been the case with our own clinical research group (cf. Webster, Konstantareas, Oxman & Mack, 1980).

The earliest basic research for assessing the information processing characteristics of autistic children was carried out by Hermelin and O'Connor (1970). Relying on neuropsychological and information processing techniques, they reported that the children did least well when required to respond to spoken instructions or to use words to respond to such instructions. Furthermore, the vast majority of autistic children were also found to be performing at the subnormal range in various problem-solving tasks which involved responsivity to sensory cues. Of particular interest, however, was the finding that despite this overall poor performance, the autistic children were relatively better on tasks involving proximal sensory input, i.e., touching, smelling and kinesthetic stimulation, than on those that involved distal receptors such as vision and hearing. In comparing vision and hearing, for example, these investigators reported that, although both modalities appeared to be impaired, it was the auditory sequential processing, i.e. temporal processing of auditory input that seemed to be particularly deficient. Of course, it is well known that the autistic children are peculiarly responding to sound, in that they either seek out some sounds or try to avoid others, but this peculiarity is as yet poorly understood. Furthermore, compared to normal, autistic children appear to suffer from more frequent and prolonged ear infections, hence they may also have physical problems in the auditory modality (Konstantareas & Homatidis, 1985).

On the relatively poorer processing and performance with auditory input, additional information is also available in the work of Tubbs. Tubbs (1966) reported that the psychotic (autistic) children's performance on the auditory decoding and association subscales of the ITPA was far below norms as compared to the performance of both normal controls and children who were defined by her as being subnormal. In addition, there were no differences in the visual area between normal and autistic children. Replication and extention of this work by Prior (1977) revealed a more complex picture. Specifically, the high functioning autistic children appeared to have this discrepancy between auditory and visual processing, favoring the visual. Members of the lower functioning subgroup were uniformly depressed in their performance on both the visual and the auditory decoding subscales. Yet, the low functioning children were not inferior to their higher functioning counterparts on the visual closure and visual sequential memory subtests. This would indicate that even the lower functioning children have some strengths in the visual area at least.

More recently, Hermelin (1976) has summarised pertinent findings and argued that the apparent advantage of autistic children in certain modalities such as the tactile-kinesthetic or the visual and their difficulty with the auditory is not due to sensory channel advantages or deficits per se, as originally thought, but rather stems from their coding problems. Autistic children apparently are better able to code visually, spacially or kinesthetically and are much worse in dealing with the coding of temporal-sequential information such as the auditory. Specific auditory channels are not differentially impaired in these children then, as it was originally proposed. Rather, Hermelin argues, their encoding capacities and their ability to restructure information and place it in the short-term, non-modality-specific abstract memory store are impaired. The children instead use an extended form of the uncoded immediate memory storage which leads to good retention of material that requires little coding and depends on specific item retention. This characteristic can also accommodate recall for objects with precise position in space such as visually presented sequences. However, information that requires recoding, and on which rules for organisation have to be imposed, cannot be adequately processed. Thus, processing of auditory information, such as information provided in spoken language, which requires decoding and recoding, may tax the autistic children's processing capacities to such an extent that they cannot deal with it at all, unless very simple rules are required such as in a chain of repetitions or alternations, e.g., "one-two-one-two" or "horse-spoon-horse-spoon" where they can do rather well (Hermelin, 1976).

In summary, the above findings although not conclusive since they were carried out mainly with higher functioning autistic children, suggest that tactile, kinesthetic and perhaps visual abilities are not as impaired in the autistic child as are his/her auditory skills, primarily because the latter demand more processing and elaboration. It is noteworthy to stress that although speech is also used, it is the tactile, kinesthetic and the visual modes on which therapists are primarily concentrating in teaching simultaneous communication to these children. On the basis of all available evidence on the information processing characteristics of this population, a number of reviewers have in fact proposed that autistic children have sustained damage to the left cerebral hemisphere (responsible for processing of verbal language, analytic functions and sequencing) while their right hemisphere (suitable for processing visuospatial information, music and gestalt forms) is relatively less severely affected (cf. Blackstock, 1978; Oxman & Konstantareas, 1981; Prior & Bradshaw, 1979; Tanguay, 1975).

Further evidence as to the auditory peculiarities and disturbances in autistic children appears in Condon (1975). He postulates that communication exists at different levels of analysis, not just at the level of the spoken word; furthermore, that a great deal of communicative signals emitted or received are not intentional. Ever since birth, the neonate's body moves in precise synchrony with the articulatory pattern of adult speech, a phenomenon which is termed "entrainment". Furthermore, that movement is precise to one twenty-fourth of a second (24 frames of moving film), so that as the adult begins to speak, the neonate's body begins to move in precise synchrony and stops moving in equally precise synchrony with the very last phonemic unit of the adult's speech pattern. The naked eye is apparently unable to detect the phenomenon, but through motion-picture, frame-by-frame analysis, the synchrony can be seen in its startling precision (Condon & Sander, 1974). For Condon, there are actually two kinds of microkinetic synchrony: "self-synchrony", the relationship between the individual's speech and his or her own body movements and "interactional synchrony", the precise correspondence between the listener's movements and the articulatory structure of the speaker's utterances. A person's body then moves in exact synchrony with the phenemic aspects of another's utterance. The minute the first person stops speaking, the body of the other stops moving as well. This bodily entrainment persists until adult life in all normal individuals. Moreover, it is not only linguistic sounds but also other auditory stimuli which have been found to yield interactional synchrony, provided that the individual is attentive (Condon, 1975).

This rhythmicity and precision in dealing with auditory input is apparently severely disturbed in some dysfunctional children and adults, i.e., the body movement patterns of these individuals are dyssynchronous with the structure of their own auditory input or that of other people. Reactivity to speech for such children, particularly those of the autistic subgroup, was found by Condon to be delayed abnormally in the more severe cases by up to a full second, i.e., twenty-four frames of moving film. For many of these children, the body movement repeated itself in a reverberatory fashion, two or more times to a single auditory signal as though the sound was actually repeated more than once. This is what Condon calls "multiple entrainment". Even more fascinating, the duration of the delayed response to the stimulus was found by Condon (1978) to be characteristic of any given child studied; this delay was always the same, regardless of the stimulus or the situation considered. Condon, however, has not obtained evidence that the child hears the sound in a delayed fashion, although he speculates that it is possible that he does. The child will sometimes move his body *as though* he hears the sound, but it is not known whether the sound is sensed, processed and coded. This can potentially be documented by further research relying on electric evoked potentials or by other means.

Attempts to replicate Condon's findings have met only with very limited success thus far. Oxman, Webster and Konstantareas (1978), reported an unsuccessful attempt to replicate the "Condon effect". Basically what we attempted to do was to add a control group of normal children and to expose both groups to specific auditory stimuli, and film the children's reactions. We analysed the film using Condon's techniques. What we found was that the autistic children were more motoric and jerky in their overall movements compared to their normal counterparts, but we were unable to replicate either the double response to sound phenomenon or the constant inter-response interval that Condon postulates to exist in autistic individuals. However, the fact remains that, if independently replicated, Condon's observations may help us to understand and better appreciate how autistic individuals perceive their auditory world and particularly the spoken world. They may have a very distorted and perhaps disturbed auditory universe, and one that does not seem to correspond smoothly to their own movements and reactions. Seen in this light, a number of specific peculiarities, distortions, or selective responsivity to spoken words by autistic children, particularly their difficulty in decoding and encoding sequenced auditory input.

C. Developmental and Motivational Features of Autistic Children

One of the major lacunae in our assessment and particularly in our treatment of the autistic child is in understanding his/her state of developmental readiness. We have attempted to expose children of diverse levels of developmental skill, for example, to the same communication training approach, be it speech, simultaneous communication or other symbol systems, frequently paying scant attention to the child's level of cognitive, linguistic, motoric and social functioning, to mention the main areas. Take the case of an 8 year-old, low functioning child, for example, who presents with severe mental retardation and an estimated communication age of 11 months or less. It is unlikely that such a child will be responsive to any of the currently available communication training systems and should indeed be treated as an 11 month-old in the area of communication. Yet, this is not what we do in actual practice. Although gestures, shared attention and turn-taking training, among other techniques, may be best suited to the needs of such a child, we may demand that he be exposed to speech training. As we move on to the third decade of systematic communication training, we clearly need to develop a more sensitive and knowledgeable approach to intervention, taking all existing evidence into account.

Research evidence from normal child development should be our main guide in meeting this goal. In an excellent volume on the topic of action and gesture as the forerunners and basis of spoken language (Lock, 1978), a number of psycholinguists from a variety of perspectives provide some important data on the rootedness of language in early action-gesture sequences. First, Clark (1978) offers an account of the transition from action to gesture in early communication. He outlines how this process unfolds through three sequential phases, without clear demarcation points in between. The first phase apparently involves the child's direct action, being developed and coordinated with the action of others into stable social/communicative structures, e.g. the sequence of giving an infant a bath. In the second phase, the child's own gestures serve a communication function, e.g. the child's pointing to a cookie while looking back and forth from the cookie to her mother. In this phase the child demonstrates that she has learned what it is to communicate as a separate activity under her control. The third phase involves communication structures which are now mediated through arbitrary sounds. These structures evolve in some fashion from the child's ability to communicate via the gestures she acquired in the second phase. Clark argues that spoken language evolves both ontogenetically and phylogenetically through gestures. He contends that the "gesture" has a meaning and form directly related to the "action-in-the-world" from which it derives.

A comparable position is put forth by Ingram (1978) who relies more specifically on Piagetian theory. He briefly traces sensorimotor intelligence and language correspondences for each of the six substages of the sensorimotor period, using data from Piaget's own children. The first words, in the case of Jackeline (Piaget's oldest child), occurred during stage 5 of the sensorimotor period (1-1:4 yrs), while during stage 6 (1:4 to 1:6 or 2.0 yrs) the first instance of deferred imitation occurred; that is, the first words were emitted by the child, without an immediately preceding demonstration by the adult, or without the object's immediate, concrete presence. As well, it was during this phase that the first references to past events occurred. Thus, by the last stage of the sensorimotor period, corresponding to the end of the second year of life, language evolves fully and it is utilised by the child in an attempt to represent the world. Comparable data have been provided by Piaget (summarised in Ingram, 1978) on Lucienne, his second child, although in her case the onset of language was even later, and on Laurent the third child, who displayed a similar pattern of early language development as his two sisters.

In a comparable vein, Carter (1978) describes the systematic emergence of such abstract determinates as "the" from the actual, gestural pointing at an object. Looking for parallelisms and correspondences between the emergence of cognition and language, she outlines eight prelinguistic, communicative schemata, taking place between the 12-16 month of life in the case of David, a middle class American child of college-educated parents. Each of Carter's schemas consists of a gesture and the sound produced by the child, mainly while he gestured. Based on systematically collected observational data on David, Carter shows how the schema "Request of Object", for example, involves reaching towards the object (gesture) while uttering a sound with an "m"-initial (vocalisation) to get the receiver's help in obtaining the object. For the schema "Pleasure/Surprise/Recognition", a smile (gesture) is accompanied by breathy "h" sounds, such as "oh" "ah" "ha" to express pleasure in someone's appearance, etc.

If cognition and language are intimately linked, an autistic child's cognitive ability should be carefully assessed, along with his/her other developmental skills, prior to devising a suitable communication training strategy for that child. In the example of the 8 year-old whose communication ability is equivalent to 11 months, it would be important to determine, through conventional psychometric and nonconventional psychological tests, his cognitive and communicative abilities. In our assessment work we have found Piagetian tasks extremely relevant in this respect. Tests for object permanence, operational causality, imitation of gestures or of vocalisation and symbolic play, although not yet standardised, provide invaluable insights into a child's level of linguistic readiness. Combined with more conventional instruments, particularly for the higher functioning children, e.g. the Leiter International Performance Scale (Leiter, 1969), the Reynell Developmental Language Scales (Reynell, 1977) and the Peabody Picture Vocabulary Test (Dunn, 1965), among others, they can lead us to the best intervention recommendations for that child's level of functioning at assessment time. If a child's cognitive ability is below the 5th substage of the sensorimotor period, for example, it would be clearly inappropriate to expose him or her to speech training. The child could be exposed to elementary sign language and gesture training however. Such training could include 6-10 highly iconic signs, as we shall see later, which are of high functional relevance to the child, such as food or activity items. Reassessments at intervals of 6 to 12 months will subsequently determine which of the available strategies could be used most for that stage.

Aside from cognitive and developmental considerations, autistic children display peculiarities and interests uniquely their own. Indeed lack of interest or diminished interest in how they impact on others or how they influence them may be the hallmark of the "autistic" condition. Furthermore, particularly for the lower functioning subgroup, motivation tends to pivot around the immediate context and the here and now, with what appears to be a minimal concern about the future. Under these circumstances, conventional views as to what might constitute motivators for autistic individuals are in most cases irrelevant. Many autistic children will satisfy need states by goal-directed movements aimed toward a coveted object rather than by requesting it from others through conventionalised linguistic means. This goal-directed reaching has in fact been considered to be one of the key factors underlying spontaneity in communication via sign language as contrasted to traditional speech training (Schaeffer, 1978). Much as normal infants, autistic children of low cognitive ability reach for and grasp objects they desire and push away objects they dislike. They clearly know what objects or people can do and actively attempt to reach for them or make them perform desired acts. They can touch one's hand or push it in the direction of an object they themselves cannot reach or they can pull an adult by the hand and take him to a desired location. In effect they use their hands to "ask" for others' help in achieving their goals. It is this motivation, coupled with goal-directed movement, which those of us who have used simultaneous communication training have capitalised upon to teach the children to communicate through sign (cf. Bonvillian & Nelson, 1978; Creedon, 1973; Konstantareas et al, 1977, 1979; Schaeffer, Kollinzas, Musil & McDowell, 1977). This tendency of many autistic children to be motoric and active, and in many instances indeed hyperkinetic, is one of their most compelling presenting characteristics.

To the extent that sign language relies on motor movement of arms, hands and face, it can be easily adapted to this tendency, as in fact it has been already adapted in the simultaneous communication training programs. It is a well known fact that, with very few exceptions, autistic children, as indeed many other neurologically impaired individuals, are not particularly interested in deciphering written material or in attempting to imitate intricate hand or mouth movements (DeMyer et al, 1981). In fact, in vain did we attempt during a pilot project to expose autistic children to blissymbolics, a pictographic language relying on symbols (Bliss, 1965). The children pushed the cards with the symbols from view and withdrew from the table on which they were placed. This of course is not specific to blissymbolics as many psychometrists or speech pathologists would readily attest. Attempting to engage an autistic child in paper and pencil tasks can be extremely taxing to both the child and the teacher, and can generate considerable frustration and ill will in both parties. Small wonder that traditionally trained teachers find the task of educating an autistic child not just a challenge but an impossibility. The children do not fulfill the teacher's expectations as to the cardinal rule of on seat behaviour and paying attention to detail, such as traditional teaching approaches require. By contrast, autistic children can be guided to function quite adequately when the physical plane of interaction is broader and when no restrictions are imposed on the child's movements in space or his sitting plan. Sign language can be easily adapted to broad movements and this may account for its apparent success (Carr, 1979; Konstantareas, 1982). For some writers this property of signs, which allows for goal-oriented movements may also account for the observed tendency of autistic children to employ their signs after simultaneous training much more generatively and spontaneously than they employ words after speech training (Schaeffer, 1978). Signs are after all an extension of the children's natural movements in space and time and do not impose excessive restrictions on them.

In summary thus far, sign language appears to possess properties relevant to both the lower developmental levels of the children, i.e., their sensorimotor and concrete intelligence, and their motivational tendencies to be active by attempting to obtain objects in a goal-directed and motoric mode. Let us next examine in more detail and more specifically the properties of sign language which make it uniquely suitable to the information processing, developmental and motivational characteristics of autistic and indeed of other dysfunctional children.

D. Characteristics of Sign Language

There are certain features of sign language that appear to render it particularly well-suited to the peculiarities and deficits of autistic children, some of whose characteristics we have just reviewed. Let us briefly consider the nature and properties of signs that might make them suitable for training with this population. First, sign language has had a very long and fruitful history. It has probably been used by the deaf for as long as spoken language has been employed by the hearing, although we may never know this fact, since the origins of both languages are shrouded in mystery. Following a phylogenetic frame of reference, Hewes (1973) has argued that, as they stood erect, members of our species were also starting to gesture, moving their extremities in various intentional, goal-related directions. This was protolanguage, the original form of language that our ancestors must have utilised. According to Hewes, vocal output was subsequently superimposed on these early gestures due to its adaptive value. By making sounds in the darkness some members of the species could get across to their band points of direct relevance to survival such as the presence of predators, of game, etc. In effect, according to this argument, vocalisation, originally a mutation present in some individuals, became an adaptive capacity which was progressively selected for in groups that utilised it successfully, and was then passed on to their progeny. Hewes' point is that gesture antidates vocal output and speech in man, and that gestures have been our earliest means of communication. Many clinicians who have utilised gestural communication, ourselves included, have intimated that many of the shyer autistic children who would previously be totally unwilling to approach others were more willing to express themselves through sign, once signs were introduced to them. Thus signs may be a more natural and spontaneous mode of expressing intent, particularly for the lower functioning, cognitively less advanced autistic children. Signs, being merely an extension of motoric movements, may also be easier for these autistic children to use. As already mentioned, although the children may not spontaneously vocalise, they do reach for desirable objects. The signs for *come, go, give, want* can be considered to be natural extensions of spontaneous, reaching, self-directing gestures.

An important additional feature of sign language is its iconicity. Iconicity is derived from the Greek word icon, i.e., image, and denotes the relationship between a sign and the object, state or activity it signifies. Iconicity is expressed in a variety of ways such as: (a) by performing an abbreviated imitation of a characteristic part of the referent, as for the signs *eat* or *write;* (b) by outlining in the air the object referred to, as for *house* or *box;* (c) by evoking a property or state, as for *fat;* and (d) by mimicking a property or state in a fragmentary fashion, as for *sleep*. Students of sign language have looked upon iconicity with considerable interest, if not always agreement, and have commented on its relevance to both the understanding of sign language's original derivation from pantomime and particularly its learnability (Stokoe et al, 1965; Wescott, 1971). Many hearing individuals, children and adults alike, laugh aloud with delight at the cleverness of some of the signs, once their meaning is explained to them. The signs for *snail, worm, turtle, dance* and *banana* are obvious cases in point. Iconic signs also provide a good opportunity for exercising wit in sign language, "iconic wit", something that fingerspelling, for example, rarely allows.

Although many people have commented on and studied the iconicity of sign language (e.g. Bellugi & Klima, 1976; Hoemann, 1975; Mandel, 1977), Brown's (1977) work on the early stages of acquisition of signs is most relevant for our purposes here. On the basis of two simple but ingenious experiments, Brown (1977) demonstrated persuasively that, with hearing children at least, iconic signs are easier to learn and recall than are noniconic signs. In considering iconicity in this case Brown stesses that he means "perceived iconicity" which is "time-bound", "culture-bound", "age-bound", and generally "experience-bound". Thus he uses an operational definition of perceived similarity rather than a formal, a priori objective similarity based on a precisely defined physical resemblance between a sign and its referent. In fact, some debate has taken place in the literature regarding the extent to which American Sign Language (ASL) is in fact iconic. Stokoe (1960), for example, places most of his emphasis on the symbolic rather than iconic aspects of sign language. For him, although signs may be iconic, what is crucial is that they are highly specific and symbolic to refer to object classes. Elsewhere (Stokoe et al, 1965), he estimates that 25% of signs in the dictionary of American Sign Language (ASL) are iconic while Wescott (1971) found that of the remaining 75%, about two-thirds were derivations from iconic signs. To test whether ASL is in fact iconic, Bellugi and Klima (1976) employed the most demanding test of iconicity, "transparency", i.e., the ability of a naive hearing person to guess the English equivalent of the sign from seeing the sign alone. For 81 of the 90 signs they used, not a single hearing adult could guess its spoken English equivalent. However, as Brown cogently points out, in first language instruction, whether of speech or of ASL and regardless of normal child, retarded child or a chimpanzee, never is the learner asked to be able to guess the meaning of the referent in isolation. The usual way is to provide the sign and to point to an instance of the class of objects named e.g., *egg, car, cookie, juice, etc.* There is little doubt that, when the child is reaching for a banana and sees a sign that resembles it (peeling an imaginary banana with the right hand, using the index finger of the left as the imaginary fruit), he is more likely to see the resemblance between the sign and the signified. In fact, in the Bellugi and Klima (1976) study, in addition to the transparency, another less demanding test of iconicity, "translucency", yielded much more promising results. Translucency refers to the degree to which a subject can discern a relationship between a sign and its referent after having been presented with both, such as in the case of the afore-mentioned sign for banana. Using the translucency test of iconicity, Bellugi and Klima found that at least 50% of the 90 signs could be seen as having some connections to their referents. It is of course translucency that comes closer to the usual learning context in which children are exposed to a language.

Even more important, Brown (1977) stresses that, in perusing the lists used with both Washoe (Gardner & Gardner, 1969) and Ted, the autistic boy who was exposed to ASL (Bonvillian & Nelson, 1978), he found that the vast majority of the signs acquired were in fact iconic. It is quite interesting that in Brown's own study of learning and recall of signs by 4½ year-old hearing children, the iconic signs employed tended to belong to the Basic Object Level. Brown refers to the work of Rosch, Mervis, Gray, Johnson and Boyes-Braem (1976) who discuss three levels of abstraction: the highest, which they call the Superordinate level, and which includes terms such as, *tool, musical instrument, furniture,* etc. the middle or Basic Object Level, which includes terms such as *piano, drum, chair, socks,* etc., and the Subordinate Level which includes such terms as *grand piano, Mackintosh apples, small yellow drum, kitchen chair, kneesocks,* etc. Rosch et al (1976) found that subjects could list far more characteristic attributes and movements for terms at the Basic Object Level than at either the more abstract Superordinate Level or the more concrete Subordinate Level. Of course, as indicated earlier, characteristic attributes of objects as well as characteristic movements performed in connection with them are the basic sources of iconicity in ASL and likely in other sign languages as well. In fact almost all iconic signs in Brown's own list belonged to the Basic Object Level of abstraction while the noniconic signs did not.

Clearly then, in early language acquisition children are more likely to acquire terms at the Basic Object Level which is also the more iconic and the easier to grasp. A perusal of our own sign lists on the 20 autistic children we exposed to sign language in our program over a five-year-period leaves little doubt that we in fact, never having the benefit of formally knowing the three levels of abstraction just presented, also chose to employ sign-word combinations at the Basic Object Level. Most of them were highly iconic sign-words for food items, clothing and activity items. It appears then that iconicity, defined as translucency, is a very crucial property of sign language which happens to be relevant to the introduction of a new system of communication. Parenthetically, it is worth perusing more systematically other data from existing published studies of sign language acquisition either in normal but deaf children or in autistic children, to clarify whether in fact their lists contain items at the Basic Object Level. The iconicity of sign language, furthermore, appears to relate to the motivational and motoric preferences of autistic children described in the earlier section and may account for the well-documented effectiveness of sign language with this population. Brown (1977) estimates that for autistic and retarded children about the first 400 words will be easier to acquire in sign language than in spoken language. This contention has received support in an explicitly set out attempt to investigate it. Relying on the Ontario Sign Language, a close variant of ASL, Konstantareas, Oxman and Webster (1978) chose 30 iconic and 30 noniconic signs out of a total of 126. Iconicity was rated by 41 college students and 25 first-graders. The ratings of the two groups were significantly correlated, yet in cases of discrepancy the children's ratings were used. Five autistic children served as subjects. The signs and their corresponding words were presented and paired with the referents drawn on 15 x 22 cm white cardboard cards. Training proceeded through the year along three categories: Reproductive or Imitative, Receptive and Elicited or Expressive, the scheme we have employed in all our training and research (cf. Konstantareas et al, 1979; Konstantareas & Leibovitz, 1981). Iconic signs, the result of interest here, were clearly easier to acquire than noniconic signs. This was particularly true of signs corresponding to verbs and adjectives, all of which had extensive sensori-motor elements associated with them.

In addition to iconicity, other properties of sign language are relevant to its learnability. One such property is speed of production. Bellugi and Fischer (1972), relying on fluent users of both speech and sign language, have reported that sign language requires at least twice as long as spoken language to produce, with fingerspelling taking even longer. When the fluent speaker-signers were asked to employ simultaneous communication, the mode normally employed with language-impaired children, it was speech which had to be slowed down until the signing was completed. If dysfunctional children have difficulties in processing input, as we have argued earlier, slower rate of presentation should clearly facilitate processing. In this connection, signs can also be deliberately held up longer to facilitate acquisition, a technique we have utilised extensively in our training of autistic children.

Another characteristic of sign language, compared to spoken languages is that, in so far as it relies primarily on hand movements and hands are amenable to direct manipulation, it can be easier to train an individual to use it. Compared to the tongue, lips, mouth and the even less accessible oral cavity structures on which we rely to produce speech, one can mold a child's hands into signs. Thus, by virtue of its reliance on accessible parts of the body, sign language appears to be easier to shape than spoken language. In this connection it is worth mentioning that in fact the first sounds and words which have been trained in speech programs have relied on vowel and consonant phonemes which could be visible and exaggerated by the therapists. Examples would be the labial consonants "m" and "n" and the open vowels "o" "a" "e" (Lovaas et al, 1966). Thus even spoken language training capitalises on some manual molding but certainly to a much more limited extent than it is possible with sign language.

Finally, sign language is far less redundant than spoken language (Bellugi & Fischer, 1972). It retains content words such as nouns, adjectives and verbs but does not use functors such as the copula, articles or prepositions. In ASL, for example, the 14-word sentence "It is against the law to drive on the left side of the road" is reduced to four words, "Illegal drive left side". Thus, the information is preserved in a condensed form. If sign language is an economical, low redundancy language, it could be better suited to the needs of children who have difficulty in processing complex information. Indeed, although Signed English has been the variant employed in simultaneous communication training programs, it is word order that is mainly adhered to rather than content and word number. Thus in asking Leslie, one of our autistic pupils, for example, to "Please close the door", we would sign and say "Leslie close door please" rather than "Would you like to close the door please, Leslie?" This approach we arrived at through trial and error because it fitted in smoothly and easily with the rhythm of our movements and interactions with the children as we went about our daily routines. The lack of redundancy in sign language may then be a compensatory mechanism for its slower rate of articulation. Yet a priori it appears to fit well with the information processing requirements of autistic children, particularly of the more severely delayed among them. Specific evidence is still needed however, on whether learnability of sign language is in fact linked to its lack of redundancy, its lower processing speed or both.

To summarise, sign language has some special properties which appear to meet the needs of autistic and indeed other populations of dysfunctional children. First, it is iconic, particularly for signs relevant to Basic Object Level items, i.e., those which are usually first presented in language training. Such signs have visible, real world exemplars. The pairing between the exemplar and its iconic sign provides the child with much needed assistance in early language acquisition. Second, sign language and its accompanying speech are presented at a slower rate than speech, hence they allow for longer processing time. Third, as they rely on hand movements which are accessible to others, signs are easier to teach to children with low motivation or ability at spontaneous initiation of communication. Finally, by being less redundant, sign language imposes a lower processing load on the autistic child's limited memory capacities.

That there is a considerable goodness of fit between the properties of the system and the population's needs becomes clearer when we turn to a brief summary of evidence on the use of sign, along with speech, in training autistic children to communicate.

IMPLEMENTATION OF SIMULTANEOUS COMMUNICATION

Since 1973 approximately 20 case studies and reports on group work on the use of simultaneous or total communication have appeared in the literature (e.g. Creedon, 1973; Konstantareas et al, 1979; Miller & Miller, 1973; Schaeffer et al, 1977). In some instances the explicit goal of training was speech acquisition (e.g. Creedon, 1973; Schaeffer et al, 1977) while in others it was more modest, being restricted to the attainment of communication in sign, speech or both (e.g. Bonvillian & Nelson, 1978; Fulwiler & Fouts, 1976; Konstantareas et al, 1977, 1979). Selective reviews of this work, most of which have included little explicit research on variables relevant to implementation, have already appeared (Bonvillian & Nelson, 1978; Carr, 1979; Kiernan, 1983; Konstantareas, 1981).

The most compelling result from these studies has been the considerable success of simultaneous communication in helping many, particularly the older mute or minimally vocal autistic children to communicate expressively for the first time in their lives. Receptively, of course, many of these children did have spoken language understanding. It was in the expressive domain where they encountered most of their difficulties. Thus, as it is explained in many of the reports, extensive previous exposure to speech training or computer-aided instruction, and so forth, led to no apparent change in the children's expressive abilities. By contrast, exposure to signs and words sometimes for only a few weeks (Konstantareas et al, 1977) led not only to elementary expressive labeling, but to relatively complex language (Creedon, 1973; Fulwiler & Fouts, 1976; Konstantareas et al, 1979; Schaeffer et al, 1977). In terms of CA, the youngest child has been 4 years-old (Creedon, 1973), while most children were between 5-9 years of age, and some were as old as 23 (Carr, 1979). Modes of training and testing ranged from the strict within-subject design (Carr, 1979) to quasi-factorial designs (Konstantareas et al, 1977, 1979) to psycholinguistic case studies (Bonvillian & Nelson, 1976; Fulwiler & Fouts, 1976). This diversity of subject characteristics and methodologies has the advantage of allowing us to draw inferences as to the applicability of the techniques to a large range of language-impaired children. On the negative side, as already stated, very little systematic research has been carried out on variables crucial to the implementation of this approach. Space limitations preclude a fair coverage of what has appeared in the literature thus far. Suffice it to discuss briefly three themes which have attracted some attention in the available reviews.

First, let us consider the issue of whether simultaneous communication can have a positive impact on the autistic child's many other presenting difficulties. Available evidence has been generally in favor of the view that simultaneous communication has a positive influence. As the children become more adept at communication, they are easier to manage, appear more aware of other people in their environment and tend to be less preoccupied with stereotypical and self-stimulatory behaviours. Practically all available reports converge on this point. However, to the extent that in addition to the communication training, other intervention strategies are also employed, e.g. gross and fine motor skills development, peer interaction exercises, control of self-stimulatory behaviours, etc., one cannot attribute gains exclusively to the simultaneous communication training (see also Carr, 1979). Ethical and treatment considerations make a systematic evaluation of the effect of the communication training alone rather problematic. Indeed the issue itself may be a pseudo issue in that we need not judge generalisation of the training to other areas of functioning as being the criterion for success of simultaneous communication. We may have to be satisfied with generalisation across different communication categories only. Any generalisation to other behaviours may then be an additional bonus.

A second question involves the possible negative impact of simultaneous communication on the nonverbal children's chances to speak. In an early study, Oxman, Konstantareas and Leibovitz (1979) provided a negative answer to this question. Indeed the exact opposite appears to be true. Many autistic children come to speak after exposure to simultaneous communication (Creedon, 1973; Konstantareas, 1984; Konstantareas et al, 1979; Miller & Miller, 1973). Furthermore, more recently an explicit comparison of oral and total communication for teaching expressive labels to three echolalic autistic children showed the total or simultaneous communication approach to be superior to the oral approach (Barrera & Sulzer-Azaroff, 1983). This result is consistent with Brown's (1977) argument, discussed earlier, as to the relative advantage of sign language in early communication acquisition, regardless of the child's ability to speak. It also runs counter to arguments that autistic children who have the ability at vocal imitation are more responsive to spoken language input (Carr, 1979).

Finally, and related to the previous question, is the issue of who is the best candidate for exposure to simultaneous communication training. As it was indicated earlier, very low functioning children may not be good candidates for exposure to formal sign language and speech training, because of their low overall cognitive ability. In their case prelinguistic turn-taking, shared attention training and simple gesturing may be the first suitable intervention strategy. However, for children of higher cognitive functioning but who present with language difficulties, simultaneous communication may be the best avenue for early communication training. Informed with a good understanding of pragmatic issues, such training could then proceed to exclusive spoken language for those children who begin to speak (cf. Schaeffer et al, 1977) or it can continue with simultaneous communication, for those who cannot. Available evidence clarly points to this conclusion, although we certainly need additional research before we can be reassured that it is valid.

CONCLUSION

The main argument presented in this review has been that traditional views as to what constitutes an optimal communication strategy with autistic and other severely dysfunctional children need to be re-evaluated on an ongoing basis. Information from as diverse areas as psycholinguistics, developmental psychology, information processing and memory, neuro-psychology, kinetics and sign language research, among others, should be included in designing therapeutic programs for these children. In addition, of course, inferences drawn from research in these areas should be examined in the context of implementation studies. Additional research is also needed on most of the issues addressed in this review. For instance, we need to know more as to which of the available techniques is best suited to children of different cognitive, linguistic and social deficits. We need more information on optimal modes of training, regardless of training modality. Further, we require research on the longitudinal or process aspects of training and certainly we need follow-up research. At present there is no systematic long-term follow-up of simultaneous communication programs, assessing the effect of the intervention with children at different levels of linguistic or cognitive readiness. Finally, we require additional work on the complexity of linguistic ability attainable through the use of either the oral or the simultaneous communication approach. Is it correct to assume, for example, that sign language is more likely than speech training to result in spontaneity as Schaeffer (1978) has argued? Although his argument has an intuitive appeal it has to be put to a systematic test. Despite these and other unresolved issues in this challenging multidisciplinary area, we could take some pride in the progress that has been achieved to date. We have certainly moved a long way from the simple S-R paradigm where we began twenty years ago.

ACKNOWLEDGEMENTS

The research reported in this review was supported in part under National Health Development Project No. 606-1240-44.

Address all correspondence to Dr. Mary Konstantareas, Child and Family Studies Centre, Clarke Institute of Psychiatry, 250 College Street, Toronto, Ontario, Canada, M5T 1R8.

I would like to acknowledge with gratitude the contribution of Drs. Chris D. Webster and Joel Oxman, both excellent colleagues and warm and caring human beings. A word of thanks to Mrs. A. Blackman and Mrs. S. Leibovitz-Bojm for their competent research support and to Ms. Sheila McCormick for her patient and cheerful typing. My special appreciation to the autistic children and their families without whose input this work would not have been carried out.

References

Barrera, R.D. & Sulzer-Azaroff, B. (1983). An alternative treatment comparison of oral and total communication training programs with echolalic autistic children. *Journal of Applied Behavior Analysis, 16,* 379-394.

Bartak, L. & Rutter, M. (1976). Differences between mentally retarded and normally intelligent autistic children. *Journal of Autism and Childhood Schizophrenia, 6,* 109-120.

Bartak, L., Rutter, M. & Cox, A. (1975). A comparative study of infantile autism and specific developmental receptive language disorder: I. The children. *British Journal of Psychiatry, 126,* 127-145.

Bellugi, U. & Fischer, S. (1972). A comparison of sign language and spoken language. *Cognition, 1,* 173-200.

Bellugi, U. & Klima, E.S. (1976). Two faces of sign: Iconic and abstract. *Annals of the New York Academy of Sciences, 280,* 514-538.

Blackstock, E.G. (1978). Cerebral asymmetry and the development of early infantile autism. *Journal of Autism and Childhood Schizophrenia, 8,* 339-353.

Bliss, C. (1965). *Semantography.* Sydney, Australia: Semantography Publications.

Bonvillian, J.D. & Nelson, K.E. (1978). Development of sign language in autistic children and other language-handicapped individuals. In P. Siple (Ed.), *Understanding language through sign language research.* New York: Academic Press.

Bonvillian, J.D. & Nelson, K.E. (1976). Sign language acquisition in a mute autistic boy. *Journal of Speech and Hearing Disorders, 41,* 339-347.

Brown, R.W. (1977, May). *Why are signed languages easier to learn than Spoken languages?* Keynote address National Symposium on Sign Language Research and Teaching, Chicago.

Carr, E.G. (1979). Teaching autistic children to use sign language: Some research issues. *Journal of Autism and Developmental Disorders, 9,* 345-359.

Carter, A.L. (1978). From sensorimotor vocalization to words: A case study of the evolution of attention-directing communication in the first year. In A. Lock (Ed.), *Action, gesture and symbol: The emergence of language.* London: Academic Press.

Clark, R.A. (1978). The transition from action to gesture. In A. Lock (Ed.), *Action, gesture and symbol: The emergence of language.* London: Academic Press.

Condon, W.S. (1975). Multiple response to sound in dysfunctional children. *Journal of Autism and Childhood Schizophrenia, 5,* 37-56.

Condon, W.S. (1978, May). Asynchrony and communicational disorders. Paper presented at the Research Symposium of the Canadian Society for Autistic Children, Vancouver.

Condon, W.S. & Sander, L.W. (1974). Neonate movement is synchronized with adult speed: Interactional participation and language acquisition. *Science, 183,* 99-101.

Creedon, M.P. (1973, March). *Language development in nonverbal autistic children using a simultaneous communication system.* Paper presented at the meeting of the Society for Research in Child Development, Philadelphia.

DeMyer, M.K. (1976). The nature of the neuropsychological disability in autistic children. In E. Schopler and R. Reichler (Eds.), *Psychopathology and child development.* New York: Plenum Press.

DeMyer, M.K., Hingtgen, J.K. & Jackson, R.K. (1981). Infantile autism reviewed: A decade of research. *Schizophrenia Bulletin, 7,* 388-451.

Dunn, L.M. (1965). *Peabody Picture Vocabulary Test.* Circle Pines, Minnesota: American Guidance Service, Inc.

Eccles, J. (1975, May). *Language development and neurological theory.* Invited Address, Brock University, Conference on Language Canada, St. Catharines, Ont.

Fay, W.H. & Schuler, A.L. (1980). *Emerging language in autistic children.* Baltimore: University Park Press.

Fulwiler, R.L. & Fouts, R.S. (1976). Acquisition of American Sign Language by a non-communicating autistic child. *Journal of Autism and Childhood Schizophrenia, 6,* 43-51.

Gardner, R.A. & Gardner, B.T. (1969). Teaching sign language to a chimpanzee. *Science, 165,* 664-672.

Gardner, R.A. & Gardner, B.T. (1975). Early signs of language in child and chimpanzee. *Science, 187,* 752-753.

Goetz, L., Schuler, A. & Sailor, W. (1979). Teaching functional speech to the severely handicapped: Current issues. *Journal of Autism and Developmental Disorders, 9,* 325-343.

Hayes, C. (1951). *The ape in our house.* New York: Harper.

Hermelin, B. (1976). Coding and the sense modalities. In L. Wing (Ed.), *Early childhood autism* (2nd ed.). Oxford: Pergamon Press.

Hermelin, B. & O'Connor, N. (1970). *Psychological experiments with autistic children.* Oxford: Pergamon Press.

Hewes, G.H. (1973). Primate communication and the gestural origin of language. *Current Anthropology, 14,* 5-24.

Hingtgen, J. & Churchill, D. (1969). Identification of perceptual limitations in mute autistic children. *Archives of General Psychiatry, 21,* 68-71.

Hoemann, H.W. (1975). The transparency of meaning of sign language gestures. *Sign Language Studies, 6-9,* 151-168.

Ingram, D. (1978). Sensori-motor intelligence and language development. In A. Lock (Ed.), *Action, gesture and symbol: The emergence of language.* London: Academic Press.

Kanner, L. (1943). Autistic disturbances of affective contact. *Nervous Child, 2,* 217-250.

Kellogg, W.N. (1968). Communication and language in the home-raised chimpanzee. *Science, 162,* 423-427.

Kiernan, C. (1983). The use of nonvocal communication techniques with autistic individuals. *Journal of Child Psychology and Psychiatry, 24,* 339-375.

Konstantareas, M.M. (1981). Developing new avenues of communication. In M.M. Konstantareas, E.G. Blackstock and C.D. Webster (Eds.), *Autism: A primer.* Montreal: The Quebec Society for Autistic Children.

Konstantareas, M.M. (1982). Variability of linguistic impairment in autism: Its relevance to intervention. *B.C. Journal of Special Education, 6,* 231-247.

Konstantareas, M.M. (1984). Sign language as a communication prosthesis with language-impaired children. *Journal of Autism and Developmental Disorders, 14,* 9-25.

Konstantareas, M.M. (in press). Autistic children exposed to simultaneous communication training: A follow-up. *Journal of Autism and Developmental Disorders.*

Konstantareas, M.M. & Homatidis, S. (1985). *Incidence of ear infections in autistic and normal children.* Manuscript submitted for publication.

Konstantareas, M.M. & Leibovitz, S.F. (1981). Early communication acquisition by autistic children: Signing and mouthing versus signing and speaking. *Sign Language Studies, 31,* 135-154.

Konstantareas, M.M., Oxman, J. & Webster, C.D. (1977). Simultaneous communication with autistic and other severely dysfunctional nonverbal children. *Journal of Communication Disorders, 10,* 267-282.

Konstantareas, M.M., Oxman, J. & Webster, C.D. (1978). Iconicity: Effects on the acquisition of sign language by autistic and other severely dysfunctional children. In P. Siple (Ed.), *Understanding language through sign language research.* New York: Academic Press.

Konstantareas, M.M., Webster, C.D. & Oxman, J. (1979). Manual language acquisition and its influence on other areas of functioning in four autistic and autistic-like children. *Journal of Child Psychology and Psychiatry, 20,* 337-350.

Leiter, R. (1969). *The Leiter International Performance Scale.* Chicago: Stoelting Company.

Lock, A. (Ed.) (1978). *Action, gesture and symbol: The emergence of language.* London: Academic Press.

Lovaas, O.I., Berberich, J.P., Perloff, B.F. & Schaeffer, B. (1966). Acquisition of imitative speech by schizophrenic children. *Science, 151,* 705-707.

Lovaas, O.I., Koegel, R., Simmons, J.Q. & Long, J.S. (1973). Some generalization and follow-up measures on autistic children in behavior therapy. *Journal of Applied Behavior Analysis, 6,* 131-166.

Lovaas, O.I. & Schreibman, L. (1971). Stimulus overselectivity of autistic children in a two stimulus situation. *Behaviour Research and Therapy, 9,* 305-310.

Mack, J.E., Webster, C.D. & Gokcen, I. (1980). Where are they now and how are they faring: Follow-up of 51 severely handicapped speech-deficient children four years after an operant-based program. In C.D. Webster, M.M. Konstantareas, J. Oxman and J.E. Mack (Eds.), *Autism: New directions in research and education.* New York: Pergamon Press.

Mandel, M.A. (1977, June). *Iconicity of signs and their learnability by non-signers.* Paper presented at the National Symposium on Sign Language Research and Teaching. Chicago.

Miller, A. & Miller, E.E. (1973). Cognitive-developmental training with elevated boards and sign language. *Journal of Autism and Childhood Schizophrenia, 3,* 65-85.

Oxman, J. & Konstantareas, M.M. (1981). On the nature and variability of linguistic impairment in autism. *Clinical Psychology Review, 1,* 337-352.

Oxman, J., Webster, C.D. & Konstantareas, M.M. (1978). Condon's multiple-response phenomenon in severely dysfunctional children: An attempt at replication. *Journal of Autism and Childhood Schizophrenia, 8*, 395-402.

Oxman, J., Konstantareas, M.M. & Leibovitz, S.F. (1979). Simultaneous communication training and vocal responding in nonverbal autistic and autistic-like children. *International Journal of Rehabilitation Research, 2,* 394-396.

Piaget, J. (1970). The developmental psychology of Jean Piaget. In P. Mussen (Ed.), *Carmichael's manual of child psychology (Vol. 1).* Toronto: John Wiley & Sons.

Premack, D. (1971). Language in chimpanzees. *Science, 172,* 808-822.

Prior, M.R. (1977). Psycholinguistic disabilities of autistic and retarded children. *Journal of Mental Deficiency Research, 21,* 37-45.

Prior, M.R. (1979). Cognitive abilities and disabilities in infantile autism: A review. *Journal of Abnormal Child Psychology, 7,* 357-380.

Prior, M.P. & Bradshaw, J.L. (1979). Hemisphere functioning in autistic children. *Cortex, 15,* 73-81.
Reynell, J.K. (1977). *Manual for the Reynell Developmental Language Scales* (Revised). England: The NFER-Nelson Publishing Company.
Rosch, E., Mervis, C.B., Gray, W., Johnson, D. & Boyes-Braem, P. (1976). Basic objects in natural categories. *Cognitive Psychology, 8,* 382-439.
Schaeffer, B. (1978). Teaching spontaneous sign language to nonverbal children: Theory and method. *Sign Language Studies, 21,* 317-352.
Schaeffer, B., Kollinzas, G., Musil, A. & McDowell, P. (1977). Spontaneous verbal language for autistic children through signed speech. *Sign Language Studies, 17,* 287-328.
Schell, R.E., Stark, J. & Giddan, J. (1967). Development of language behavior in an autistic child. *Journal of Speech and Hearing Disorders, 32,* 51-64.
Stokoe, W.C. (1960). Sign language structure: An outline of the visual communication systems of the American deaf. In *Studies in linguistics:* Occasional papers: No. 8. Buffalo, N.Y.: University of Buffalo Press.
Stokoe, W.C., Casterline, D. & Croneberg, C. (1965). *A dictionary of American Sign Language: On linguistic principles.* Washington, D.C.: Gallaudet College Press.
Tanguay, P. (1975). Clinical and electrophysiological research. In E. Ritvo (Ed.), *Autism, diagnosis, current research and management.* New York: Spectrum.
Tubbs, V.K. (1966). Types of linguistic disability in psychotic children. *Journal of Mental Deficiency Research, 10,* 230-240.
Webster, C.D., Konstantareas, M.M., Oxman, J. & Mack, J. (Eds.) (1980). *Autism: New directions in research and education.* New York: Pergamon Press.
Wescott, R. (1971). Linguistic iconism. *Language, 47,* 416-428.

SECTION 3

THE DEVELOPMENT OF FINE MOTOR SKILLS

THE FORMATION OF THE FINGER GRIP DURING PREHENSION A CORTICALLY-MEDIATED VISUO-MOTOR PATTERN

M. Jeannerod

1. INTRODUCTION

Formation of the finger grip during the action of grasping a visual object involves two main functional requirements, the fulfilment of which will determine the quality of the grasp. First, the grip must be adapted to the size, shape and use of the object to be grasped. Second, the relative timing of the finger movements must be coordinated with that of the other component of prehension by which the hand is transported at the spatial location of the object. Thus, a study of grip formation during prehension has to take into account, not only the motor pattern in itself as it is obtained by discrete finger posturing, but also its change over time until prehension is actually achieved. Simple observation of prehension movements shows that finger posturing anticipates the real grasp and occurs during transportation of the hand. This hand "shaping" (of which grip formation is the most representative aspect) is therefore related to purely visuomotor mechanisms, that is, mechanisms that are independent from manipulation itself. Manipulation, which occurs after the object has been grasped, relates to coordination between finger movements and tactile and kinesthetic inputs: this aspect will not be considered in the present paper. Visually guided prehension movements have received relatively little attention, partly because the large number of degrees of freedom involved in such movements makes their experimental approach difficult. Until recently only global descriptions have been given, based on presence or absence of grip formation, or on time to perform a grasping task.

The role of neural structures in grip formation, and particularly the role of cerebral cortex, has been investigated in monkeys following experimental lesions and in man under pathological conditions. One of the most generally accepted facts from these studies is the critical importance of the corticospinal tract in the control of discrete finger movements. This notion was first introduced by Tower (1940) in monkeys and later confirmed by Lawrence and Kuypers (1968) and Woolsey et al (1972), who showed that section of the pyramidal tract produces a long-lasting, if not permanent, inability to perform independent finger movements, as in grasping small pieces of food. The degree of recovery from this deficit has been quantified by Chapman and Wiesendanger (1982) in monkeys following unilateral section of the pyramidal tract at the pontine level. The animals' performance was scored in a Kluver board task, i.e., the number of pellets of food extracted from holes of different sizes and the time needed for clearing the board, were measured for each hand. The strategy utilised by the animals for grasping the pellets was found to be changed after pyramidotomy when the hand contralateral to the lesion was tested. Animals first used all four fingers for extracting the food, a strategy that was efficient only for the larger holes. At a later stage (30 to 40 days after surgery), monkeys regained the ability to pry out the pellets from the smaller holes by using either the thumb or the index finger. Once extracted, the pellets could be grasped between the opposed thumb and index finger, but this precision grip remained weak and clumsy and the food was eventually dropped before reaching the mouth. Partial recovery of grip formation in the Chapman and Wiesendanger experiment might have been explained by incompleteness of the pyramidal tract lesions (Chapman & Wiesendanger, 1982). In fact, other experiments have shown that monkeys with a complete unilateral ablation of cortical area 4 performed during infancy never acquired a precision grip when tested later in adulthood (Lawrence & Hopkins, 1972; Passingham et al, 1978). Precision grip in monkeys normally develops around the 8th postnatal month, i.e., by the time when maturation of the corticospinal tract is completed as judged from the formation of corticomotoneuronal synapses (Kuypers, 1962) and the level of excitability of motoneurons by motor cortex stimulation (Felix & Wiesendanger, 1971). Effects of lesions on finger movements in monkeys confirm evidence accumulated in anatomical and physiological experiments for the predominant, if not exclusive, cortical involvement in the control of finger muscles (e.g., Philips & Porter, 1977; For a recent confirmation of these findings, see Muir, 1985)

It has been found possible to dissociate, in the action of grasping, between mechanisms responsible for grip formation and those that account for carrying the hand at the object location. Observations in monkeys with complete split-brain have shown that these animals are able to intercept very efficiently a moving object with either arm when vision is restricted to one eye (and therefore, to one hemisphere). By contrast, they can orient and shape their fingers according to the object size only with the hand on the side opposite to the stimulated eye (and hemisphere). This result (Trevarthen, 1965) indicates that the visuomotor apparatus for reaching (presumably located at the brainstem level) remains undivided by the split, although the visuomotor apparatus controlling prehension (presumably located at the hemispheric level) governs each hand independently. The dichtomoty between levels of visuomotor control for proximal and distal components of prehension has been confirmed by Brinkman and Kuypers (1973), also in experiments with split-brain monkeys. In these experiments, animals were tested monocularly with an improved version of the Kluver board, where information necessary for extraction of food pellets was restricted to visual cues only. Extraction of the pellets, which required formation of a finger grip, was possible only with the hand contralateral to the open eye. The other hand could reach to the board, explore it tactually, but not shape according to the visual aspect of the food target. In another series of experiments also using split-brain monkeys, Haaxma and Kuypers (1975) showed that proper control of the hand contralateral to the open eye became inefficient if a deep parieto-occipital leucotomy was made within the corresponding hemisphere. The authors had used a more refined food target such that extraction of the food pellets required not only precision grip formation but also correct orientation of the plane of the thumb and index fingers. Haaxma and Kuypers interpreted their results as reflecting intra-hemispheric disconnection between occipital cortex and motor centres in the frontal lobe. Although this interpretation may be basically correct, one has to consider the fact that the parieto-occipital leucotomy performed in these experiments in fact involved posterior parietal cortical areas that have been shown to be critical for visuomotor control (e.g. Hyvärinen & Poranen, 1974). Monkeys with posterior parietal lesions (Hartje & Ettlinger, 1973; Hyvärinen, 1982), or even with lesions restricted to area 7 (Faugier-Grimaud et al, 1978), make large errors in reaching for food with their arm contralateral to th lesion. In addition, these lesioned animals are unable to correctly shape their fingers during prehension. Instead, they tend to approach the object with fully extended fingers (Faugier-Grimaud et al, 1978).

In man, arguments similar to those developed from monkey experiments, can be used for relating the digital component of prehesion to cortical function. Behavioural studies of the development of prehension in babies by Halverson (1931) have shown that finger posturing is lacking during reaching at visual objects until the age of approximately 20 weeks. Inaccurate posturing is then observed but it is not until the age of 36 to 52 weeks that precision grip can be formed. More recent work, however, has shown that infants were able to make use of visual information for crude finger posturing earlier than previously suspected. According to Bruner and Koslowski, 1972), infants 10 to 22 weeks of age may show coarsely adapted hand movements when they are presented with small graspable visual objects within reach. The same is not observed for objects of a larger size, exceeding the grasping capability of the hand. Von Hofsten (1979) has shown that even younger infants may intercept the trajectory of moving objects and come in contact with them. However, these reaching movements are effected with a widely open hand without evidence for grip formation. It is only when the object has been touched that crude prehensile movements of the fingers can be observed. Fine finger movements resembling grip formation have in fact been observed as early as the first postnatal days. These movements, however, are very slow, and do not seem to be related to the presence of a visual object (Bower et al, 1970; Trevarthen, 1982). They might in fact correspond to "reflex" activation of the hand motor system, rather than to visuomotor activation.

It is tempting to relate the developmental time course of finger movements in children to the maturation of motor pathways. It is known that pyramidal fibers continue to increase in diameter up to somatic maturity. In addition, it has been shown that the pyramidal tract myelinates relatively late in man: myelination increases up to the 8th postnatal month, and seems to be complete around the age of one year (Yakovev & Lecours, 1967) or even 2 years (Langworthy, 1933). These results indicate that consistent formation of a precision grip during prehension of visual objects would be contemporary with the existence of a functional corticospinal tract, although more data are still needed for establishing a precise anatomo-functional correlation.

The effects of brain lesions on finger grip formation in man have been less systematically investigated. The available clinical descriptions, however, provide evidence for dependence of discrete finger movements on cortical mechanisms. Patients with hemiplegia following stroke, for instance, may finally recover the shoulder-elbow synergy for transporting the hand near an object, provided the shoulder is passively supported against gravity (see Lough et al, 1984). Finger movements, however, seem to remain indefinitely clumsy: during prehension, they do not shape in anticipation to the grasp, which is achieved with the palmar surface of the whole hand instead of the fingertips.

Similarly, subjects with surgical section of the corpus callosum or lesions interrupting callosal transfer, show typical impairments in finger movements when they are properly examined. Gazzaniga et al (1967), have examined finger movements in split-brain patients who were requested to reproduce hand and finger postures presented as outlines flashed on one side of the visual field, so that only one hemisphere was stimulated at each presentation. Patients could easily reproduce finger postures with their hand contralateral to the stimulated hemisphere, although their hand ipsilateral to the stimulated hemisphere usually failed except for the simplest postures. This result was interpreted by Gazzaniga et al (1967) as a demonstration of the fact that ipsilateral motor control is at its worst in tasks in which the hemisphere is required to direct individual movements of the fingers. Subsequent work in monkeys by Brinkman and Kuypers (1973) (see above) has amply confirmed the validity of this interpretation.

Finally, lesions of the posterior parietal areas also produce, among other deficits, a decorrelation of finger movements from visual input. According to Tzavaras and Masure (1975) and Perenin and Vighetto (1983), subjects with such lesions misshape their hand when they have to achieve specific visuomotor tasks (e.g. a variant of the Haaxma and Kuypers task) requiring accura grip formation and orientation (see below). The aim of the present paper was to reinvestigate the problem of the neurological substrate involved in grip formation during prehension of visual objects in man. The pattern of grip will be first described in normal subjects with the help of a quantifiable technique. Then, the same technique will be applied to the description of prehension in a group of patients selected for the locus of their lesions. The effects of these lesions on grip formation will be interpreted under the light of a hypothesis involving the duality of mechanisms controlling prehension movements.

2. METHODS

This study is based on the study of films of prehension movements directed at three-dimensional graspable objects. The degree of visual feedback from the moving hand during prehension was controlled by way of an apparatus consisting of a box resting on a table, and divided horizontally into two equal compartments by a smireflecting mirror (Fig. 1). Subjects were seated in front of the box with their forehead resting on the front panel. They looked through a window within the upper compartment and placed their hand under study in the lower compartment. Target objects were placed in the lower compartment along the subject's sagittal axis. These were small solid objects, such as a sphere, a cube, or a vertical rod. Distance from the body could be varied (e.g., 25, 32, or 40 cm). Two experimental situations were used. In the control situation (Visual feedback condition), subjects could see the lower compartment through the mirror and therefore, they could see both the target object and their moving hand. In the other situation (No visual feedback condition), vision of the hand was prevented by inserting a mask below the mirror, so that the lower compartment was no longer visible. In the latter situation, target objects had to be displayed from the top of the upper compartment (Fig. 1). Since the mirror was placed half-way between the target display and the table, subjects saw in the mirror a virtual image of the objects, projecting at the table level. Another object identical to that seen in the mirror was placed directly on the table in exact coincidence with the virtual image. Thus, subjects reached for the virtual object below the mirror without seeing their hand, and met the second, real, object at the expected location. During the experiment, subjects had to place their hand under study on a starting block near the body axis, with the forearm in the prone position and the fingers semiflexed. They were required to perform rapid and accurate movements, to grasp the target-object as precisely as possible, and to carry it near the starting block. No formal time

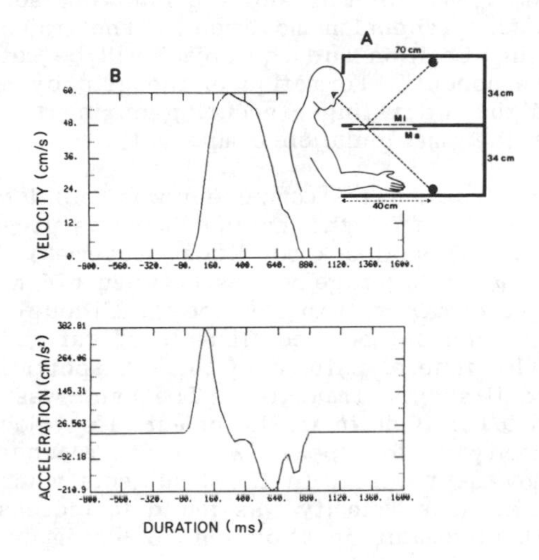

Fig. 1. A) Apparatus for measuring prehension movements. Mi: two-way mirror. Ma: Mask. Condition represented here is No-visual-feedback condition (From Jeannerod, 1984). B) velocity and acceleration profiles of arm during a single prehension movement. Target placed at 32cm from body. No-visual feed-back condition. Total movement duration: 800ms. Time to velocity peak: 280ms. Onset of reacceleration: 600ms. Curves have been smoothed by using a least square polynomial approximation. Frequency cut-off: 5Hz.

constraint was given. At the beginning of each trial a new object was displayed, while the subjects kept their eyes closed. At an acoustic signal they opened their eyes and had to wait 2 to 5 s until a small light was turned on in front of them, before performing the reaching movement.

The radial aspect of the subject's hand was filmed with a cine-camera running at 50 frames per s. Data were processed by projecting frame by frame the image of the movement on a screen with a 1 to 1 magnification. Duration of the movement was measured as the number of frames between the first detectable arm displacement, and contact with the target object. Position of anatomical details on the wrist was plotted over successive frames. Distance between successive positions gave a measure of the instantaneous tangential velocity of the arm trajectory. From the same frames, the relative positions of the tip of the index finger and the tip of the thumb were also plotted. This allowed measuring the size of the finger grip and its change over time. Due to the resting posture of the hand and the shape of the objects, no rotation of the wrist occured during the movement.

3. RESULTS.

A. Prehension movements in normal adult subjects

This desciption is partly drawn from a study of prehension in 7 young adults (Jeannerod, 1984). In this and the following sections, two components will be described for prehension movements. The trajectory of the arm between the starting position and the object will be referred to as the "transportation component". Formation of the grip by combined movements of the thumb and the index finger occuring during the arm movement will be referred to as the "manipulation component".

Transportation component. This component was found to be little affected by whether visual feedback from the moving limb was present or not (Jeannerod, 1984). In the No visual feedback condition, movement duration was found to vary across subjects (average values between 674 ms and 1013 ms for a target located at 40 cm away from the body), although it remained relatively constant for each given subject (coefficients of variation were within 10% in most subjects). The general pattern of the transportation component was that of a reverted U-shaped trajectory. The hand was first raised from the support and then lowered down to the object. Its velocity profile involved a fast rise of velocity up to a peak, which was reached at an average value of 308 ms from movement onset. In the 3 subjects where this was tested, the amplitude of the peak velocity was found to increase linearly with target distance, although movement duration tended to remain constant.

Deceleration of the arm trajectory was marked by a discontinuity where tangential velocity tended to become constant or even to reincrease before the movement was stopped (Fig. 1, upper diagram). Although the peak on the acceleration graph, corresponding to this discontinuity (Fig. 1, lower diagram) rarely reached positive values of acceleration, it was nevertheless likely to represent reacceleration of the arm partly damped by inertia of the limb. The time of occurence of the discontinuity (measured at the lowest point on the acceleration graph) consistently corresponded to 70% to 80% of total movement duration. One of the possible interpretations for reacceleration of the arm movement at the vicinity of the target could be a visual correction for undershooting. This interpretation does not seem likely, however, because reaccelerations were still observed in movements executed in the absence of visual feedback. This result (Jeannerod, 1984) suggests that visual feedback from the moving limb, when present, can be incorporated within the pre-existing structure of the movement, without being constrained to act at a particular time of its trajectory.

Manipulation component. Grip formation took place during transportation of the hand at the object location. The resting position imposed on the subject's hand before performing the movements implied semiflexion of the fingers. As the arm was displaced, the fingers began to stretch and the grip size increased rapidly up to a maximum. At this time, the fingers were flexed again and the grip size was reduced in order to match the size of the object. The size of the maximum grip aperture was proportional to the anticipated size of the object. An example of this behaviour is given in Figure 2, where grip size is compared in 2 subjects (Subjects 1 and 2 of Jeannerod, 1984) during movements aiming objects of different sizes (see also Table 1). This biphasic pattern of grip formation (extension followed by flexion of the fingers, see Jeannerod, 1981) was confirmed by Wing and Fraser (1983). According to the latter authors, only the index finger would contribute in grip formation, although the position of the thumb would remain invariant throughout the movement. Complete and accurate grip formation was observed in the absence of visual feedback from the hand. No significant difference in the values of maximum grip size and final grip size before contact with the object were found between the Visual feedback and the No visual feed-

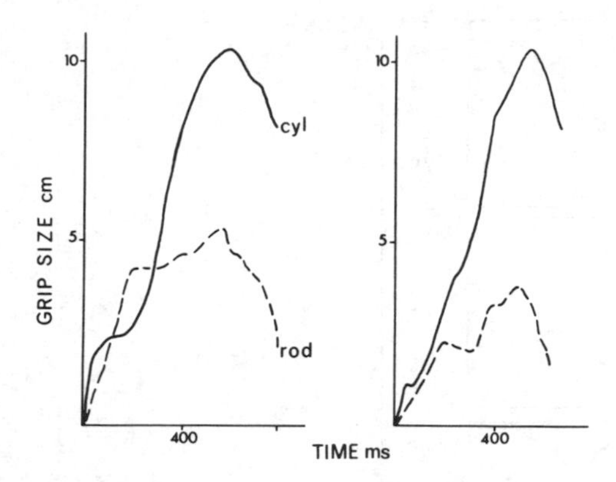

Fig. 2. Change in grip size (cm over time, ms) in 2 different subjects reaching either for a small object (a 2mm dia., 10cm long Rod) or a large object (a 55cm dia., 10cm long Cylinder). Dashed lines correspond to movements aiming at the Rod. Solid line, at the Cylinder (From Jeannerod, 1981).

Table 1. Mean value (in mm) of maximum and final grip size (before contact) as a function of object size and visual feedback condition, in two subjects. Numbers in parenthesis are SDs.

	ROD		CYLINDER	
	Visual feedback	No Visual feedback	Visual feedback	No Visual feedback
Maximum grip size	31.9 (4.7)	34.7 (7.7)	74.6 (3.0)	80.2 (4.3)
Final grip size	13.3 (1.9)	12.6 (2.9)	58.1 (2.4)	57.7 (6.3)

back conditions (Table 1). Although the transportation and the manipulation components appeared to be relatively independent from each other, they shared a common time course. This point, which is essential for understanding the coordination of the two components, can be exemplified by the fact that, for each prehension movement, the time occurrences of the re-acceleration of the arm and the maximum grip size were strongly correlated to each other (Jeannerod, 1984). Figure 3 demonstrates this relation in one subject. This figure shows the average profiles of acceleration of the arm, and the averaged profiles of grip size corresponding to the same movements as a function of time (Fig. 3, left), and a regression analysis of the arm re-accelerations with respect to maximum grip sizes (Fig. 3, right).

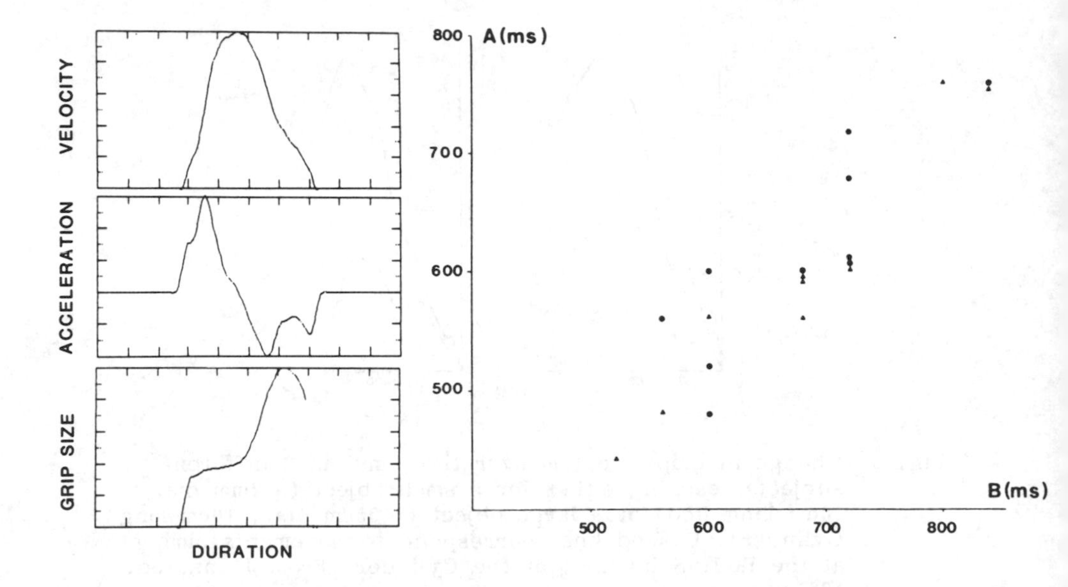

Fig. 3. Time relation between the two components of prehension. Left: averaged velocity and acceleration profiles of 20 transportation components in one subject, and of the grip size of the 20 corresponding maniuplation components. No-visual-feedback condition.
Right: plot of the time occurence of maximum grip size (B, ms) versus onset of reacceleration of transportation component (A, ms) for the same movements. Data from subject 7 of Jeannerod (1984).

B. Prehension movements in children with infant hemiplegia

Infant hemiplegia is a disease of unknown origin associated with malformation and/or lack of maturation at the cortical level within one hemisphere. It consists in spastic palsy of the limbs on one side, sometimes accompanied by mild mental retardation. Interestingly, the hemiplegia is usually not noticed until the age of about 40 weeks, i.e., around the time where the hand becomes normally engaged in prehensile activities. At this early stage, the only noticeable deficit is disuse of the affected hand in manipulation normally requiring both hands. Spasticity may appear at a later stage (see Goutieres et al, 1972 for review). I have examined finger movements during prehension in two such patients aged 23 months (Patient 1, Mag) and 5 years (Patient 2, Gis), respectively. In the younger patient, the affected (right) hand remained unused as long as the normal hand was not attached. It was only then that the right hand could be teased, though with difficulty, to grasp objects. Figure 4, redrawn from film shows comparative records of grasping of a prong from a pegboard with either hand, in the Visual feedback condition. The normal hand (Fig. 4a) appeared to shape uncompletely with respect to the object, though the finger extension-flexion pattern was nonetheless clearly present. In addition, contact of the hand with the object triggered an immediate posturing of the fingers which ensured accurate grasping. By contrast, the affected hand remained exaggerately stretched throughtout the duration of the movement, without any evidence for grip formation (Fig. 4b). Some posturing of the fingers occured after contact with the object, resulting in a very uncorrect and clumsy grasp.

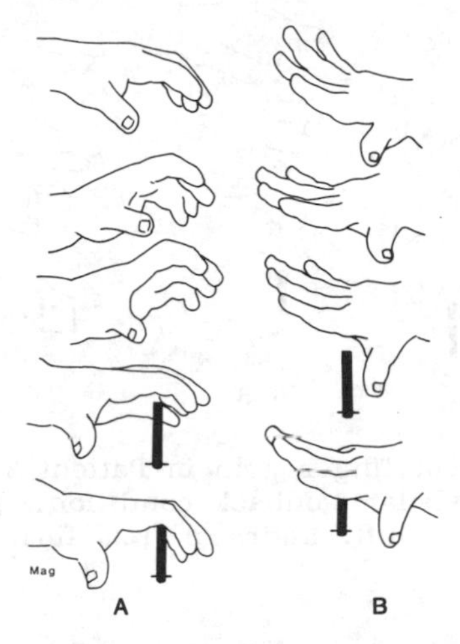

Fig. 4. Pattern of finger grip in Patient 1 (Mag), during reaching in the visual-feedback condition. A: normal hand. B: affected hand. Redrawn from film.

In the other child (Patient 2), the affected hand could be used spontaneously, partly as a result of training and rehabilitation procedures continued for several years. Better cooperation of this patient allowed more complete analysis of her prehension movements. With her normal hand, she performed correct and accurate grips with a fully developed, adult-like pattern. This point is illustrated by the example given in Figure 5a, and by the graphical analysis of another movement represented in Figure 6a. Prehension with the affected hand differed from that of the normal hand only for what concerned the pattern of grip formation. In the 3 examples shown in Figure 5b, c, and d, finger posturing appears abnormal. The index finger is exaggerately extended and flexes incompletely, if at all, before contact with the object. In the 2 other examples analysed graphically in Figure 6b and c, no finger grip formation can be detected, although the velocity profiles corresponding to the transportation components appear relatively similar to those of the normal hand (Fig. 6a). The lack, or the abnormal character of grip formation with the affected hand resulted in awkward and clumsy grasps of the objects which were occasionally dropped from the hand.

Lesions of the motor part of cerebral cortex, which seem to represent the major brain damage in infant hemiplegia affects the output stage of the grip formation mechanism. Although the effects of these lesions clearly confirm cortical dependence of finger movements, they do not provide information as to visuomotor control mechanisms that contribute to hand shaping. These mechanisms are studied in the following two sections.

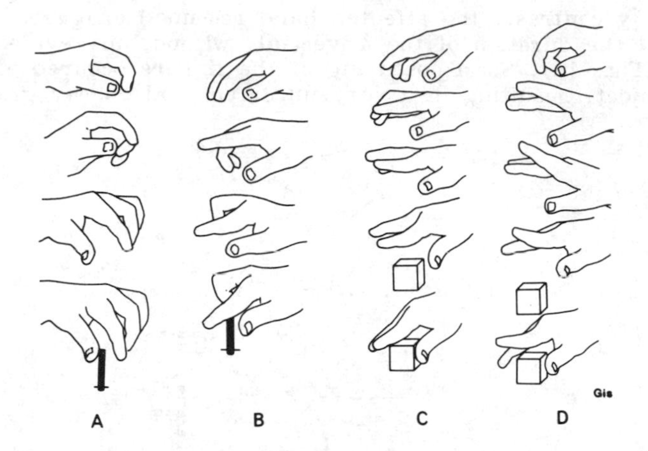

Fig. 5. Pattern of finger grip in Patient 2 (Gis), during reaching in the visual-feedback condition. A: normal hand. B, C, D: affected hand. Redrawn from film.

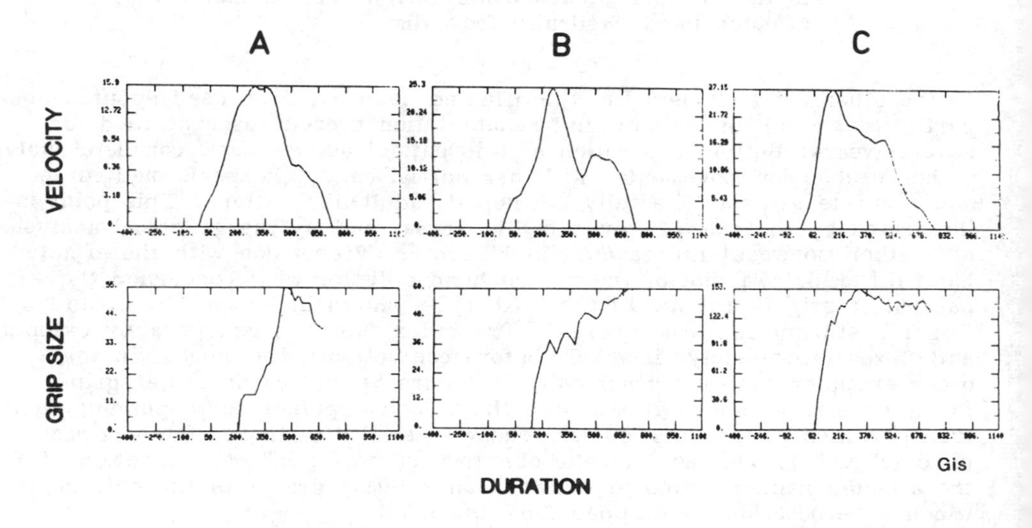

Fig. 6. Change in velocity of the transportation component and grip size of the manipulation component in individual prehension movements as a function of movement duration in Patient 2 (Gis). A: normal hand. B, C: affected hand. Visual-feedback condition. Maximum grip size: A= 55mm, B= 60mm, C= 153mm.

C. Prehension movements in patients with posterior parietal lesions

Posterior parietal lesions, e.g., lesions involving the inferior parietal lobule and the surrounding areas, are known to produce a complex clinical syndrome, more frequently observed when the cerebral hemisphere non-dominant for language is affected. This syndrome includes cognitive and sensorimotor disorders in behaving within immediate surrounding space. Reaching behaviour appears to be affected specially when the patients are examined in the No-visual feedback condition. Patients tend to misdirect the reaching movements of their arm contralateral to the lesion, so that they miss the targets (the so-called "optic ataxia", Balint, 1909; Carcin et al, 1967). It has been recently shown that such misreaches usually result from a systematic error whereby the affected hand is directed too far toward the side of the lesion (Perenin & Vighetto, 1983, see Jeannerod, 1986). The other impairment in visuomotor behaviour following posterior parietal lesions, which is directly relevant to the present topic, is inadequate hand and finger posturing (Perenin & Vighetto, 1983; Tzavaras & Masure, 1975). Prehension movements were examined in two patients with lesions involving the posterior parietal areas. In both cases, neurological examination ascertained the absence of somatosensory deficit. Patient 3 (Biz). In this case, the lesion was located within the posterior parietal areas of the left hemisphere.

Transportation component of prehension movements: With his hand ipsilateral to the lesion, the patient performed accurate reaches in both the Visual feedback and the No visual feedback conditions. This is documented in Figure 7 (left) showing the points on the palmar surface of the left hand

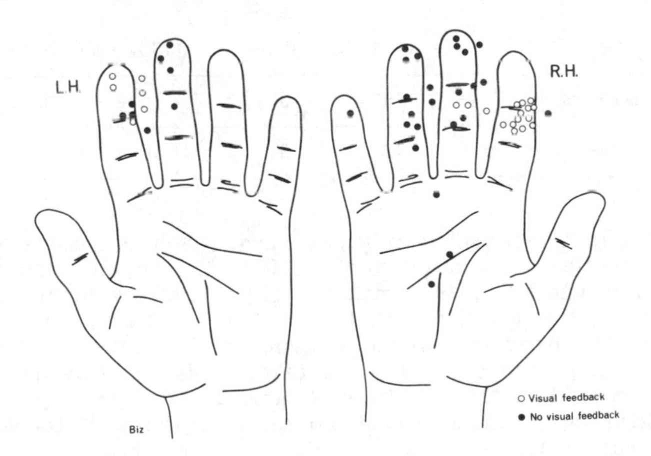

Fig. 7. Points of contact with object during prehension in Patient 3 (Biz). L.H.: left, normal hand. R.H.: right, affected hand. Open circles: visual feedback condition. Black dots: no-visual-feedback condition. Points located between 2 fingers indicate simultaneous contact with the 2 fingers. Data reconstructed from film.

which came in contact with the object at the end of the arm trajectory. In both conditions of visual feedback, these points appear to be located on the palmar surface of the tip of the index and third fingers, as one should expect for an accuracte reach of a small object. The velocity profile of the left arm trajectory in the No visual feedback condition was not entirely normal in that it involved a time to peak velocity somewhat too long with respect to total movement duration (Table 2). This increased time was due to stepwise increase in velocity during the acceleration phase of the movements (Fig. 8a), instead of the usual sharp rise in velocity. With his hand contralateral to the lesion, the patient behaved in a strikingly different way whether visual feedback was available or not during the movement. In the Visual feedback condition, reaching was as accurate as with the normal hand, and the points of contact with the object were restricted to the index finger (Fig. 7 right). Total duration of the movement was increased (Table 2).

Table 2. Averaged movement parameters during prehension in subject Biz (Patient 3). Duration and time to velocity peak are in ms. Maximum and final grip size (before contact) are in mm. Numbers in parenthesis are SDs.

	NORMAL HAND		AFFECTED HAND			
	No Visual feedback		Visual feedback		No Visual feedback	
Duration	740	(120)	1125	(86.6)	1212	(236)
Time to Velocity peak	410	(105.1)	585	(104.6)	564	(137.8)
Maximum grip size	69.7	(5.1)	70.2	(5.4)	89.2	(8.6)
Final grip size	42.0	(6.3)	50.1	(4.0)	66.4	(9.1)

In the No visual feedback condition, large reaching errors appeared, the hand being systematically deviated to the left of the object, that is, to the side of the lesion. Points of contact with the object were widespread over the palmar surface of the third and fourth fingers. In addition, occasional contacts with the palm of the hand indicate a tendency of the patient to overshoot the object position in the sagittal plane (Fig. 7 right). Movement duration was further increased in this condition (Table 2), due to longer deceleration phases which were marked by sharp reaccelerations of the movement before the stop (Fig. 8c).

Pattern of grip formation: With his hand ipsilateral to the lesion, Patient 3 performed normal grips, including in the No visual feedback condition (Table 2 and Fig. 9a). By contrast, the hand contralateral to the lesion showed, in the Visual feedback condition, an incomplete shaping where all the fingers were stretched, with little evidence for grip formation until late in the movement (Figs. 8b and 9b). Finger closure was incomplete (terminal grip size was too large with resepct to object size, see Table 2). In the No visual condition, grip formation was completely inaccurate. The fingers opened widely, and did not close sufficiently in order to accommodate size of the object (Table 2 and Figs. 8c and 9c).

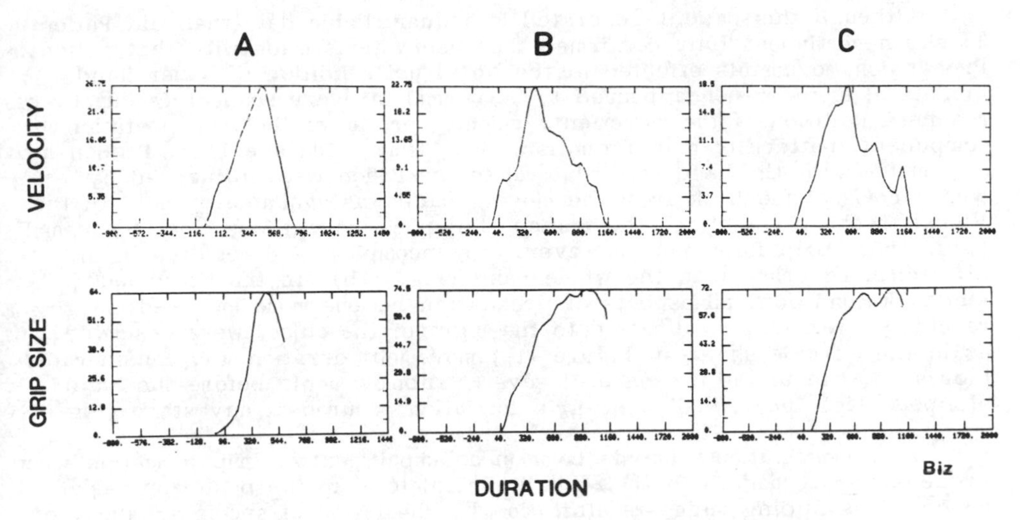

Fig. 8. Change in velocity of the transportation component and grip size of the manipulation component in individual prehension movements as a function of movement duration in Patient 3 (Biz). A: normal hand, no-visual-feedback condition. B, C: affected hand, in the visual-feedback and no-visual-feedback conditions, respectively. Maximum grip size: A= 64 mm, B= 74.5mm, C= 72mm.

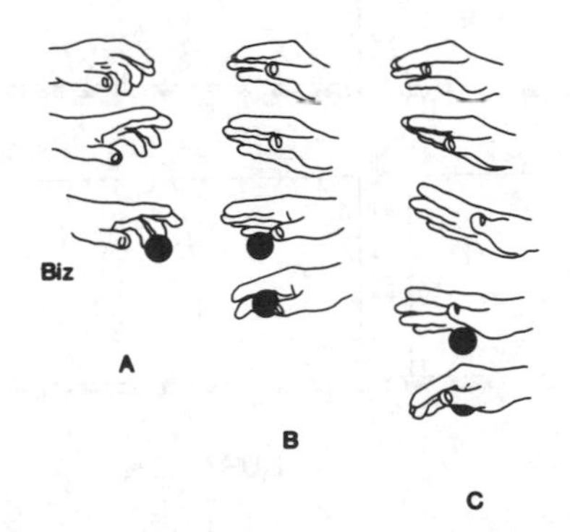

Fig. 9. Pattern of finger grip in Patient 3 (Biz) during reaching. A: normal hand, no-visual-feedback condition. B, C: affected hand in the visual-feedback and no-visual-feedback conditions, respectively. Redrawn from film.

Patient 4 (Tho). In this case, the lesion was located within the posterior parietal areas of the right hemisphere.

Although this patient generated less quantifiable data than did Patient 3, she nevertheless fully confirmed the observations made with that patient. Prehension movements effected in the No visual condition with her hand ipsilateral to the lesion appeared to be normal in every respect (accuracy of reaches, duration of the movement, velocity profile of the transportation component, pattern of grip formation. See Figures 10a and 11a). Prehension movements with the hand contralateral to the lesion were influenced by whether visual feedback from the moving hand was available or not. In the Visual feedback condition, the transportation component was close to normal (Fig. 10b); Grip formation, however, was incomplete and resulted in undifferentiated grasp with the whole hand (Fig. 11b). In the No visual feedback condition, all aspects of prehension became more impaired: large reaching errors always directed to the right of the object were observed, as in the example shown in Figure 11c; movement duration was considerably increased, due to the presence of several submovements before the hand stopped (Fig. 10c); finally, no grip formation occured at any stage (Fig. 11c).

These two patients had in common an impairment of grip formation when prehension was made with their hand contralateral to the posterior parietal lesion. This finding suggests alteration by the lesion of specific visuomotor mechanisms for adjustment of finger posture to the object shape. In addition, the observations made on these patients show that direct visual control of the hand during prehension only partly substitutes for the defective visuomotor mechanisms.

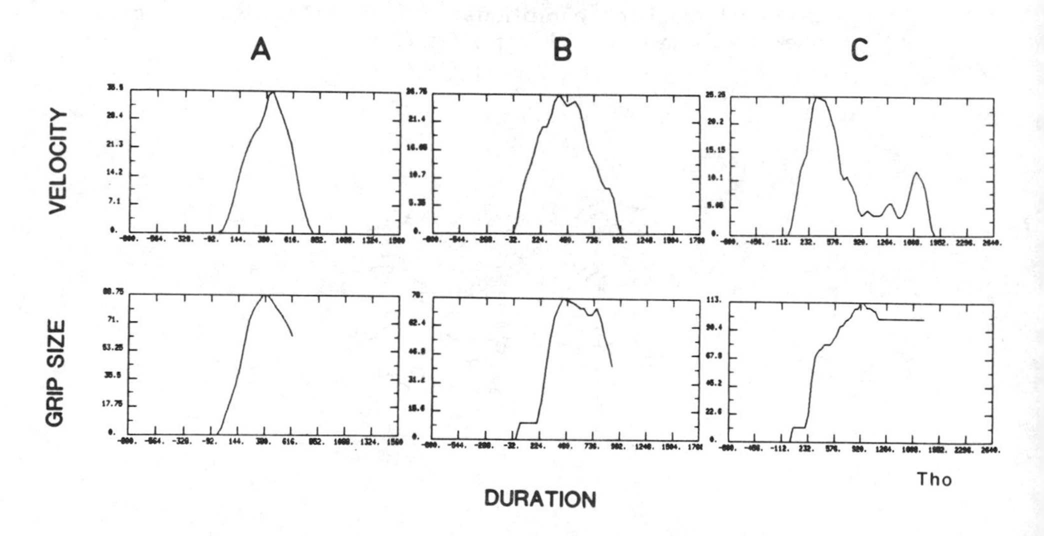

Fig. 10. Change in velocity of the transportation component and grip size of the manipulation components as a function of movement duration in Patient 4 (Tho). A: normal hand, no-visual-feedback condition. B, C: affected hand in the visual-feedback and no-visual-feedback conditions, respectively. Maximum grip size: A= 88.75mm, B= 78mm, C= 113mm.

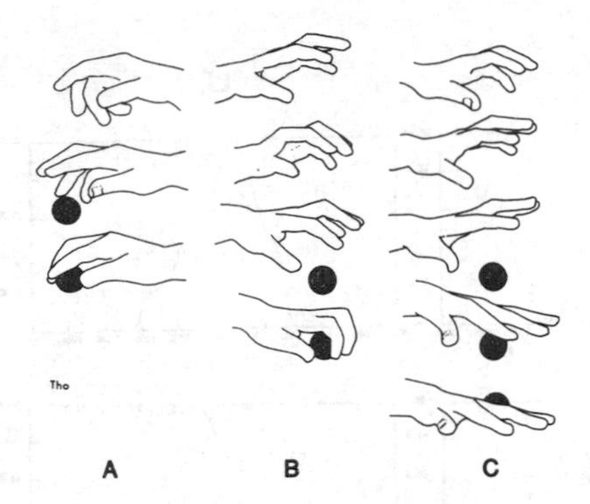

Fig. 11. Pattern of finger grip in Patient 4 (Tho) during reaching. A: normal hand, no-visual-feedback condition. B, C: affected hand in the visual-feedback and no-visual-feedback conditions, respectively. Redrawn from film.

D. Prehension movements in patients with lesions of the somatosensory pathways

Patient 5: (Tah). This patient was a 37 year old man who underwent a severe head injury with a fracture of the occipital bone. CT scan revealed the presence of a bone fragment protruding in the right anterolateral quadrant of the medulla. This fragment was likely to have destroyed the lemniscal sensory pathways at this level. When he was first examined, the patient presented a mild hemiparesis of right upper and lower limbs, and a complete loss of stereognosis and position sense of the same side. The loss of tactile sensation was less complete. Six months after the trauma, i.e., when the film of prehension movements was made, the hemiparesis had completely cleared, although the sensory deficit remained unchanged. A specific component of the somatosensory evoked potential in response to stimulation of the right hand was permanently abolished (for a complete description, see Mauguiere et al, 1983).

Prehension movements performed by the patient's hand contralateral to the lesion (the "normal", left hand) were normal in every respect. Mean values of the maximum grip size and final grip size before contact for that hand in the No visual feedback condition, are given in Table 3. Movements performed by the hand ipsilateral to the lesion (the "affected", right hand) differed whether visual feedback was available or not during the movements. In the Visual feedback condition, duration of the movements was found significantly longer than with the normal hand (Table 3), and finger posturing was such that accurate grasps were performed (Figs. 12a, 13a). The normal character of finger grip formation with that hand is obviously critical for assessing the integrity of the pyramidal tract in this patient. In the No visual feedback condition, by contrast, prehension movements were deeply altered. Not only was movement duration exaggerately long (Table 3), but also finger grip was either absent or incomplete. The first movement recorded in the No visual feedback condition showed a complete lack of grip formation (Figs. 12b, 13b). In subsequent movements incorrect grip formation was observed, with exaggerated opening of the index and third fingers and incomplete finger closure (Table 3, Figs. 12c, 13c).

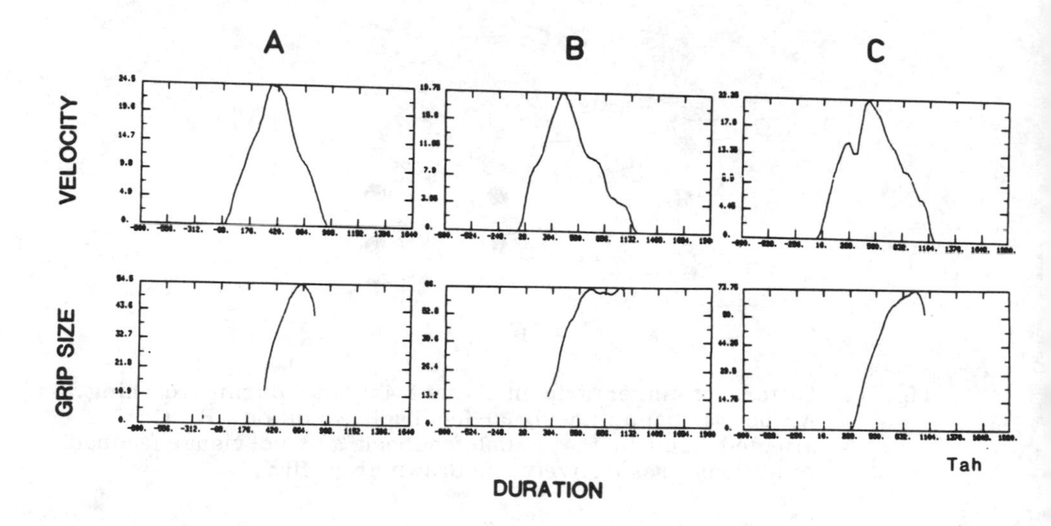

Figure 12. Change in velocity of the transportation component and grip size of the manipulation component as a function of movement duration in Patient 5 (Tah). A: affected hand, visual-feedback condition. B, C: affected hand, no-visual-feedback condition. Movement represented in B is the first movement recorded in the no-visual-feedback condition. Maximum grip size: A= 54.5mm, B= 66mm, C= 73.7mm.

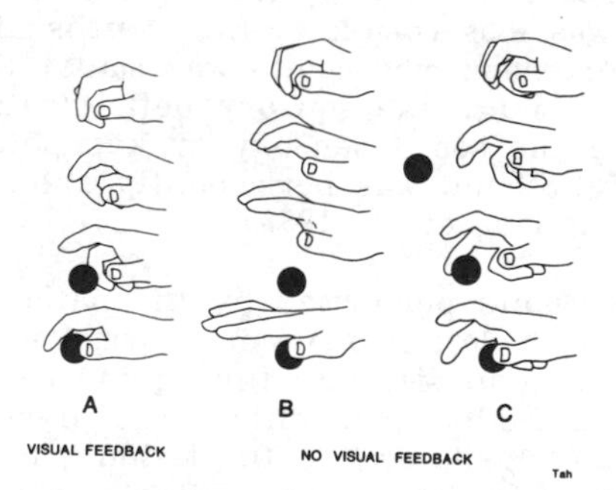

Fig. 13. Pattern of finger grip during reaching in Patient 5 (Tah). A: affected hand, visual-feedback condition. B, C: affected hand, no-visual-feedback condition. Movement represented in B is the first movement recorded in the no-visual-feedback condition. Redrawn from film.

Patient 6: (R.S.). The observations made with Patient 5 were replicated in another patient, for whom a complete clinical description has been published elsewhere (Jeannerod et al, 1984). R.S. presented a complete anaesthesia of th right hand and forearm following a large lesion of the anterior part of the

Table 3. Average movement parameters during prehension in subject Tah (Patient 5). Duration and time to velocity peak are in ms; maximum and final grip size (before contact) are in ms; Numbers in parenthesis are SDs.

	NORMAL HAND	AFFECTED HAND	
	No Visual feedback	Visual feedback	No Visual feedback
Duration	560	925 (105.6)	1096 (188.8)
Time to Velocity peak	300	370 (63.2)	400 (101.9)
Maximum grip size	54.0 (1.7)	51.0 (5.4)	74.3 (5.6)
Final grip size	46.0 (3.6)	34.7 (6.5)	62.7 (13.1)

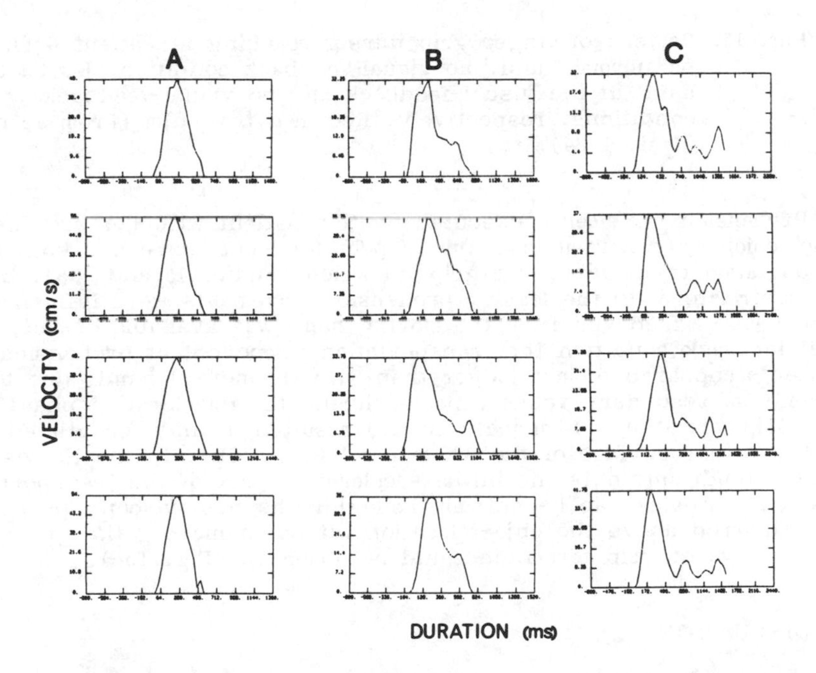

Fig. 14. Change in velocity of the transportation component as a function of movement duration in Patient 6 (R.S.). A: normal hand, no-visual-feedback condition. B, C: affected hand in the visual-feedback and no-visual-feedback conditions, respectively. Four movements are shown in each condition.

left parietal lobe (somatosensory strip), which had spared the motor cortex.

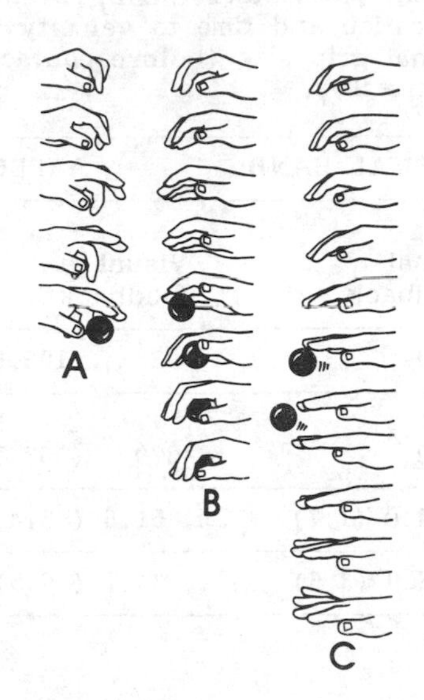

Fig. 15. Pattern of finger grip during reaching in Patient 6 (R.S.). A: normal hand, no-visual-feedback condition. B, C: affected hand in the visual-feedback and no-visual-feedback conditions, respectively. Redrawn from film (From Jeannerod et al, 1984).

Prehension movements executed by this patient with her arm ipsilateral to the lesion were normal in every respect for what concerned both the transportation components and grip formation (Figs. 14a and 15a). With her hand contralateral to the lesion, prehension movements were influenced by whether visual feedback from the moving hand was available or not. In the Visual feedback condition the transportation component of prehension movements appeared to last longer than with the normal hand, due to the occurence of secondary velocity peaks during the deceleration phase (Fig. 14b). Grip formation was inaccurate and resulted in undifferentiated grasps with the palmar surface of the whole hand (Fig. 15b). In the No visual feedback condition, only the initial acceleration part of the transportation components appeared to be normal. Following the first velocity peak, the hand wandered above the object location without achieving the grasp (Fig. 14c). No sign of grip formation could be observed (Fig. 15c).

4. DISCUSSION

A. Visuomotor channels

The present results on impairment of grip formation following cortical lesions (Patients 1, 2, 3, 4, 6) seem to provide arguments as to the hypothesis of "visuomotor channels" previously formulated by Jeannerod and Biguer (1982). Briefly stated, this hypothesis postulates that visuomotor mechanisms are structured in a modular way, in order to cope with the similarly modular organisation of the visual system itself. Although objects may be perceived visually as phenomenal entities, visual pathways are known to detect features, not objects. Therefore, objects are decomposed at the sensory level into elemental features like size, shape, position in space, by way of specific activation of different visual pathways. Visual pathways are conceived here as the input limb of specialised input-output structures or visuomotor channels, each of which extracts a limited number of parameters from the visual world and generates the corresponding motor responses. Accordingly, processing, within a given visual pathway, of the spatial location of the object to be grasped, will activate at the other end of the channel, those muscles which are relevant to carrying the hand at the object location, i.e., proximal arm muscles. Processing, within another visual pathway of shape or size of the object will feed into muscles of more distal segments. Experimental data obtained in animals, as summarised in the Introduction section of the present paper, clearly support the notion of visuomotor subsystems which, when activated in parallel, would account for execution of actions involving several musculoskeletal segments, like prehension. In addition, these experimental data together with the present results in man, justify the role attributed to cerebral cortex as a structural basis for those channels involving the most distal segments.

The hypothesis of parallel visuomotor channels governing the two components of prehension, however, should not contradict the notions of a single act and a unified percept. It could be further speculated that visuomotor channels represent selective pathways for the input-output information flow related to each component; but that the action of prehension as a whole is also represented by another program governing its integrated aspect, in other words the coordination between its components. Accordingly, the musculo-skeletal segments related to the action of prehension, in addition to their differential involvement in independent channels, would also be constrained as a motor ensemble (the "coordinative structure" concept, Kugler et al, 1980). The coordinative structure related to prehension would obey a specific set of rules, hierarchically higher than those of the channels, and coordinating the activity of the channels in the time domain (Arbib, 1981; Jeannerod, 1981). This explanation is compatible with the results of the study of prehension in normal subjects, showing temporal coordination of the two components. The explanation is also compatible with the observation made in lesioned subjects, showing that impairment in grip formation is consistently associated with alteration of the other, proximal, component. This is clearly true for Patients 2, 3, 4, 5, and 6, where the transportation component of the arm affected by the lesion was abnormal in the No visual feedback condition.

B. Interactions between visual and somatosensory inputs at the cortical level

The present results can also be interpreted as reflecting interaction between visual and somatosensory inputs in the control of visually goal-directed actions. This interaction seems to be clearly demonstrated by observations made in Patients 5 and 6. Patient 5, although his lesion was restricted to somatosensory pathways at the medullar level, nevertheless proved to be unable to correctly adapt his fingers to the visual shape of the objects with his affected hand. This result is confirmatory of experimental data in monkeys showing loss of grip formation, following peripheral deafferentation of the arm by section of the corresponding dorsal roots (e.g., Liu & Chambers, 1971). Because the processing of visual information concerning object shape obviously could not have been affected by such peripheral lesions, one has to assume that the defect in grip formation reflected the impossibility for visual information to be integrated with somatosensory information (of tactile and/or proprioceptive origin) concerning finger posture and movements. Furthermore, the fact that interruption of the somatosensory information flow at the cortical level produced the same effects on grip formation as interruption at the peripheral level (as from the observations made with Patient 6), indicates that only the parts of that information that transfer through the cortex is critical for grip formation.

The site for interaction between these two inputs can be suspected from anatomical work in monkey, describing connections of posterior parietal areas, and specially area 7 located within the inferior parietal lobule (see Humphrey, 1979; Hyvärinen, 1982 for review) Area 7 is known to receive abundant visual input from both cortical and subcortical sources. In addition, area 7 is the last member in a chain linking the higher order processing of somatosensory information to motor output (Jones & Powell, 1970). It is therefore quite conceivable that a lesion at this level could disconnect from each other visual and somatosensory informations, critical for the patterning of visually goal-directed movements. This hypothesis would explain the relative similarity, for what concerns grip formation, between patients with posterior parietal lesions and patients with interruption of somatosensory pathways at lower levels (Jeannerod, 1986).

ACKNOWLEDGEMENTS

Part of this work was presented in the Annual Lecture of the European Brain and Behaviour Society, Strasbourg, September, 1984 and is being published in Behavioural Brain Research (1986). Thanks are due to Dr. C. Bérard (L'Escale, Centre Hospitalier Lyon-Sud) for allowing me to examine the two patients with infant hemiplegia. Dr. M.T. Perenin (Laboratoire de Neuropsychologie Experimentale, INSERM U 94), drew my attention to Patients 3 and 4.

Wing, A.M. & Fraser, C. (1983). The contribution of the thumb to reaching movements. *Quarterly Journal of Experimental Psychology, 35A,* 297-309.
Woolsey, C.N., Gorska, T., Wetzel, A., Erickson, T.C., Earls, F.J. & Allman, J.M. (1972). Complete unilateral section of the pyramidal tract at the medullary level in Macaca Mulatta. *Brain Research, 40,* 119-123.
Yakovev, P.I. & Lecours, A.R. (1967). The myelogenetic cyles of regional maturation of the brain. In A. Minkowski (Ed.), *Regional Development of the Brain in Early Life*. Oxford: Blackwell.

References

Arbib, M.A. (1981). Perceptual structures and distributed motor control. In V.B. Brooks (Ed.), *Motor Control, Handbook of Physiology, Vol. 2, Part 2,* pp. 1449-1480.

Balint, R. (1909). Seelenhamung des "Schauens", optische Ataxie, raümlische Störung des Aufmerksamkeit. *Mschr. Psychiatr. Neurol., 25,* 51-81.

Bower, T.G.R., Brougton, J.M. & Moore, M.K. (1970). The coordination of visual and tactual inputs in infants. *Perception and Psychophysics, 8,* 51-53.

Brinkman, J. & Kuypers, H.G.J.M. (1973). Cerebral control of contralateral and ipsilateral arm, hand and finger movements in the split-brain rhesus monkey. *Brain, 96,* 653-674.

Bruner, J.S. & Koslowski, B. (1972). Visually pre-adapted constituents of manipulatory action. *Perception, 1,* 3-14.

Chapman, E. & Wiesendanger, M. (1982). Recovery of function following unilateral lesions of the bulbar pyramid in the monkey. *Electroenceph. clin. Neurophysiology,* 374-387.

Faugier-Grimaud, S., Frenois, C. & Stein, D.G. (1978). Effects of posterior parietal lesions on visually guided behaviour in the monkey. *Neuropsychologia, 16,* 151-168.

Felix, D. & Wiesendanger, M. (1971). Pyramidal and nonpyramidal motor cortical effects on distal forelimb muscles of monkeys. *Experimental Brain Research, 12,* 81-91.

Garcin, R., Rondot, P. & Recondo, J. de. (1967). Ataxie optique localisée aux deux hémichamps visuels homonymes gauches. *Rev. neurol., 116,* 707-714.

Gazzaniga, M.S., Bogen, J.E. & Sperry, R.W. (1967). Dyspraxia following division of the cerebral commissures. *Arch. Neurol., 16,* 606-612.

Goutieres, F., Challamel, M.J., Aicardi, J. & Gilly, R. (1972). Les hémiplégies congénitales. Sémiologie, étiologie et pronostic. *Arch. franc. Pédiat., 29,* 839-851.

Haaxma, H. & Kuypers, H.G.J.M. (1975). Intrahemispheric cortical connections and visual guidance of hand and finger movements in the rhesus monkey. *Brain, 98,* 239-260.

Halverson, H.M. (1931). An experimental study of prehension in infants by means of systematic cinema records. *Genet. Psychol. Monogr., 10,* 110-286.

Hartje, W. & Ettlinger, G. (1973). Reaching in light and dark after unilateral posterior parietal ablations in the monkey. *Cortex, 9,* 346-354.

Hofsten, C. von. (1979). Development of visually directed reaching: the approach phase. *Journal of Human Movement Studies, 6,* 160-178.

Humphrey, D.R. (1979). On the cortical control of visually directed reaching. Contributions by nonprecentral areas. In R.E. Talbot and D.R. Humphrey (Eds.), *Posture and Movement.* New York: Raven Press.

Hyvärinen, J. (1982). *The Parietal Cortex of Monkey and Man.* Berlin: Springer Verlag.

Hyvärinen, J. & Poranen, A. (1974). Function of the parietal associative area 7 as revealed from cellular discharges in alert monkeys. *Brain, 97,* 673-692.

Jeannerod, M. (1981). Intersegmental coordination during reaching at natural visual objects. In J. Long and A. Baddeley (Eds.), *Attention and Performance, Vol. 9.* Hillsdale: Erlbaum.

Jeannerod, M. (1984). The timing of natural prehension movements. *Journal of Motor Behavior, 16,* 235-254.

Jeannerod, M. (1986). Mechanisms of visuomotor coordination. A study in normal and brain-damaged subjects. *Neuropsychologia* (in press).

Jeannerod, M. & Biguer, B. (1982). Visuomotor mechanisms in reaching within extrapersonal space. In D. Ingle, M. Goodale and R. Mansfield (Eds.), *Advances in the Analysis of Visual Behaviour.* Boston: MIT Press.

Jeannerod, M., Michel, F. & Prablanc, C. (1984). The control of hand movements in a case of hemianaesthesia following a parietal lesion. *Brain, 107,* 899-920.

Jones, E.G. & Powell, T.P.S. (1970). An anatomical study of converging sensory pathways within the cerebral cortex of the monkey. *Brain, 93,* 793-820.

Kugler, P.N., Kelso, J.A.S. & Turvey, M.T. (1980). On the concept of coordinative structures as dissipative structures. I. Theoretical lines of convergence. In G.E. Stelmach and J. Requin (Eds.), *Tutorials in Motor Behavior.* Amsterdam: North-Holland.

Kuypers, H.G.J.M. (1962). Corticospinal connections: postnatal development in rhesus monkey. *Science, 138,* 678-680.

Lamotte, R.H. & Acuna, C. (1978). Defects in accuracy of reaching after removal of posterior parictal cortex in monkeys. *Brain Research, 139,* 309-326.

Langworthy, O.R. (1933). Development of behavior patterns and myelinization of the nervous system in the human fetus and infant. *Contributions to Embryology of the Carnegie Institution, 24,* 1-58.

Lawrence, D.G. & Kuypers, H.G.J.M. (1968). The functional organization of the motor system in the monkey. I. The effects of bilateral pyramidal lesions. *Brain, 91,* 1-14.

Lawrence, D.G. & Hopkins, D.A. (1972). Development aspects of pyramidal control in the rhesus monkey. *Brain Research, 40,* 117-118.

Liu, C.N. & Chambers, W.W. 81971). A study of cerebellar dyskinesia in the bilaterally deafferented forelimbs of the monkey (Macaca mulatta and Macaca speciosa). *Acta Neurobiol. exp., 31,* 363-389.

Lough, S., Wing, A.M., Fraser, C. & Jenner, J.R. (1984). Measurement of recovery of function in the hemiparetic upper limb following stroke: a preliminary report. *Human Movement Science, 3,* 347-256.

Mauguiere, F., Courjon, J. & Schott, B. (1983). Dissociation of early SEP components in unilateral traumatic section of the lower medulla. *Neurol., 13,* 309-313.

Muir, R.B. (1985). Small hand muscles in precision grip: a corticospinal prerogative? *Experimental Brain Research, 10,* 155-174.

Passingham, R., Perry, H. & Wilkinson, F. (1978). Failure to develop a precision grip in monkeys with unilateral neocortical lesions made in infancy. *Brain Research, 145,* 410-414.

Perenin, M.T. & Vighetto, A. (1983). Optic ataxia: a specific disorder in visuomotor coordination. In A. Hein and M. Jeannerod (Eds.), *Spatially Oriented Behavior.* New York: Springer.

Phillips, C.G. & Porter, R. (1977). *Corticospinal Neurones. Their Role in Movement.* New York: Academic Press.

Trevarthen, C.B. (1965). Functional interactions between the cerebral hemispheres in the monkey. In E.G. Ettlinger (Ed.), *Functions of the Corpus Callosum.* London: Ciba Foundation, Churchill.

Trevarthen, C.B. (1982). Basic patterns of psychogenetic change in infancy. In T.B. Bever (Ed.), *Dips in learning.* Hillsdale: Erlbaum.

Tower, S.S. (1940). Pyramidal lesion in the monkey. *Brain, 63,* 36-90.

Tzavaras, A. & Masure, M.C. (1975). Aspects différents de l'ataxie optique selon la latéralisation hémisphérique de la lésion. *Lyon med., 236,* 673-683.

HANDWRITING DISTURBANCES: DEVELOPMENTAL TRENDS

J.P. Wann

1. INTRODUCTION

There is sometimes a tendency for handwriting to be viewed as a rather esoteric area of developmental research. Handwriting has, in common with everyday tasks of prehension and locomotion, the advantage of surmounting the problems of learning and ecological validity presented by the use of novel, complex-motor tasks with children. In contrast to more natural behaviours "emerging" earlier in development however, the control of handwriting cannot be assigned to purpose-designed phylogenic structures. Whether skill acquisition entails a process of recruiting and refining natural control structures, or a more traditional process of program building, a fine motor task with constraints on spatial accuracy, that receives time and emphasis within the education system would seem an ideal focus for study.

1.1. Facets of the task

The acquisition of cursive handwriting not only provides a significant hurdle to most children, but a conspicuous stumbling block to some. Despite a plethora of research into the dynamics of mature handwriting, there has been few attempts to apply such advanced techniques to the development of handwriting in children. Research with children exhibiting writing difficulties, in particular, has generally been restricted to the analysis of the graphic product and assessment through additional fine motor tasks, rather than an appraisal of the movements 'in process'. Given such a population, the range of possible problems is wide. Figure 1 depicts a model cataloguing some of the factors pertinent to form control and their possible lines of influence. Naturally this cannot be considered as fully comprehensive, nor can it depict all lines of influence between its members. It may, for instance be argued that regulation of feedback should link into the control of individual movements, and (with kinaesthetic awareness) to the control of force. In this respect a truer, though less practical alternative would be to replace this 'writing wheel' with a 'graphic globe'.

The influence of many of the listed areas upon handwriting performance has been charted by a number of researchers. In the afferent domain Sovik (1979, 1981) has been foremost in emphasising the development of feedback control and its influence upon writing quality, while Lazlo and Bairstow (1983) demonstrated a remarkable increase in the copying performance of children after "kinaesthetic training". The links between hand preference, posture and cerebral organisation are less clear. The Levy and Reid (1978) model linking cerebral organisation and posture has been strongly challenged by the work of Weber (1983), although Todor (1980) has linked writing posture to sequential processing ability. Such tenuous relationships however, should

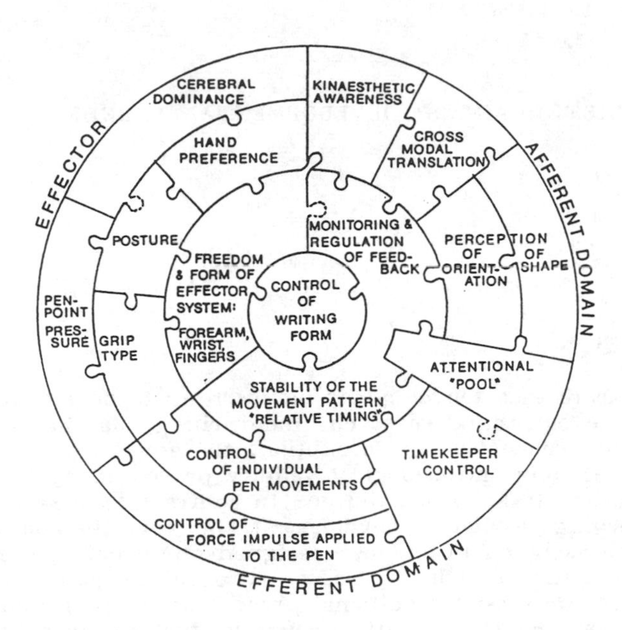

Fig. 1. Factors pertinent to the control of handwriting form and possible lines of influence (nodes).

be considered as supplementary to the direct influence of the effector as a mechanical link-system, the freedom and constraints of which will interact with the nature of the task. The scarcity of comprehensive data on the dynamics of the link-system and the need to reassess some of the assumptions made about it, are discussed in a later section of this paper. Some appraisal of developmental trends in grip however, have been attempted. Ziviani (1983) catalogued age-related changes in the degree of finger flexion and forearm pronation in childrens penholds. Both of these factors are likely to dictate whether shifts of the pen, particularly along the page, must be effected predominantly by the fingers, wrist or forearm. Although such developmental trends were not found by Sassoon, Nimmo-Smith & Wing (1985), other findings such as a reduction in speed with a "hand on edge" grip, support the notion of postural influence in writing production. A further salient but poorly documented relationship is that of grip and penpoint pressure. Kao (1983) has been foremost in charting intra-task and inter-task variations in writing pressure with adult subjects. Kao (1979) also summarised the influence of writing instruments and made some observations of the grip-pressure relationship. To date, however, few studies have followed the early lead of Harris and Rarick (1958) in exploring pen pressure as a dependent variable in handwriting development, or the effect that the 'maturity' of grip may have on penpoint pressure. Normal (perpendicular) force is a critical factor in determining the inertia and damping characteristics of the pen, and hence the planar force required to produce writing strokes. The differentiation and control of conflicting forces must be seen as a major feature in skill development and in handwriting in particular. It is such kinetic control, the nature of pen movements and the stability of childrens movement pattern, that this paper addresses. Where possible an integrated appraisal of the findings is attempted, although it should be emphasised that the primary goal of the following research was an assessment of differences in childrens motor control in a complex fine-motor task, rather than a treatise of handwriting per se.

2. QUANTITATIVE APPRAISAL OF HANDWRITING DIFFICULTIES

In many education systems, cursive handwriting is introduced during primary school, to children between the ages of 8 and 11 years. Where children exhibit difficulty in acquiring cursive script, their checkered progress may well be indicative of accumulated difficulties in fine motor control, rather than specific to the demands of the cursive task. It is likely that such children have 'stuttered' if not 'stumbled' at similar fine motor hurdles prior to their identification as poor writers. The choice of this developmental phase therefore is primarily a pragmatic one. It is a time when each child is required to modify, link and phase patterns of precise movement, not only with the spatial accuracy required by previous printing skills, but with some degree of fluency and speed. Such a critical period serves to highlight difficulties that may well have been present, though less evident, during the acquisition of elementary phases of movement in printing or drawing (see Nihei, 1983).

The following studies focused on children who had been practising cursive handwriting for 5 months (Australian primary school grade 4, mean age 109 months), and those with just under 17 months experience (grade 5, mean age 123 months). Handwriting samples were collected from the children (n= 197), and the Rubin and Henderson (1982) protocol used to assess the relative quality of script, in terms of the constancy of letter size, form and legibility. This enabled the 10th and 90th percentiles to be identified as those children displaying advanced and retarded handwriting acquisition, with respect to their peers. The final sample size was 32 children (8 of each standard from each grade), matched on age, experience and non-verbal (non-graphic) I.Q. Obviously such a sample allows appraisal of trends across age (experience), although the primary concern was that of consistent trends within age, between children of different writing standard.

2.1. Writing time as a dependent variable in handwriting assessment

Writing time or writing speed has been used as a dependent variable in both handwriting scales and research, (Sassoon et al, 1985; Sovik, 1979). Its choice would seem logical, if one accepts the main goals of written communication to be legibility and speed (Suen, 1983). From a developmental perspective, speed of manipulative movement has been a pertinent variable for use in motor assessment (see Keogh and Sugden, 1985 for a comprehensive review). Some contrasts should be drawn however, between speed on a peg-board task or tapping, and cursive handwriting. In the former the child's maximum speed is assessed over a relatively short period, where as it is seldom the case that a child (or adult) is asked to write at a maximum rate, but rather maintain a reasonable, and comfortable rate of progress. Rubin and Henderson (1982) calculated writing speed (number of letters written in minutes), for good and poor writers in junior school and found no differences in speed or any correlation between speed and quality. Our own analysis (Wann & Jones, in press) concentrated on a more micro-level, measuring precise movement times for letters and words written at preferred pace by good and poor writers. Each child performed eight trials of five letters (a, o, n, v, w) and four trials of two words (nun, nine) after unrestricted practice, on an x, y digitiser (ultrasound, 100 Hz sampling rate, 0.2 mm resolution). After smoothing at 5 Hz (second-order Butterworth filter), writing duration was calculated by searching the absolute velocity profile.

In confirmation of the findings of Rubin and Henderson (1982), no significant differences were found in absolute writing time between good and poor writers. Poor writers, however, were significantly more variable (at $p < .01$), from trial to trial in the time taken to complete identical letter tasks.

An obvious criticism of the above findings is that neither discrete letters of single words constitute a continuous writing task. Good and poor writers, however, took similar times to perform full cursive forms (some complete with joining strokes). If when imbedded in text, some children take an extended duration to perform a series of letters (or words), then the additional delay is due to the addition of context. As such extended writing time may be more a measure of lexical or parallel processing ability than purely of motor ability. Older children in both groups, however, did write significantly faster than younger children. This finding agrees with Athenes (1984) who observed no significant effect of handedness, posture or sex on the writing time of children, but did observe age effects. Although natural writing speed may increase with age and experience, the available evidence suggests that it should not be considered as a direct indication of competence. A variable providing a more reliable indication of writing difficulties was variability in writing time, across repeated trials of the same task.

2.2. The occurrence of intra-letter pauses

The incidence of pauses or 'breaks' in the writing stroke would seem, on the basis of teachers reports, to be a salient factor in identifying childrens writing difficulties. At the time of writing there appears to have been no detailed quantitative assessments of such a factor in childrens writing. Most letter forms require that a number of form-related pauses occur at points of inflexion. With adult writers these normally result in sharp dips in the velocity profile, of no appreciable duration. In childrens writing these may become pauses of an extended duration. In addition arcs of high curvature, that are marked by smooth troughs in an adult profile, may become additional pause locations during trials by children, Figure 2.

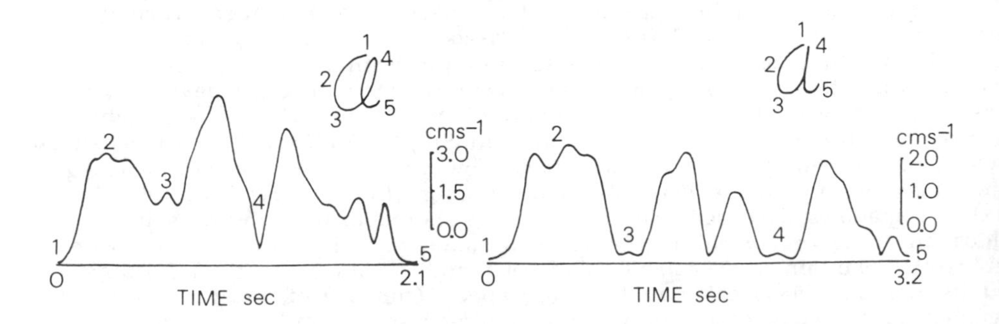

Fig. 2. Form related features in the velocity profile of a letter *a*, written by an adult (left) and a 10 year-old (right). Redrawn from original data.

A search of the velocity profiles for writing trials by good and poor writers by Wann and Jones (in press), highlighted a number of significant contrasts in pause occurrence between good and poor writers. A greater number of pauses was not purely indicative of poorer writers. Amongst younger (grade 4) children, a higher incidence of short duration pauses (mean 87 msec), marked the performance of good writers whereas fewer pauses of an extended duration (mean 122 msec) were typical of poorer writers. Generally pause duration proved the most reliable indicator of differences in writing standard, with poor writers from both grades taking significantly longer pauses ($p < 0.01$).

2.3. The selection of diagnostic variables

Qualitative scales for the assessment of handwriting have been undergoing review and revision since early in the twentieth century. In developmental assessment, however, it is desirable that suitable qualitative appraisal should be supplemented by quantitative observations indicative of motor competence in pen control. Spatial accuracy is closely tied to legibility, and Sovik (1979) observed a high correlation between accuracy on a copying task and writing quality, mental age and visuo-motor integration scores. During freehand writing however, accuracy is a redundant variable due to the lack of a criterion path, hence only the extent of movement (letter height) may be measured. Our own results suggest that, in an unstressed situation, both good and poor writers can achieve a criterion height for letters, and although the coefficient of variation across trials was slightly greater for poor writers, this trend was not significant. An ideal measure of spatial accuracy during freehand would be a quantitative appraisal of consistency of letter shape across trials, although the need for complex computational procedures takes it rather beyond the reaches of the applied setting.

In the time domain, writing speed has been questioned by a number of researchers, and variability in writing time would seem a more favourable alternative. A greater number of short duration pauses may be taken by novice but competent writers, possibly to enable greater visual control, although longer breaks in the writing stroke do seem indicative of poor quality writers. The measurement of writing time variability, pause duration and possibly variation in letter height or width, would seem to have diagnostic potential in handwriting assessment. In addition to these, stroke organisation (Nihei, 1983) during the manuscript to cursive transition, and the control of pen pressure (Harris & Rarick, 1959) would seem to be promising areas of investigation, in order to realise the full potential of handwriting appraisal in developmental assessment.

3. THE STABILITY OF THE MOVEMENT PATTERN

The demonstration by Viviani and Terzuolo (1980), that mature handwriting can retain an "invariant structure" across changes in size and speed of execution, has almost become motor control 'folklore'. Although data was presented from only an extremely small sample, its agreement with earlier observations by other workers made its findings both enticing and plausible. There is undoubtedly a need to reconfirm the pervasive assumptions that have emerged from this work. The extent to which an invariant structure is evident within stages of handwriting development, would shed light on both the nature of skill acquisition and the validity of the "homothetic" hypothesis.

3.1. Relative Timing

The measurement of writing time and pause duration have already highlighted some instabilities in the writing performance of poorer quality writers. The issue of relative timing, is whether a common structure underlies the patterning of the composite movements of a task, across repeated trials that may vary in total duration. Figure 3 illustrates repeated trials (unscaled) of the letter *a* performed by children varying in writing competence. Inspection of Figure 3 suggests that, allowing for differences

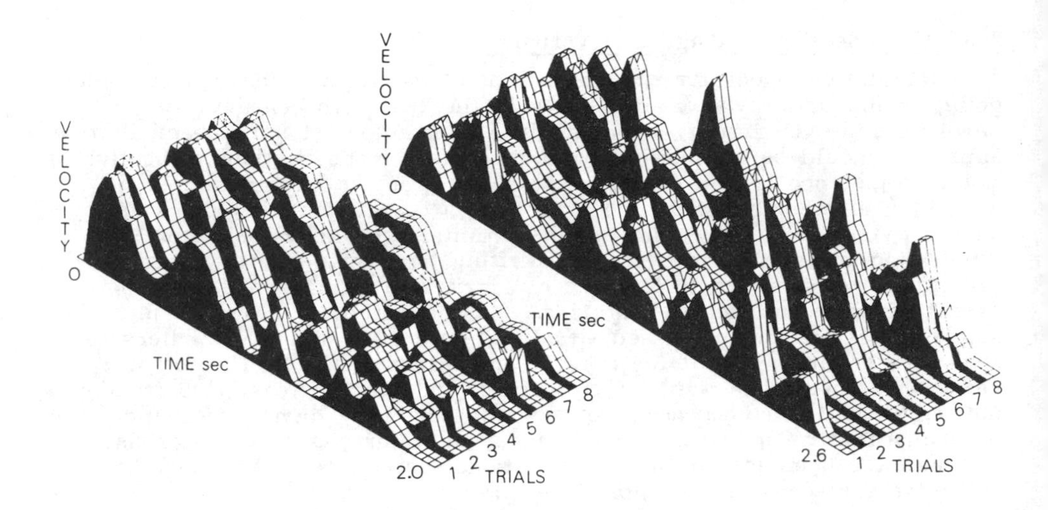

Fig. 3. Velocity profiles for repeated trials of the letter *a*; those of a good writer (left) displaying some correspondence between feature form and peak location; whereas trials by a poor writer (right) are of a more disparate organisation. (All profiles unscaled).

in overall duration, the composite movements performed by a good quality writer have some similarities of form and relative duration. A similar pattern however, is not evident for trials by a poor writer. To provide a more quantitative appraisal, childrens trials on each task were scaled to a common time-base. The scaling procedure merely expressed each time point as a percentage of the series length, then for computational simplicity, multiplied by a constant (the common duration). This should not be confused with Viviani and Terzuolo's (1980) "Homothetic transformation" which was criticised by Gentner (1982). Scaled series were then cross-correlated to find the maximum correspondence and the lag (phase shift) at which it occurred.

In contrast to the synchronisation coefficient of Morasso (1983), the value of the cross-correlation coefficient is not purely dependent upon the relative temporal location of movement features, but also the height (velocity) and slope (acceleration) of respective movements. Taking this into account, the finding that trials by poor writers in grade 5 exhibited significantly lower correspondence and greater phase shift (Wann & Jones, in press), should be interpreted as indicative of greater variability in the timing of the onset, duration and level of force, rather than a measure of temporal synchrony. This qualification does not degrade the notion of relative timing within the analysis, but rather provides a more comprehensive assessment of movement stability, in terms of rates of displacement, rather than a feature alignment procedure which may overlook significant differences in the time-histories of the movements. Differences in correspondence were not evident amongst 'novice' (grade 4) writers although phase shift was significantly higher for poor writers in this grade.

The findings were essentially supportive of the invariant timing hypothesis of Viviani and Terzuolo (1980), and suggested that poor writers lacked the stability in generating movements, that is apparently a feature of more mature handwriting.

3.2. Rhythm

Temporal stability within a repetitive task (rather than across trials) may be reflected in the rhythm of the movement. The nature of many cursive tasks is not only repetitive (in the vertical plane), but mature cursive script often appears to have a high rhythmic content. Hollerbach (1980) demonstrated through simulation, that it is possible to generate cursive forms by modulating the relative phase of orthogonal oscillations. While a direct application of the Hollerbach perspective to human performance is fraught with problems, it would seem a plausible notion that repetitive components of a task may be oscillatory in nature, with more discrete shifts being superimposed. This also highlights the possibility that repetitive features of a well learned task may be controlled by something equivalent to the pattern generators proposed for gait movements (Grillner, 1981).

It is apparent that infants possess the 'hardware' to generate rhythmic patterns of movement (Thelen & Fisher, 1983). Studies by Smoll (1975) however, indicated that children progressively acquire the ability to maintain rhythmic movements of the upper limbs. It is possible that children exhibiting delayed writing acquisition may not be able to generate or harness suitable rhythmic movements, to enable progression towards rapid, fluid script. This hypothesis was examined using childrens trials on the words *nun* and *nine*. Both words are composed predominantly of transverse strokes and lend themselves towards the use of short rhythmic oscillations in the vertical plane. The periodogram of the vertical displacement data was calculated for each trial, and the principle peaks (dominant frequencies) identified. Variability in the dominant frequencies across trials and cross-spectral estimates were calculated, and the strength of the principle peak assessed by expressing it as a percentage of the total signal energy (up to 5Hz).

No significant differences were evident in the ability of good or poor writers to produce rhythmic pen movements in the vertical direction. The children had not been prompted to concentrate on such a feature, but merely instructed, as for the other tasks, to write at a normal comfortable pace. The periodogram of such movement indicated that the vertical shifts for most children were strongly rhythmic, suggesting that rhythmic generation in itself was not a problem. This concurred with the findings of Thomassen and Teulings (1983), who observed that children as young as seven had little difficulty in performing simple looped strokes. It would seem that the presence of a writing rhythm does not preculde the possibility of instability in motor output, possibly due to the poor phasing of vertical and horizontal pen movements. On a more theoretical note, the finding that many vertical strokes had similar frequency components would seem to lend weight to a more Bernsteinian perspective for the control of such movements. The notion that such tasks can be partialled into orthogonal repetitive, and discrete progressive/regressive components however, has not received empirical support. Thomassen and Teulings (1983) have demonstrated the phasing of a horizontal progression into a stationary oscillation is an unlikely strategy for letter formation. Further work however, is warranted on this issue.

4. THE REFINEMENT OF INDIVIDUAL MOVEMENTS

Although the physical appearance of cursive script is of a continuous running line, most writing tasks can be broken down to a series of discrete pen shifts which in practice are linked and phased to provide a smooth, fluent product. This is not to argue that such discrete shifts are the unit of production in handwriting, but rather that such sub-components may be useful units of analysis. The pertinent question is whether the more 'global' differences in childrens writing performance, highlighted by cross-correlation techniques, can in part be accounted for by the childrens ability to control smaller discrete aspects of the tasks.

4.1. The maturity of movement patterns

Hay (1979, 1984) identified three types of displacement pattern within childrens aimed reaching movements. Type I "Ballistic" patterns are marked by rapid acceleration and deceleration, and a high peak velocity, these were more evident amongst younger children (5 years). With children of 7 and 9 years, type III "step" and "ramp" movements were evident, with a number of small intra-movement steps, or a slow gradual acceleration phase (ramp) being used, apparently to aid greater use of feedback. By the age of 11, type II patterns predominated, with smooth acceleration and deceleration phases contributing to a 'mature' bell-shaped velocity profile.

If a writing task is considered as a series of composite 'aiming' movements, where the goal may be to project the pen between the upper and lower bounds of letter height or to follow a specific curved trajectory, it is possible that the application of categories similar to those identified by Hay (1979, 1984) may highlight salient differences in the childrens mode of pen control. The discreteness of composite pen-shifts within a writing task is arguable. There is evidence from adult writing that the kinematics of an individual stroke are subject to contextual influence from neighbouring segments (Greer & Green, 1983). If however, the incidence of each pattern type is averaged over all segments of a task, and over repeated trials, then the findings describe consistent trends in each childs mode of achievement of individual pen-strokes.

Writing trials by good and poor writers on *v* and *w* were analysed, as these tasks were the most congruent with the notion of a series of composite 'aimed' segments, and under normal circumstances all segments are of a similar form. "Ballistic", "ramp" and "step" patterns were identified on the basis of high peak velocity and acceleration/deceleration, low peak velocity and acceleration, and a high number of intra-movement steps, respectively. The qualification of 'high' and 'low' was based upon the 16th and 84th percentiles, respectively, of total writing distribution across subjects for each variable. Figure 4, illustrates the form of type I and type III patterns, as well as the frequency of occurrence for each pattern type with repeated trials of v and w.

The frequency breakdown of pattern types across groups indicated that although there was no significant differences between younger grade 4 children (concurring with the findings of the cross-correlational analysis),

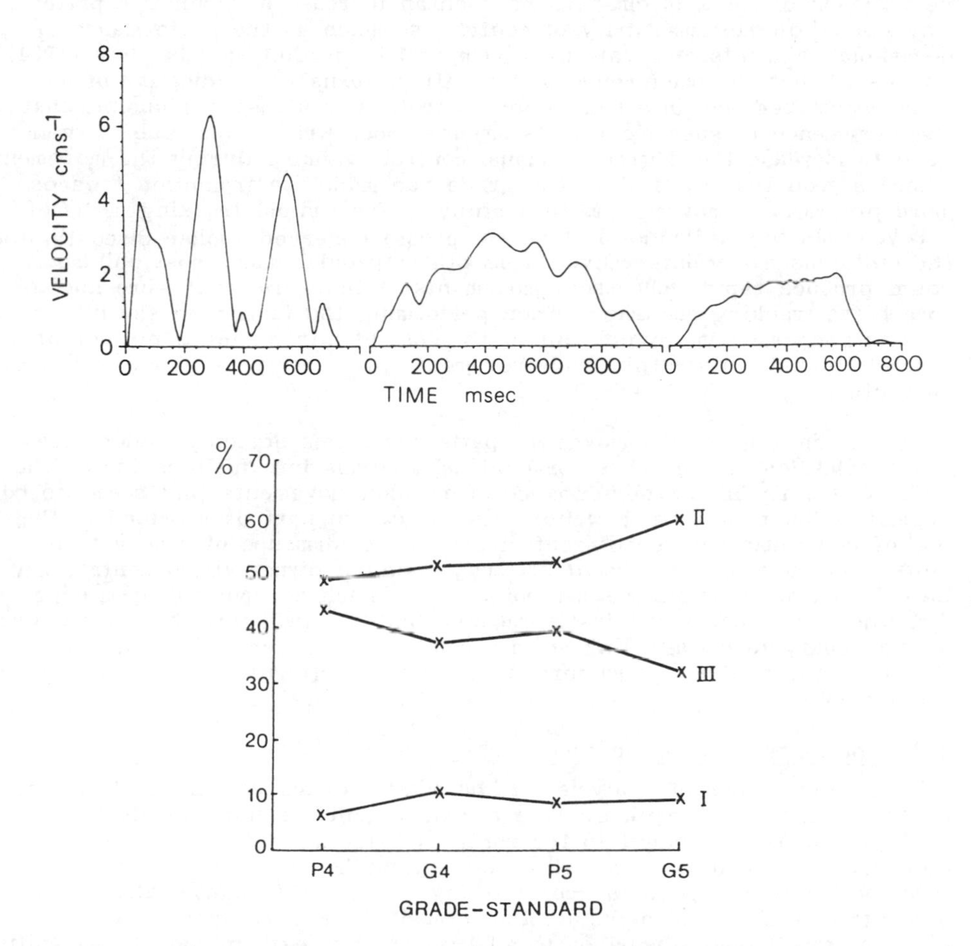

Fig. 4. Upper: Examples of movement patterns similar to those identified by Hay (1979); left to right, a series of type I "ballistic" movements, a type III "step" and one example of a type III "ramp" pattern. (All redrawn from original writing trials by children).
Lower: Frequency of type I, type II (mature) and type III patterns across grade (4, 5) and standard (good, poor).

good writers in grade 5 used significantly more 'mature' movement patterns than poor quality writers of the same age. A breakdown of the type III frequencies indicated that there was little difference between good and poor writers in the incidence of "step" patterns but that the degraded type II percentages of poor writers was due to a preponderance of "ramp" movements. A slight anomaly was the higher incidence of "ballistic" movements amongst good quality writers. It should be noted, however, that generally all children used low velocity movements as compared to adults, hence the criterion values for the identification of ballistic movements were below what might be observed during normal adult writing (e.g. peak velocity cut off of 3.86 cms^{-1}). As such an increase in "ballistic" patterns may not be due to immaturity of control, so much as the performance of occasional segments at a rate more comparable to adult speeds. Hay (1984), suggested that the occurrence of type III patterns was indicative of a reliance on feedback information for control. It would seem plausible that the prevalence of such movements amongst poor writers was due to their need to increase the degree of visual control available during the movement, whereas good writers of the same grade had made the transition towards more programmed movements. In a study of the manual tracking skills of 5-9 year old boys, Mounoud et al (in press) observed similar discontinuities i the childrens movements: Given a smooth sinusoidal task, most children could produce rapid (600 msec) movements of this form, but were not able to achieve tracking accuracy. When performing the task more slowly, tracking accuracy improved, but at the cost of introducing a number of discrete adjustments within each movement, presumably to allow visual error correction.

The findings of the movement pattern analysis not only underscores the conclusions of the cross-correlational analysis but qualifies them. The lack of stability in the performance of complex movements that seems to be typical of the poor quality writers tested, can in part be ascribed to their use of less mature modes of control for the performance of composite pen shifts. The use of a movement strategy enabling direct visual control may be effective in completing some motor tasks, such as printing or tracing, but where the goal is not just form but fluidity, it will introduce a constraint on the ability to serially link segments into refined cursive script. Fuller details of the analysis procedure for movement patterns can be found in Wann (1985).

4.2. The control of kinetic cost

A second level of analysis for the control of simple pen shifts is the control of force and impulse. To a certain extent, as indicated in Figure 1, such control is antecedent to the control of movement form, in that the ability to control force may well dictate the ability to control form. In practice however, the influence of timing (e.g. onset, and relative duration of contractions) will also dictate the form of movement. Such influence is not the case if one subscribes to a "mass-spring" explanation of pen-shifts effected through the regulation of stiffness, in a self-equilibrating system. The difficulty in accounting for the various movement types* with such a model however, leads one to conclude that either the model is not appropriate or that due to other constraints, children have yet to effect such a simple

---

* It would be possible to propose mass-spring explanations for "step" and "ramp" movements using pre-computed torques from a poorly structured "motion blackboard" (see Hinton, 1984). The distinction between a series of length-tension adjustments and a series of agonist bursts however, seems rather too fine, given the present state of developmental research.

method of control. Because the relationship of force control to movement form control is a complex one, the analysis of kinetic costs was not aimed at providing explanations of the latter so much as an insight into the extent to which good and poor writers appear to be optimising certain kinetic features.

Skilled motor behaviours are often described as "smooth" or "effortless", and in the daily performance of many motor acts, it would seem that low energy expenditure may be equated with proficiency. Broer and Zernicke (1979) suggest that "good form is not a set pattern but rather the movement or movements which accomplish the purpose with the least expenditure of energy" (p. 29). From an analytic point of view this should not be taken too literally. Developmentally a reduction in energy expenditure does not necessarily mean better form, but as a general trend over development it would seem to have some diagnostic merit.

Nelson (1983) lists distance, time, force, impulse, energy and jerk as possible "performance objectives" for optimisation during movement. Within a given script size, movement distance is a constraint (primary goal), hence maximum-distance should not really be considered as an objective to be modulated. A minimum-time criterion would seem more applicable to explosive sports than handwriting. The analysis of the movement times for individual pen-strokes did not indicate that good writers completed such movements significantly faster than poor writers, given a mean movement time of 432 msec for movements of less than 12 mm it would seem presumptuous to propose that minimum-time was a goal being adopted by good quality writers.

The minimisation of force and impulse is of direct relevance for the control of pen movements and as a general trend in development. Keogh and Sugden (1985) suggest that "children often need to reduce their general and normal force...inhibition in this sense may be the fundamental problem in movement development" (p. 96). A selective integral procedure was used with displacement derivatives for the composite movements of v and w, to yield estimates of total planar force and everage impulse (Wann, 1985). Nelson's (1983) procedure for estimating energy cost was rejected in favour of a total power estimate which Ayoub & Walvekar, i.e.; Ayoub, Ayoub & Walvekar (1974) suggested was "the most suitable mechanical criterion which is sensitive to changes in motion characteristics" (p. 593). All three estimates supported the hypothesis that poor writers tend to produce more forceful, kinetically costly movements. The greater impulse and power cost for the movements of poorer writers could to a large degree, be accounted for by an increase in force levels. While these estimates were not corrected for inter-subject variations in pen-pressure, an analysis of pressure variation using line thickness, suggested that such trends would be unchanged, or at best mildly reinforced by such corrections. These findings strengthen the notion that poorer writers have some difficulty in producing individual pen strokes and that part of the difficulty experienced by such children may be in the control of overforceful movements.

The analysis of jerk (rate of change of acceleration) for the childrens movements also served to highlight control difficulties. As movement control increases, higher derivatives are generally reduced and smoothness of execution marks skilled performance. Hogan (1984) and Flash and Hogan (1985) have suggested the reduction of jerk may be a suitable goal for dictating the organisation of voluntary arm movements. Significantly higher jerk costs for movements performed by poorer writers would seem to indicate a lack of sensitivity to, or inability to modulate, this feature of movement, which in turn may be seen as dependent upon the ability to control force levels.

The application of such an analysis is very much in its infancy. A greater volume of data and reliable estimates of individual variations in normal force are required, before conclusions can be drawn about the extent to which the development of pen control (or the control of other limb movements) can be charted throughout development in terms of the control of force, impulse, power or jerk.

5. TIMEKEEPER CONTROL AND THE NATURE OF TIMING

All of the previous levels of analysis have, to some extent, been dependent upon the ability of the child to initiate or terminate events within some temporal context. Just as pause duration is dictated by the timing of the cessation and subsequent onset of movement, so impulse is dictated by the timing of contractions. A lack of control in producing temporally spaced events amongst poor writers, while not accounting for all the previous findings, could be seen as a major factor in producing degraded performance.

Events occurring within handwriting are generally self paced rather than linked to external stimuli. To test each childs ability to generate self paced responses, a simple tapping task was devised. In the first condition children were asked to tap at a rate of their own choosing upon a metal plate which produced an audio 'bleep' for the period the key was depressed. It was emphasised that they should tap as regular a beat as possible, and were given demonstrations of regular and irregular beats. All children then performed five trials of tapping for 15 seconds, with the final two trials being recorded. A second condition followed an identical procedure but required the children to tap between two 2 cm wide targets which were 8 cm apart. Data were recorded as an analog audio pulse which was subsequently digitised at 200 Hz.

If some children experience difficulty in timing phases of a complex motor task it may be the case that a general timing deficit can be highlighted through the use of purer tests of timekeeper control. The two conditions were used to examine; the initiation of very small movements of almost negligible duration, and the timing of similar simple movements which required the execution and temporal prediction of a short trajectory between two keys. Both key-down, and key-up phases were analysed in addition to the overall tapping period (time between the start of successive key depressions), as it seemed plausible that some children may use an extended key-down period prior to execution of a movement, or use variable key-up periods if experiencing difficulty with the task. An analysis of task differences revealed a predictable increase in the key-up duration for the task requiring travel, $F(1,92) = 20.129$, $p < 0.01$, when this was combined with a slight decrease in keydown duration however, the tapping period was not significantly longer (Table 1).

Older (grade 5) children tapped significantly quicker than grade 4 children, $F(1,28) = 7.054$, $p < 0.01$, although there were no significant differences in tapping rate between good and poor writers (Table 2).

The most useful measure for the analysis of suspected timing difficulties

Table 1. Mean duration (msec) for phases of two tapping conditions performed by primary school children.

TAPPING PHASE[a]	TAPPING CONDITION	
	Implace	Travel
Keydown	114	109
Keyup	249	294
Tap period	364	414

[a] Due to rounding errors during log transformations, the mean tapping period does not equal the sum of the mean keydown and keyup phases.

in self-paced movements would seem to be the coefficient of variation for each phase duration, (standard deviation as a percentage of the mean). Despite being a measure of variability in relative timing, however, there were no significant differences in the variability of tapping performance.

Table 2. Mean duration (msec) for tapping phases performed by primary school children.

GROUP	TAPPING PHASE[a]		
	Keydown	Keyup	Period
Grade 4	121	289	418
Grade 5	102	253	373
Good writers	102	291	408
Poor writers	122	270	400

between good and poor quality writers (Table 3). Given a consistent finding that motor performance differences were predominantly evident between grade 5 writers it is prudent to examine the data for this subgroup. Table 3 indicates that, although not significant, there was a trend across all tapping phases for poor writers to be more variable. Identical findings emerged when the analysis was rechecked using absolute rather than mean adjusted variance values.

Given the lack of any salient findings, one must question the validity of the approach. The results are essentially supportive of the findings from the rhythmic analysis of writing movements, in that given a suitable task, all children were able to produce accurately timed rhythmic movements. The question must be raised as to whether traditional tapping paradigms are effective in highlighting the nature of the timing required by complex motor acts. Where a problem of 'timing' is inferred from the observation of movements kinematics, there is often confusion as to how this equates to time perception, timekeeper control (Wing, 1980), or the timing of muscle bursts (Wallace, 1981). The findings of the previous analyses indicate that although children may not differ in their peformance of a simple 'timing' task, they may still exhibit strong differences in their ability to generate controlled trajectories. Explanations of the latter feature need not include

Table 3. Coefficients of variation for tapping phases performed by primary school children

GROUP	TAPPING PHASE Keydown	Keyup	Period
Good writers	0.2258	0.1564	0.1089
Poor writers	0.2738	0.1512	0.1004
Good writers grade 5	0.2278	0.1374	0.0872
Poor writers grade 5	0.2851	0.1484	0.1038

extensive temporal specifications. Flash and Hogan (1985) have demonstrated that the minimisation of jerk will result in velocity profiles typical of those seen in mature performance. The active avoidance of high jerk costs, along with some overall speed parameter, will serve to dictate much of the inter-segment timing within a complex trajectory. Other constraints are necessary to fully model behaviour, but the broad concept of intra-movement timing dictated by the systems sensitivity to kinematic/kinetic functions is appealling as an alternative to more specific time representations within a motor program.

6. HANDWRITING ACQUISITION: A MOTOR CONTROL PERSPECTIVE

As with many developmental 'difficulties' a vagueness of definition as to what constitutes handwriting difficulties has prevented a reliable assessment of their incidence. As previously mentioned the primary goals of handwriting have been stated to be legibility and speed (Suen, 1983). I would however, argue against directly equating low legibility with writing problems. The direct application of this relation, according to a popular myth, would classify the whole of the medical fraternity as having writing difficulties. It is obvious that a large number of motor-competent adults have poorly legible writing, due to choice, carelessness or ignorance of the ambiguities within their script. The essence of writing difficulties lies in the source of such degraded legibility. Where an ambiguous form (e.g. an "e" with a closed-loop shape) is consistently produced, it may be assumed that attention to form may remedy the problem. When poor quality is due to variability in the size, form and orientation of letters across repetitions however, the problem may go beyond the need for greater care. The aim of this series of studies was to explore the association between differences in the script quality of children, assessed on the above features, and differences in the control of pen movements by such children. The value of such an approach is threefold. Firstly it provides some indication of quantitative measures of writing differences that may be of diagnostic use in the applied setting. Secondly it explores the hypothesis that such differences should not be attributed purely to a childs diligence, effort, or even perceptual abilities, but that genuine difficulties may exist in the ability to control pen movements. Finally, it charts ability related progressions in a fine motor skill that are of interest to the wider issues of control of upper limb movements.

The findings strongly support the notion that it is necessary to acquire stability in the patterning of the composite movements of a writing task, and that poorer quality writers exhibited delay in acquiring this feature. A more detailed analysis of individual pen strokes suggested that such variability across trials may, in part, have been due to the use of less mature movement patterns which allowed greater visual monitoring and closed-loop control. The suggestion of a need for greater feedback processing is supported by the use of longer duration pauses by poor writers. Together these observations point towards an inability on the part of poorer writers to program writing strokes for execution without extensive within-movement monitoring. If this were the sole cause of such writing difficulties, then much of this appraisal could have been replaced by an assessment of each childs ability to perform simple rapid aiming movements. It must be emphasised however, that proficiency is dependent not only on the control of individual movements, but on the linking and phasing of these, as well as the efficient use of visual and kinaesthetic cues to monitor and adjust form. The control of force and the ability to reduce the jerk content of pen movements also seem to be problem areas and worthy of attention from both an applied and a theoretical perspective.

7. FUTURE DIRECTIONS

There is a need for more detailed research into the development of control of writing dynamics, particularly in respect to the control of normal force (pen pressure) and its interaction with planar movements. In developmental studies however, I would suggest there is a need to explore an avenue that has received little attention in adult studies, and monitor the control of limb movements. Work currently in progress suggests that some of the previously assumed roles of the fingers, wrist and forearm in vertical and horizontal pen displacement may be misleading. In addition initial data from adult subjects (n= 2), has suggested that some degree of invariance may be retained over proximal (wrist, forearm) joint movements, over small changes in script size (up to 80% above preferred size), with adjustments presumably being made in patterns of phalangeal extension/ flexion. The development of inter-link coordination of the writing limb is necessary for effective pen control, just as the development of throwing skills requires a refinement of patterns of upper limb coordination (Wickstrom, 1977). The influence of pen grip upon the freedom and flexibility of the effector system, also warrants investigation. Ziviani (1983) suggested that penholds may undergo developmental changes, which on preliminary inspection would appear to increase the 'degrees of freedom' and flexibility of the effector. Specifically a reduction in, proximal interphalangeal flexion and distal interphalengeal hyperextension with age, should increase the potential range of finger movements. Whereas a reduction in forearm pronation, frees the restrictions that are placed on horizontal movements by limited ulnar deviation of the wrist, and allows horizontal pen shifts by wrist extension. When children modify and refine patterns of pen movements, they do so by modulating the respective movements of the writing limb. Where difficulties arise, some account of patterns of limb movement may be of value both to developmental research and in the applied setting for remediation.

References

Athenes, S. (1984). *Adaptabilite et development de la posture manuelle dans l'ercriture.* Unpublished Masters thesis, University of Marseille.

Ayoub, M.A., Ayoub, M.M. & Walvekar, A.G. (1974). A biomechanical model for the upper extremity using optimisation techniques. *Human Factors, 16,* 585-594.

Broer, M.R. & Zernicke, R.F. (1979). *Efficiency of Human Movement.* Philadelphia: W.B. Saunders.

Flash, T. & Hogan, N. (1985). The coordination of arm movements: an experimentally confirmed mathematical model. *Journal of Neuroscience, 5,* 1688-1703.

Gentner, D.R. (1982). Evidence against a central model of timing in typing. *Journal of Experimental Psychology: Human Perception and Performance, 8,* 793-810.

Greer, K.L. & Green, D.W. (1983). Context and motor control in handwriting. *Acta Psychologica, 54,* 205-215.

Grillner, S. (1981). Control of locomotion in bipeds, tetrapods and fish: In V.B. Brooks (Ed.), *Handbook of Physiology, the Nervous System II: Motor Control.* American Physiology Society.

Harris, T.L. & Rarick, G.L. (1959). The relationship between handwriting pressure and legibility of handwriting in children and adolescents. *Journal of Experimental Education, 28,* 65-86.

Hay, L. (1979). Spatial-temporal analysis of movements in children: motor programs versus feedback in the development of reaching. *Journal of Motor Behavior, 11,* 189-200.

Hay, L. (1984). A discontinuity in the development of motor control in children. In W. Prinz and A.F. Sanders (Eds.), *Cognition and Motor Processes.* Berlin: Springer-Verlag.

Hinton, G. (1984). Parallel computations for controlling an arm. *Journal of Motor Behavior, 16,* 171-194.

Hogan, N. (1984). An organising principle for a class of voluntary movements. *Journal of Neuroscience, 4,* 2745-2754.

Hollerbach, J.M. (1981). An oscillation theory of handwriting. *Biological Cybernetics, 39,* 139-156.

Kao, H.S.R. (1979). Handwriting ergonomics. *Visible Language, 13,* 331-339.

Kao, H.S.R. (1983). Progressive motion variability in handwriting tasks. *Acta Psychologica, 54,* 149-159.

Keogh, J. & Sugden, D. (1985). *Movement Skill Development.* New York: Macmillan.

Laszlo, J.I. & Bairstow, P.J. (1983). Kinaesthesis: its measurement, training and relationship to motor control. *Quarterly Journal of Experimental Psychology, 35A,* 411-421.

Levy, J. & Reid, M. (1978). Variations in cerebral organisation as a function of handedness, hand posture in writing and sex. *Journal of Experimental Psychology: General, 107,* 119-144.

Morasso, P. (1983). Coordination aspects of arm trajectory formation. *Human Movement Science, 2,* 197-210.

Mounoud, P., Viviani, P., Hauert, C.A. & Guyon, J. (in press). Development of visuomanual tracking in 5 to 9 year olds boys. *Journal of Experimental Child Psychology.*

Nelson, W.L. (1983). Physical principles for economies of skilled movements. *Biological Cybernetics, 46,* 135-147.

Nihei, Y. (1983). Developmental change in covert principles for the organisation of strokes in drawing and handwriting. *Acta Psychologica, 54,* 221-232.

Rubin, N. & Henderson, S.E. (1982). Two sides of the same coin? Variability in instructional practices in handwriting and the problems of those who fail to learn to write. *Special Education: Forward Trends, 9,* 17-24.

Sassoon, R., Nimmo-Smith, I. & Wing, A.M. (in press). An analysis of childrens penholds. In H.S.R. Kao (Ed.), *Graphonomics: Contemporary Research in Handwriting.*

Smoll, F.L. (1975). Variability in development of spatial and temporal elements of rhythmic ability. *Perceptual and Motor Skills, 40,* 140.

Sovik, N. (1979). Some instructional parameters related to childrens copying performance. *Visible Language, 13,* 314-330.

Sovik, N. (1981). An experimental study of individualised learning/ instruction in copying, tracking and handwriting based on feedback principles. *Perceptual and Motor Skills, 53,* 195-215.

Suen, C.Y. (1983). Handwriting generation, perception and recognition. *Acta Psychologica, 54,* 295-312.

Thelen, E. & Fischer, D.M. (1983). The organisation of spontaneous by movements in newborn infants. *Journal of Motor Behavior, 15,* 353-377.

Thomassen, A.J.W.M. & Teulings, H.E. (1983). Constancy in stationary and progressive handwriting. *Acta Psychologica, 54,* 179-196.

Todor, J.I. (1980). Sequential motor ability of left-handed inverted and non-inverted writers. *Acta Psychologica, 44,* 165-173.

Viviani, P. & Terzuolo, C. (1980). Space-time invariance in learned motor skills. In G.E. Stelmach and J. Requin (Eds.), *Tutorials in Motor Behaviour.* Amsterdam: North-Holland.

Wann, J.P. Trends in the optimisation and refinement of a fine motor skill: Observations from a further analysis of the handwriting of primary school children. *Journal of Motor Behavior* (submitted Sept. 1985).

Wann, J.P. & Jones, J.G. (in press). Time invariance in handwriting: contrasts between primary school children displaying advanced or retarded handwriting acquisition. *Human Movement Science.*

Weber, A.M. (1983). Capacity to vary writing hand/posture in relation to the Levy and Reid model for control of writing. *Journal of Motor Behavior, 15,* 19-28.

Wickstrom, R.L. (1977). *Fundamental Motor Patterns,* 2nd edition. Philadelphia: Lea & Febiger.

Wing, A.M. (1980). The long and short of timing in response sequences. In G.E. Stelmach and J. Requin (Eds.), *Tutorials in Motor Behaviour.* Amsterdam: North-Holland.

Ziviani, J. (1983). Qualitative changes in dynamic tripod grip between seven and 14 years of age. *Developmental Medicine & Child Neurology, 25,* 778-782.

SECTION 4

PERCEPTUAL AND COGNITIVE CONTROL OF MOTOR BEHAVIOUR

NORMAL AND ABNORMAL REPETITIVE STEREOTYPED BEHAVIOURS

G. Berkson and R.J. Gallagher

In this paper, we address the transition between the normal repetitive behaviours of infancy and the abnormal stereotyped movements of severely handicapped children and adults. The focus of the discussion assumes that, as children grow, the environment increasingly influences their motor behaviour. We believe that the pathology of stereotyped behaviours represents a reflection not only of the pathology of the children but more particularly a failure of the child-environment interaction.

Thelen (1981, p. 245) has expressed our view quite well:

> Rhythmical stereotypes may also assume a variety of functional ends. Varying with the infant's current needs and motor capabilities, stereotyped movements may provide a means of self-stimulation,contingent control over people and objects, exercise, and communication, and probably serve other functions as well. Thus, although orginating and sometimes functioning as almost automatic "by-products" of motor maturation, stereotypies may also become instrumental behaviour.

NORMAL AND ABNORMAL STEREOTYPED BEHAVIOURS

Interest in abnormal stereotyped behaviours comes both from their similarities to and differences from the normal repetitive behaviours of infancy. It is likely that all of these repetitive behaviours are similar in that they are suppressed when the individual cognitively engages the environment. They are also similar in that they are increased when the individual is *not* engaged with the environment but is behaviourally aroused.

While there may be similarities between abnormal stereotyped behaviours and the normal repetitive behaviours of infancy, there are at least some differences. The most obvious difference is that the abnormal activities are extended in time. For instance, individual bouts are longer. As may be seen in Figure 1, one difference between the body rocking and hand-gazing of severely retarded children and of normal infants of the same developmental age is that the retarded children continue a movement longer in a bout once they have started it.

In addition to carrying it on longer within a session, abnormal stereotyped behaviours continue without much change in form for extended periods. Miller (1984) for instance, has shown that blind developmentally disabled 4-year-old to 10-year-old children continue a stereotyped behaviour without

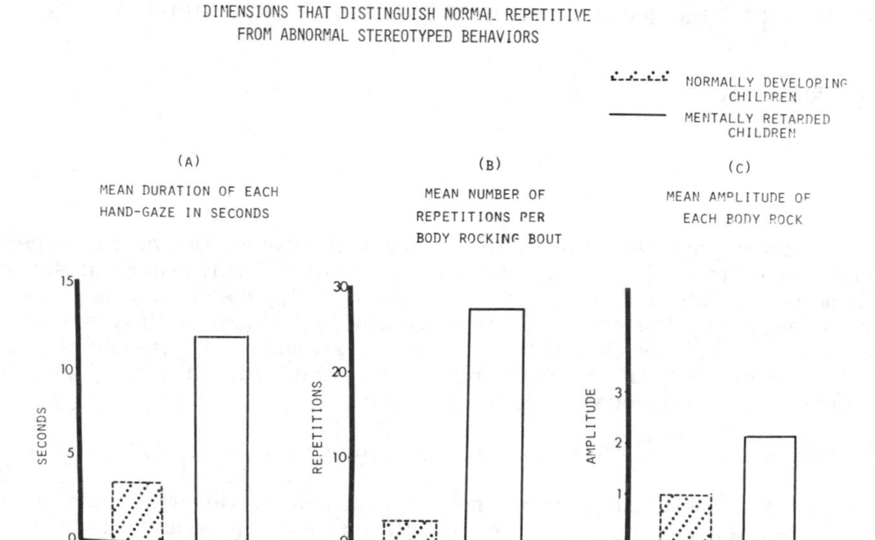

Fig. 1. Behavioural dimensions that distinguish normal repetitive from abnormal stereotyped behaviours.

significant change in form for at least two years. Also older children and adults continue to perform certain stereotyped behaviours like body-rocking well beyond the time that they supposedly promoted motor development.

The importance of the unchanging nature of abnormal stereotypy despite significant progress in general motor development is that it puts into question the hypothesis that stereotypy serves to promote motor development. The notion that stereotypy has a function in motor development comes from the observation of a coincidence in time between the various normal repetitive behaviours of infancy and various stages of motor development. The data that we alluded to above and also casual observations of stereotypy in people who walk around normally suggest that stereotypy is not necessarily connected in time with normal stages of development. This means that while it is still possible that *normal* repetitive behaviours do promote normal motor development, they may also be a consequence of motor development, be independent, and/or take on other functions later.

So much for the relationship between general motor development, on the one hand, and normal repetitive behaviours and abnormal stereotyped movements on the other. Now we turn to a consideration of the relationship between normal repetitive behaviours of infancy and abnormal stereotyped behaviours. Here another unique aspect of abnormal stereotyped behaviour becomes important. In addition to being more extended in time, abnormal stereotyped behaviours tend to be more elaborate than the normal repetitive behaviours of infancy. There are no formal studies demonstrating the greater complexity of abnormal stereotyped behaviours within and across individuals but it is likely that this is the case. It is possible that abnormal stereotyped behaviours begin as one of the normal repetitive behaviours of infancy and then become elaborated. This view is probably correct, but it should be pointed out that the longitudinal studies that would be necessary to demonstrate this progression are difficult to perform and, in fact, have not yet been accomplished. Thus, the notion that abnormal stereotyped behaviours develop out of the normal repetitive behaviours of infancy actually has no empirical basis at present. The alternative, that at least some stereotyped behaviours have another developmental course, is at least as plausible. Consider, for instance, eye-poking and elaborate forms of string-twirling. It is perhaps difficult to identify the normal infant repetitive behaviours that regularly precede these common stereotyped behaviours.

Up to this point, we have been discussing the relationships between abnormal stereotyped behaviours, the normal repetitive behaviours of infancy and general motor development. Our general points have been that abnormal stereotyped behaviours differ from normal infant repetitive behaviours in important ways and that we need more research to show how these classes of behaviour are related.

We turn now to a third way in which abnormal stereotyped behaviours differ from the normal repetitive behaviours of infancy, that is, their time course. In this section, we use a difference in time course to explore the determinants of abnormal stereotyped behaviours.

Each of the normal repetitive behaviours of infancy remains in the behaviour repertoire for a brief time, a matter of weeks (Thelen, 1979), and the behaviour class as a whole tends to disappear as the young child becomes older. Exactly the reverse seems to be true of abnormal stereotyped behaviours. As we indicated above, individual stereotyped behaviours remain in the repertoire for years. Also, as may be seen in Figure 2, there is an increment (not a decrement) in the expression of abnormal stereotyped

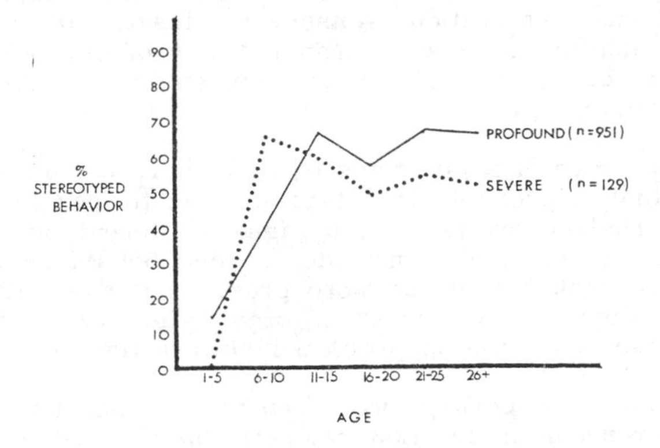

Fig. 2. The relationship between chronological age and abnormal stereotyped behaviours in severely and profoundly retarded people.

behaviours with age. This finding of an increase in the abnormal stereotyped behaviours with chronological age has been replicated in several samples (Berkson et al, 1985; Thompson & Berkson, 1985).

Of most interest is that the relationship is with chronological age specifically. In studying severely retarded children, it sometimes is possible to separate correlates of developmental age from correlates of chronological age. This is obviously not true in normal children in whom developmental and chronological age are completely confounded. However, in one study (Thompson & Berkson, 1985), developmental and chronological age were not correlated very strongly (r= .27) so that estimating possible separate correlates with abnormal stereotyped behaviours was possible. Similar to Figure 2, there was an increase of stereotyped behaviours with chronological age. At the same time, there was a negative correlation of abnormal stereotyped behaviours with developmental age (-.40), as one would expect with normal infant repetitive behaviours. In summary, then, it appears that abnormal stereotyped behaviours decline with developmental age, as do infant repetitive behaviours, but they increase with chronological age, opposite from the case with normal repetitive behaviours.

EARLY HISTORY AND ABNORMAL BEHAVIOURS

The negative correlation between developmental age and abnormal stereotyped behaviours is probably attributable to the increasing tendency to engage the environment cognitively which occurs with age in the normal child and which tends to interfere with stereotyped behaviours. However, to what can we attribute the increase in abnormal behaviours with chronological age?

We believe that the general answer to this question is that there is a disruption in the normal interaction between the child and his or her physical and/or social environment. We attribute the increase of abnormal stereotyped behaviours to a cumulative effect of a pathological child-environment interaction. We emphasise that while a pathological child-environment interaction may be a common explanation for all cases of increasing stereotypy with age, the specific causes of the problem can differ. Thus, depriving institutionalisation, maternal deprivation, sensory handicap, and autistic processes are all ways of reaching the final common pathway of deficient child-environment interaction. All of these factors have been shown to increase abnormal stereotyped behaviours.

There are several implications of this view. Let us mention just two. The first is that it probably is not productive to look for any single problem (such as maternal deprivation) as a cause of stereotyped behaviours. In fact, there are many cases of abnormal stereotyped behaviours. In any particular child, one must look for one or more problems that might be unique to the child. Thus, when one detects an *abnormal* stereotyped behaviour, one can look for an associated unique problem in interaction with the environment.

The second, and perhaps more important implication, is that analysis of the child-environment interaction problem allows a reduction of the abnormalities. It has been known for at least 25 years that providing a person with something interesting to do reduces stereotyped behaviours at the time the person is engaging in the alternative behaviour (e.g. Berkson & Davenport, 1962). However, we are really interested in doing more than reducing stereotypy momentarily. We would like to eliminate the abnormality completely in the treatment situation and also see to it that the abnormality is not expressed in situations other than that into which we intervene. The general focus of the studies that we now present is an analysis of the child-environment pathology in the early developmental period and a test of the effect of an experimental intervention in a situation different from the one in which the intervention is done.

The first study is one done several years ago with William A. Mason (Mason & Berkson, 1975). In this study, rhesus monkeys were reared from birth away from their natural mothers in isolation under two conditions. The conventional control condition was a large cage containing a furcovered surrogate-mother which remained stationary. The experimental condition was identical with the control except that the surrogate mother moved around the cage providing a ride for the infant and something for it to play with.

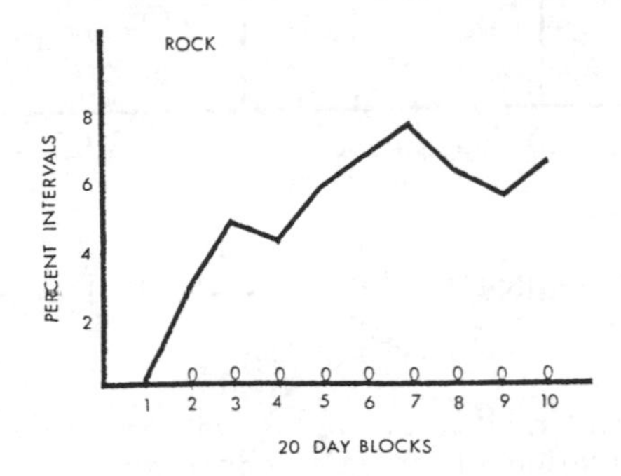

Fig. 3. Level of body rocking of monkeys reared on moving or stationary surrogate-mothers.

Figure 3 shows the results. The stationary-surrogate group showed an increment in body rocking with age in the home cage, and they showed a similar elevation of body rocking in a testing situation. At the same time, animals in the moving surrogate condition never demonstrated a significant amount of body rocking at all. This says that the body rocking which is a consequence of conventional isolation-rearing can be eliminated by "correcting" the environment.

While at first sight, this "correction" might seem to be providing "vestibular" stimulation, let us emphasise that the original paper in which this study was reported mentioned proprioceptive-kinaesthetic stimulation as a possibility and also pointed out that the moving surrogate condition evoked vigorous play. Thus, the basis of the effect is still an open question. The main point, of course, was that with a complex intervention, it was possible to eliminate an abnormal stereotyped behaviour.

EARLY INTERVENTION FOR ABNORMAL BEHAVIOURS

The next figure (Figure 4) shows the results of another intervention accomplished over several weeks with a severely retarded two-year-old institutionalised boy who engaged in hand-gazing. In this case, we increased the amount of occupational therapy he received so that someone was playing

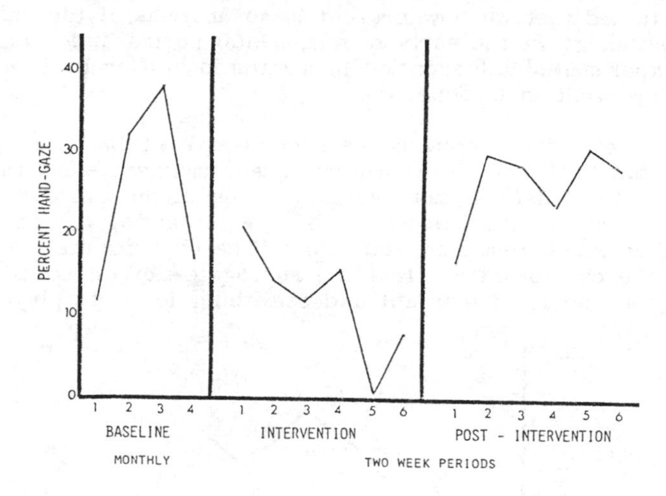

Fig. 4. The effect of general intervention on hand-gazing behaviours.

and/or carrying the child during all of his waking hours. As may be seen from a brief testing situation in which intervention was not done, there was a general decrement in hand-gazing over the weeks of intervention followed by an increment when intervention was withdrawn. This was accompanied by an increment in manipulation of toys (see Figure 5) followed by a decline.

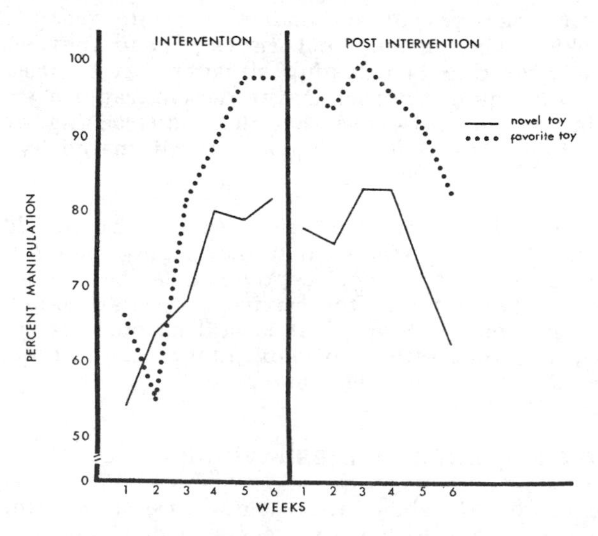

Fig. 5. The effect of general intervention on toy manipulation.

The first study with children demonstrated therefore that a generalised intensive normalisation of the environment can decrease abnormal stereotyped behaviour. In other words, these behaviours can be modified even in very handicapped children.

These studies with generalised modifications of the environment are informative in that they show that one can normalise child-environment interaction and produce a desired effect even with severely handicapped children.

Such a generalised approach may be necessary in some cases. However, there are other cases where a more focussed treatment is as effective and may be more informative. Figure 6 displays the consequences on hand-gazing of fitting a child with glasses. In this case, a mother had been told by her pediatrician that the hand-gazing of her multiply-handicapped two-year-old son was a consequence of his "cognitive delay". From casual observation, it seemed to us, instead, that he was looking at his hands because he was very near-sighted. The test of this, of course, was to have his eyes examined and, if necessary, to provide visual correction. This was done. The data in Figure 6 show that when he had glasses on, the hand-gazing was essentially eliminated. In fact, there was a dramatic change in his posture and in his visual scanning of the distant environment which apparently competed with his stereotyped behaviours.

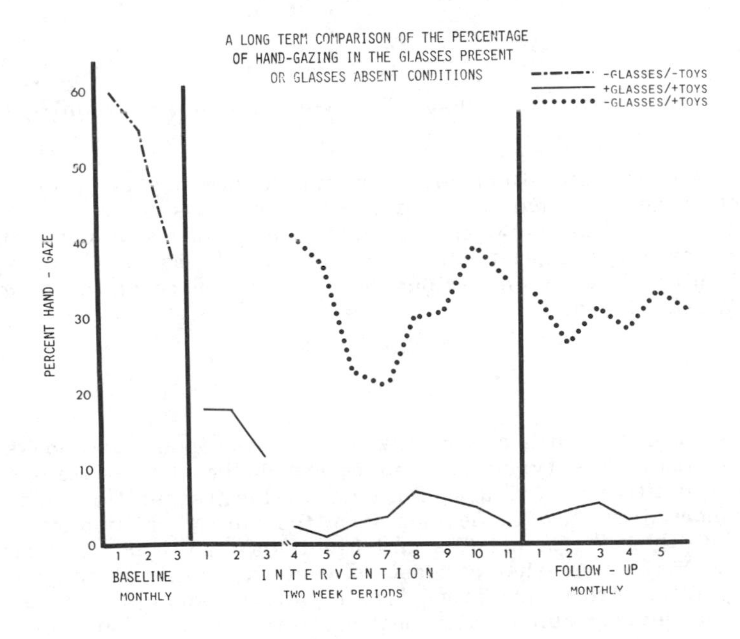

Fig. 6. The long-term effect of glasses on hand-gazing.

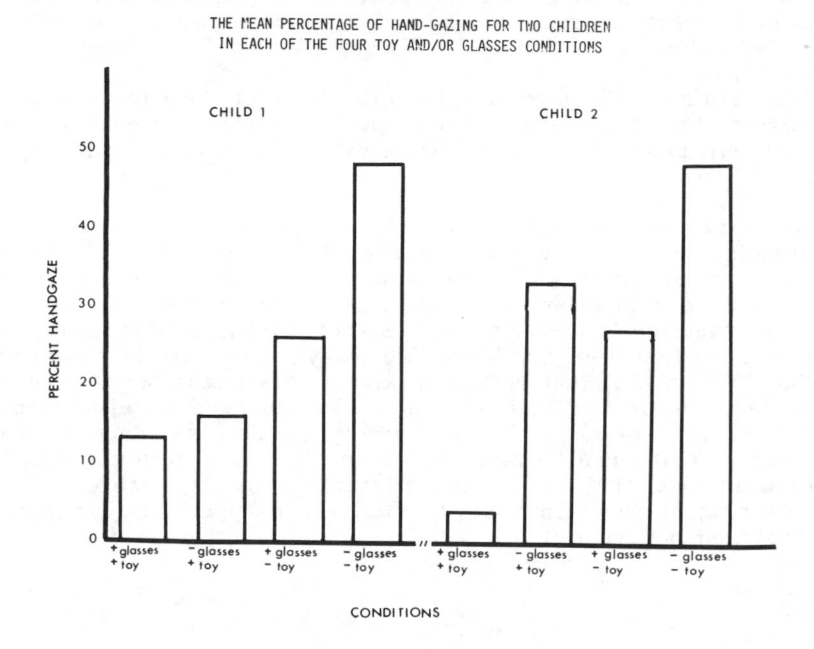

Fig. 7. The short-term effect of glasses and toys on hand-gazing.

Figure 7 shows the effects of providing toys and glasses to this child and to another severely handicapped two-year old. As may be seen, providing the conditions of normal child-environment interactions seems immediately to reduce the stereotypy dramatically and thereby informs us of the specific child-environment interaction problem that is the source of the abnormal stereotyped behaviours.

CONCLUSIONS

Let us close now with a summary of our major points. It looks as though abnormal stereotyped behaviours are different in several ways from the normal repetitive behaviours of infancy. This is consistent with the view that the abnormal movements develop from the normal behaviours and that they take on other characteristics and functions. However, it is also consistent with the view that at least some of the abnormal behaviours develop separately from the normal infant patterns. Longitudinal research examining the development of abnormal stereotyped behaviours can clarify the picture.

The prevalence of abnormal stereotyped behaviours decreases with developmental age but increases with chronological age. This suggests that while children normally engage the environment cognitively, there are a variety of conditions in which this occurs less efficiently. The result is an increase in abnormal stereotyped behaviours that ultimately dominates the behaviour repertoire.

These abnormalities can, however, be minimised with procedures that promote the child's normal interaction with the physical and social environment. Depending on the specific child, the procedures may be quite complex or very specific and simple. Above all, whether complex or simple, with many children they are within the range of current technology.

ACKNOWLEDGEMENTS

The research reported here was supported in part by a grant from the U.S. National Institute for Child Health and Human Development (HD 15008). We are indebted to the parents and children who participated in the research.

References

Berkson, G. & Davenport, R.K. Jr. (1962). Stereotyped movements of mental defectives, I: Initial survey. *American Journal of Mental Deficiency, 66,* 849-852.

Berkson, G., McQuiston, S., Jacobson, J.W., Eyman, R. & Borthwick, S. (1985). The relationship between age and stereotyped behaviours. *Mental Retardation, 23,* 31-33.

Mason, W.A. & Berkson, G. (1975). Effects of maternal reliability on the development of rocking and other behaviors in rhesus monkey: A study with artificial mothers. *Developmental Psychobiology, 8,* 197-211.

Miller, L.K. (1984). Stability of multiple stereotypies in handicapped children. Paper presented at the American Psychological Association. Toronto, Canada.

Thelen, E. (1979). Rhythmical stereotypies in normal human infants. *Animal Behaviour, 27,* 699-715.

Thelen, E. (1981). Rhythmical behavior in infancy: An ethological perspective. *Developmental Psychology, 17,* 237-257.

Thompson, T.J. & Berkson, G. (1985). Stereotyped behavior of severely disabled children in classroom and free-play settings. *American Journal of Mental Deficiency, 89,* 580-586.

INHIBITORY MECHANISMS IN CHILDREN'S SKILL DEVELOPMENT

J.I. Todor and J.C. Lazarus

We have been studying the involvement of innate neuromuscular synergies in voluntary movement. However, rather than focusing on how they might be useful building blocks for volitional acts, we have focused on situations where the synergy is undesireable, that is, when it may interfere with or be counter productive to the completion of the intended act. For example, a favorite trick of a person in our laboratory is to attempt to open her office door with a cup of coffee in the other hand. Both hands rotate, spilling the coffee.

The studies described here, address the issue of inhibiting neuromuscular synergies. However, we do propose that the developing child must also frequently inhibit other easily activated components of action, such as salient or misleading percepts or overlearned response patterns, in order to be successful on novel tasks. For, example, we have used a modified version of Piaget's Water Level Test with children of various ages (Todor & Lazarus, 1981; Todor & Lazarus, 1982; Lazarus, 1985). Briefly, the child is presented with an outline drawing of bottles tilted at various angles and asked to draw in the water line as if the bottles were half-full.

Children 6 years of age and less typically respond quickly, drawing a line perpendicular to the sides of the bottles regardless of the bottles spatial orientation. That is, they produced a response based on the overlearned view of liquids in upright containers. In the 7 to 10 year old range (and some adults), the task is more likely to be performed slowly and with a great deal of apparent effort. These ages usually can inhibit the overlearned response but are not able to produce the correct one. Responses often vary from trial to trial. By 10 years of age, the responses are more appropriate to the bottle orientation. However, periodic regressions to an earlier response pattern are observed, suggesting that an active competition between response modes is still occurring. On a number of occassions, we have observed children who started to draw the appropriate water line but then reverted to the overlearned response (seen in 6 year olds) before comple completing the trial. It is as if they were not able to sustain the inhibition of this response.

We have observed a similar behaviour when children are asked to perform a walk-slow task like that used by Constantini and Holving (1973). First, baseline measurements of normal walking rates are obtained. Then, the child is asked to walk as slowly as possible without stopping. We tested 7 to 8 year olds and found a sizeable subgroup of children who initially walk slow, for about 1/2 the distance, and then reverted to their normal pace.

The problem of inhibition is especially important when you consider that over time children exhibit marked changes in the way they perform a given task. Attempts to respond using a more sophisticated strategy often requires the inhibition of the previous response tendency. Consider another example where maturational and performance variables interact. We have attempted to look at sequencing ability in children by having them perform a single finger tapping task. In many 6 year olds you get:

a) whole hand movements or at least simultaneous movement of the second finger,

or,

b) efforts to keep the fingers from moving such as curling the fingers into a fist, or, stiffening of the fingers. In all cases the act of tapping is dramatically changed. Eric Roy (personal communication, 1985) has observed similar behaviour in adult apraxic when they attempt to do single finger tapping. The point here, is that in both the young children and the adult apraxics, ineffectual or slow finger tapping may have as much or more to do with the inability to inhibit extraneous actions as it does with co-ordinating the successive up-down-up action of the index finger.

In a series of experiments, we evaluated the type of neuromuscular synergy that has been referred to as: associated movements (Fog & Fog, 1963), synkinesis (Cambier & Dehen, 1977), motor overflow (Yensen, 1965), or mirror movements (Green, 1967). In this group Prechtl (Touwen & Prechtl, 1970), Connolly (Connolly & Stratton, 1968) and Wolff (Wolff, Gunnoe & Cohen, 1983) have all described various manifestations of this phenomenon.

We have specifically looked at the tendency for the action of the two hands to be linked. The most commonly reported linkage is one that supports simultaneous symmetrical or mirror movements. Kelso, Southard and Goodman (1979) describe a bilateral aiming task that is a good example of this linkage. Developmentally, Elliott and Connolly (1973) found young children to exhibit asymmetrical simultaneous bilateral actions at a later age than simultaneous symmetrical actions.

The consensus in the literature is that mirror movements and associated movements in general, become less frequent with increasing age. That is, these actions which are involuntary and unrelated to the purpose of the primary action, decline with age (for example, squeezing one hand and getting involuntary squeezing in the other hand). Recently, Wolff et al (1983), have argued that associated movements may be a good indicator of developmental age. Similarly, in the clinical literature, excessive associated movements are often taken to indicate a developmental delay or as a soft sign of CNS dysfunction (Cohen, Taft, Mahadeviah & Birch, 1967; Touwen & Prechtl, 1970).

With regards to the developmental trend, we have been concerned with two issues:

1) the extent to which this decrease in associated movements is maturationally regulated; and,

2) the extent to which the child's ability to appropriately direct his/her resources, including inhibition and allocation of attention, plays a role in regulating associated movements. At some age these two factors may both contribute, but, at earlier or later ages, one or the other may be the primary limiting factor.

In order to address these concerns, we had to deal with a number of related issues. First, we focused on developing a method of obtaining quantitative data (Todor & Lazarus, in press). With a few exceptions, the previously existing data comes from studies where the frequency of associated movements observed was noted across trials. Often, a subjective rating of the intensity was also made.

A second measurement concern stemmed from the fact that most previous studies did not systematically regulate the intensity of the active hand contraction. For example, Fog and Fog (1963) and others (Cohen et al, 1967; Connolly & Stratton, 1968) have reported the frequency of associated movements to decrease with increasing age on a clip pinching task. Children were asked to squeeze a bulldog clip with one hand and movements in the other hand were noted. Age differences were compared when all children used the same clip. However, when a stiffer clip was used, the frequency of associated movements went up in all ages. Since older children are typically stronger, it is highly likely that on any given clip they were performing at a lower percentage of their capacity to exert force. This factor may well have resulted in underestimating older children's associated movements.

Our apparatus was a modification of Fog and Fog's (1963) clip pinching task (see Figure 1). Two parallel steel bars were attached to a wooden platform that was secured to a desk. Strain gauges were mounted on the inner surface of the lateral bar for each hand. The output of the strain gauges were amplified, displayed on an oscilloscope, and fed into a computer for analysis. The oscilloscope displayed a horizontal line which rose in proportion to the force of the contraction of the active hand.

Each child was seated on an adjustable stool facing the apparatus described above. The forearms were positioned and secured with velcro straps to the armrests. The child was instructed to place the thumb and index finger of each hand on the outside of the squeeze bars at a standardised location. The thumbs were positioned such that they were in alignment with the radial side of the forearm, restricting the squeezing movement to flexion of the index finger. The rest of the fingers were wrapped around wooden dowels projecting from the horizontal armrests.

After determining the child's maximal volitional force (MVF) they performed a series of trials at 25, 50, 75 and 100% of their MVF. On all trials they were instructed to keep the other thumb/finger motionless. The order of hand use was counterbalanced across subject. A five minute interval occurred between the use of the hands in the reverse role.

In the first study (Todor & Lazarus, in press), forty-two 7-8 year old children were tested, half male and half female. All were right-handed.

There was a highly significant main effect due to active hand force level. The intensity of associated movements increased only slightly between 25% and 50% MVF, but increased dramatically in intensity at 75% and 100% MVF. At 100% MVF, associated movements ranged in intensity from 13.3% to 62.7% of the active hand force. Thus, for many children, the associated movements were not trivial.

In addition to looking at the relationship between active hand force and associated movements, we addressed the issue of lateral asymmetries. Most previous studies that discussed this issue report more frequent associated movements when the non-dominant left hand was active (Cohen et al, 1967; Davis, 1942; Stern, Gold, Hoin & Barocas, 1976; Touwen & Prechtl,

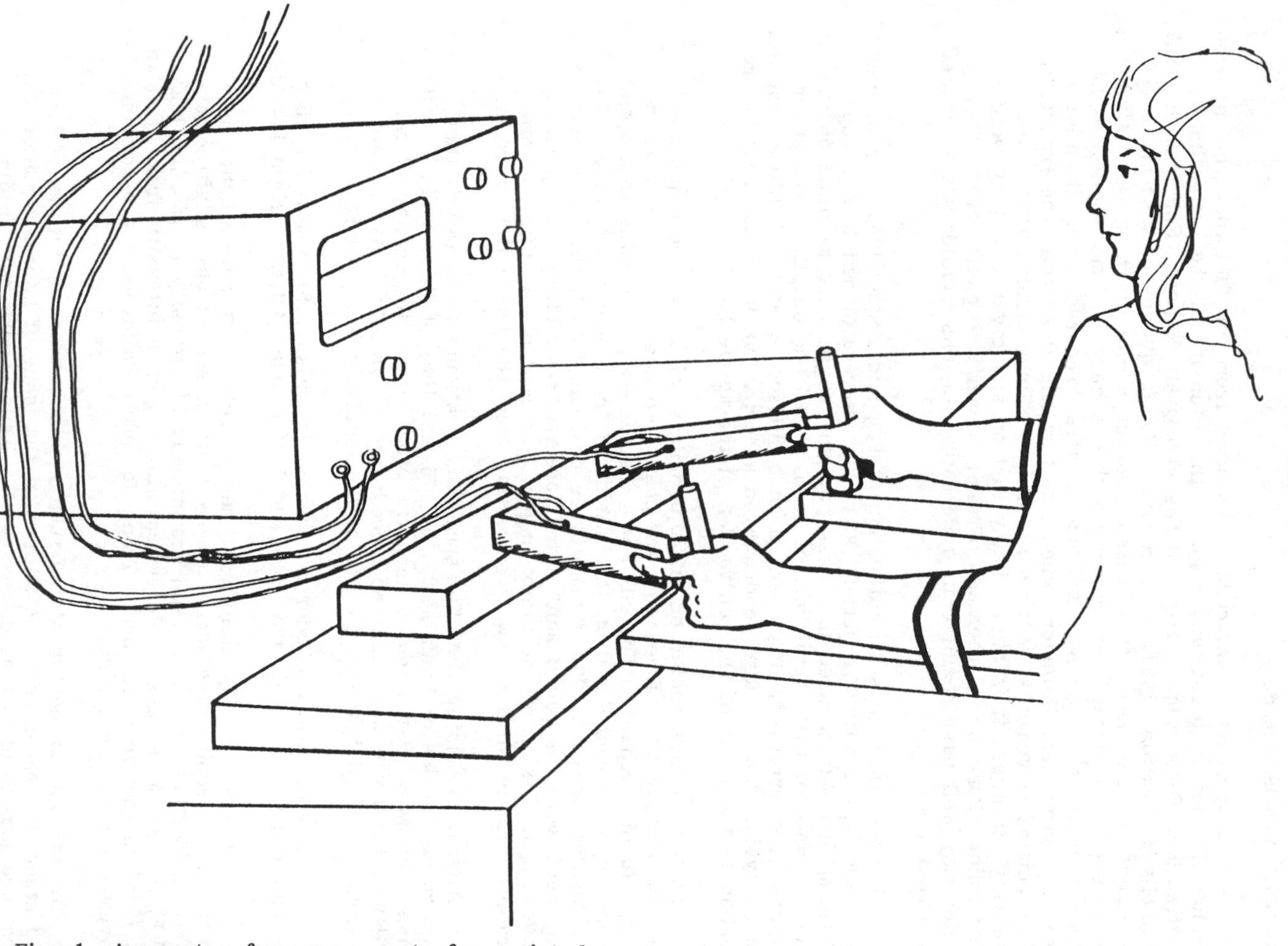

Fig. 1. Apparatus for assessment of associated movements.

1970; Wolff et al, 1983).

Our concern was rooted in the measurement issues: (1) would the asymmetry be present when the "intensity" of associated movements rather than "frequency" was the dependent measure, and, (2) since in previous studies, a standard task was used by both hands, it is conceivable that the typically weaker left hand would have been working at a higher percentage of it's MVF. If this were the case, associated movements measured in the right hand may have been inflated.

Our data support the previous findings. The associated movements were significantly more intense in the right hand when the left hand was active compared to the converse.

At least three non-independent factors may contribute to the observed lateral asymmetry. First, according to the position taken by Semmes (1968), motor activity is viewed as being more focally organised in the left hemisphere and more diffusely represented in the right. Hence, right hand activity (left hemisphere) may be structurally more resistent to spreading. Although Semmes position has not been well accepted, there does not appear to be any direct evidence to refute it. Indirect support reported by Halsey, Blavenstein, Wilson and Wills (1979) indicates that Rolandic cerebral blood flow during left hand movement was greater than blood flow during comparable right hand movements. Accordingly, the amount of blood flow is viewed as indicative of neuronal activity.

Secondly, Kimura and Archibald (1974) have argued that the left hemisphere plays a role in the motor function of both hands. Thus, when the left hand is active, neuronal activity would occur in both the right and left hemispheres, increasing the potential for spread to the motor area in the left hemisphere that controls the right hand. However, right hand movements would involve a circumscribed area restricted to the left hemisphere and primarily affect contralateral pathways to the right hand.

Finally, the differential use of the preferred right hand may lead to the development of more refined patterns of neuronal activity. This implies that left hand movements, typically being less efficient, would involve a more diffuse network of neurons, which conceivably leads to greater associated movements.

As mentioned earlier, movements of the "passive" hand off the bar were noted. These movements were typically involved extension and were often forceful. We have referred to these actions as heterologous to emphasize that the action is opposite to the active hand, i.e., extension rather than flexion.

In this experiment we did not quantify the heretologous movements, but did note their relative frequency. The fact that they occurred on 17% of the trials suggests they were not due to momentary lapses in attention to the task, but were involuntary co-contractions. For this reason we believe heterologeous movements are an alternative form of a common phenomenon.

A final issue we addressed in the first experiment was that of the order of hand use. This issue was of concern because we had previously found order effects in rapid single finger tapping that were so pronounced that they obscured the typically observed right hand superiority (Todor & Smiley-

Oyen, 1985). We were curious to see if such an effect would be present in the current task involving simple forceful flexion.

There was a significant hand by order interaction. Hand differences existed in the R/L order but not the L/R order. Since there was a significant hand difference when the data of the two orders were pooled, there appears to be both a lateral asymmetry and an order effect in the intensity of associated movements. Apparently, the order effect is sufficient to obscure hand differences in the L/R order.

One thing to note is that associated movements were greater when the hand had previously been active. Therefore, it is conceivable that a post-contraction potentiation of nerve or muscle such as that described by Hutton (1985) was operating. However, according to Hutton, these effects have not been observed to persist for more than two minutes post-contraction. In this experiment, approximately five minutes intervened between the hand being in the "active" and "passive" role. Additionally, the effect apparently persisted through a series of 3 trials and 4 levels of force.

A second potential causal factor may be the priming of a given hemisphere in a manner similar to that described by Kinsbourne (1970), albeit, in a different context. In this case, prior contraction may leave the controlling contralateral hemisphere differentially susceptible to activation, leading to enhanced associated movements. At this point, both explanations are speculative. As a first step in understanding the nature of this order effect we are attempting to replicate it using a within-subject design.

In a second set of experimens, we used the same apparatus to look at the developmental trend. In this case, we tested male children 6, 8, 10, 12 and 16 years of age, approximately 30/age. To get a measure of their best performance/least associated movements, we had all children use only their dominant right hand in the active role. To control for large age differences in strength, the dependent measure of associated movements was expressed as the percentage of the active hand's MVF.

Six year old children were found to differ from all older ages at all active hand force levels. There were no significant differences between the other age groups. Six year olds showed their greatst increase in associated movements between 50% and 75% MVF, while all older groups had their greatest increase in associated movements between 75% and 100% of their MVF. As an interesting aside, when age differences in absolute grams of force were analysed, we got a U-shaped function at 100% MVF. The 6 year olds and 16 year olds showed the most intense associated movements.

Since the magnitude of associated movements increased with increasing active hand force, one might postulate that the mechanism of inhibiting the involuntary contractions becomes progressively harder to invoke at higher exertion levels. Thus, it is conceivable that the 6 year old children differ from older children in two ways: (1) they exhibit more intense associated movements at all levels of exertion, and, (2) their process or potential for inhibiting is less effective and thus breaks down at lower exertion levels.

Considering the above and the fact that associated movements can be elicited in older children and adults, these results (Lazarus & Todor, 1983) suggest the mechanism underlying the phenomenon is still in place.

Several possibilities were considered to explain the distinct break in the intensity of associated movements between 6 years of age and older children: (1) maturation of the underlying neural mechanism is incomplete in the 6 year olds, (2) the 6 year olds have less developed mediation or cognitive control processes, and (3) the observed behavioural differences are the result of an interaction of the above two factors.

In a subsequent experiment we wanted to gain a sense of which of the two factors played the dominant role. To do this we wanted to determine the extent to which children of different ages could be made to voluntarily inhibit the contralateral co-contraction. The assumption was that if voluntary inhibition were possible, mediational processes, rather than neural maturation, would be involved.

We selected the 10 children from each age group in the previous experiment who had the most intense associated movements. They performed 3 trials at 75% MVF in each of 3 conditions. On the first set of trials control or baseline data was collected. The following instructions were given: "Keep this hand still in this position while you squeeze the other hand to make the line raise to the colored line".

The second set of trials involved enhanced sensory feedback. We connected a tone generator to the output of the "passive" hand strain gauge. As force increased the pitch of the tone changed. After the child played with the bar to hear the effect, they were instructed to perform the active hand task without making any noise with the "passive" hand.

Immediately after the second set of trials 3 more trials were performed under the baseline condition (no sensory feedback) to see if there would be a persisting benefit due to enhanced sensory feedback.

As expected, the 6 year olds exhibited more intense associated movements in the control trials than all other ages. During the enhanced sensory feedback conditions all ages appeared to improve. However, while the 6 year olds had the greatest numerical decrease, they still exhibited more associated movements than all older ages except the 8 year olds. Similarly, there was a slight trend for the children 8 years and older to regress during the post feedback trials. However, this regression was considerable, for 6 year olds, although they did not return to control levels.

This data indicates that 6 year olds do not exhibit more intense associated movements because of maturational limitations in cortical inhibition or neural maturation. Rather, age differences appear to occur because of ineffectual allocation of attention. The fact that they dropped off without the presence of sensory feedback, suggests that as a group they lacked the ability to self-direct the inhibitory process. Additionally, since the 8 year olds were in an intermediate position, the process of regulating associated movements is apparently still developing.

To determine if there was some general cognitive ability to utilise inhibitory processes, we tested all 6 year olds in the enhanced sensory feedback experiment. Prior to testing we categorised them on the Children's Embedded Figures Test (CEFT) (Karp & Konstadt, 1963). In our opinion this measure reflects the ability to inhibit salient perceptual cues. The child is presented with a drawing of a simple geometric figure and then asked to find it in a more complex figure. High performance scores on this test reflect the ability to suppress or inhibit the tendency to perceive the complex figure as a whole.

Based on CEFT performance we categorised children into 3 groups. On the control trials all groups were equal. Similarly, during the sensory feedback trials, the groups did not differ. However, during the post sensory feedback trials, the group with superior performance on the CEFT did not drop-off. Both other groups regressed.

These experiments suggest that children as young as 6 years of age are capable of inhibiting associated movements if provided with some sort of cue such as enhanced sensory feedback. Additionally, strategic or cognitive factors play a significant role in determining the extent to which children benefit from enhanced sensory feedback. However, based on the initial control trials, none of these children were spontaneously effective in inhibiting associated movements.

In summary, our experiments support the contention that an innate neuromuscular synergy facilitates involuntary symmetrical or mirror movements of the hands. In these studies, this synergy was manifest as involuntary associated movements. It did not disappear with increasing age during childhood, but rather, apparently became increasingly regulated or controlled by cognitive or attentional processes. In the age range studied, the most marked age difference occurred between the 6 and 8 year old groups. Within the 6 year olds, those children with superior ability on a cognitive test of inhibitory ability were also most able to benefit from enhanced sensory feedback.

The manifestation of associated movements was found to be affected by a number of variables. (1) The intensity of associated movements increased with increases in the force exerted by the active hand. (2) There was a marked lateral asymmetry in the intensity of associated movements. The intensity was greater in the right hand (left hand active) than the converse. (3) Associated movements were greater if the hand they were measured in had previously performed the active hand role. (4) When movements were unconstrained, involuntary heterologous, rather than homologous movements, were observed on some trials. This behaviour was affected by intensity and laterality in a similar manner to the more common homologous form of associated movements.

References

Cambier, J. & Dehen, H. (1977). Imitation synkinesis and sensory control of movement. *Neurology, 4,* 646-649.
Cohen, H.J.S., Taft, L.T., Mahadeviah, M.S. & Birch, H.G. (1967). Developmental changes in overflow in normal and abberrantly functioning children. *Journal of Pediatrics, 71,* 39-47.
Connolly, K. & Stratton, P. (1968). Developmental changes in associated movements. *Developmental Medicine and Child Neurology, 10,* 49-56.
Constantini, A.F. & Holving, K.L. (1973). The relationship of cognitive and motor repsonse inhibition to age and IQ. *Journal of Genetic Psychology, 123,* 309-319.
Davis, R.C. (1942). The pattern of muscular action in simple voluntary movement. *Journal of Experimental Psychology, 31,* 347-366.
Elliott, J. & Connolly, K.J. (1973). Hierarchical structure in skill development. In K.J. Connolly and J.S. Bruner (Eds.), *The growth of competence.* New York: Academic Press.
Fog, E. & Fog, M. (1963). Cerebral inhibition examined by associated movements. In M. Bax and R.C. MacKeith (Eds.), *Minimal Cerebral Dysfunction. Clinics in Developmental Medicine, No. 10.* London: Spastics Society/Heineman.
Green, J.B. (1967). An electromyographic study of mirror movements. *Neurology, 17,* 91-94.
Halsey, J.H., Blavenstein, V.W., Wilson, E.M. & Wills, E.H. (1979). Regional cerebral blood flow comparison of right and left hand. *Neurology, 29,* 21-28.
Hutton, R.S. (1985). Acute plasticity in spinal pathways with use: implications for training. In M. Kumamoto and P. Komi (Eds.), *Proceedings of Kyoto Satellite Symposium.* Kyoto: Yamaguchi Shoten.
Karp, S.A. & Konstadt, N.L. (1963). *Manual for the children's embedded figures test.* Brooklyn, NY: Cognitive Tests.
Kelso, J.A.S., Southard, D.L. & Goodman, D. (1979). On the nature of human interlimb co-ordination. *Science, 203,* 1029-1031.
Kimura, D. & Archibald, Y. (1974). Motor functions of the left hemisphere. *Brain, 9,* 337-350.
Kinsbourne, M. (1970). The cerebral basis of lateral asymmetries in attention. *Acta Psychologica, 33,* 193-201.
Lazarus, J.C. (1985). Age differences in the magnitude of associated movements. Unpublished doctoral dissertation, University of Michigan.
Lazarus, J.C. & Todor, J.I. (1983). Unpublished data, University of Michigan.
Roy, E.A. Personnel communication, February, 1985.
Semmes, J. (1968). Hemispheric specialization: a possible clue to mechanism. *Neuropsychologia, 6,* 11-26.
Stern, J.A., Gold, S., Hoin, H. & Barocas, V.C. (1976). Towards a more refined analysis of the "overflow" or "associated movement" phenomenon. In D.V.S. Sankar (Ed.), *Mental Health in Children.* Westbury, NY: PJD Publications, Ltd.
Todor, J.I. & Lazarus, J.C. (1981). A comparison of longitudinal and cross-sectional age differences on the Water Level Test. Unpublished study, University of Michigan.
Todor, J.I. & Lazarus, J.C. (1982). Cognitive style and the rate and mode of motor learning. Presented to the North American Society for the Psychology of Sport and Physical Activity, University Park, Maryland.
Todor, J.I. & Lazarus, J.C. (in press). Exertion level and the intensity of associated movements. *Developmental Medicine and Child Neurology.*

Todor, J.I. & Smiley-Oyen (1985). Performance differences between the hands: implications for studying disruption or limb praxis. In E.A. Roy (Ed.), *Neuropsychological studies of apraxia and related disorders.* Amsterdam: North Holland Publishing Co.

Touwen, B.C.L. & Prechtl, H.F.R. (1970). The neurological examination of the child with minor nervous dysfunction. *Clinics in Developmental Medicine, 38,* 1-105.

Wolff, P.H., Gunnoe, C.E. & Cohen, C. (1983). Associated movements as a measure of developmental age. *Developmental Medicine and Child Neurology, 25,* 417-429.

Yensen, R. (1965). A factor influencing motor overflow. *Perceptual and Motor Skills, 20,* 967-968.

SENSORY-MOTOR CONTROL AND BALANCE: A BEHAVIOURAL PERSPECTIVE

H. Williams, B. McClenaghan, D. Ward, W. Carter, C. Brown, R. Byde, D. Johnson and D. Lasalle

INTRODUCTION

Balance is an integral part of skilled movement performance of individuals of all ages. Successful performance of motor skills depends in many instances upon the individual's ability to establish and maintain balance. This is especially true for movements which involve complex manipulation and/or projection of the body. There is little doubt that for the young child, effective balance control is an important part of the foundation upon which the emergence of normal, skillful, and efficient movement or motor behaviour proceeds (Williams, 1983). It is clear, however, that the acquisition of efficient balance is a widespread problem for large numbers of children of pre-school and elementary school age.

Behaviourally, balance may be viewed as on overt manifestation of the nervous system's solution to the problem of assuming and maintaining an appropriate relationship between the body's centre of gravity and its base of support. Neurophysiologically, balance involves complex, and as yet far from completely understood, interactions among vestibular, proprioceptive, visual and motor systems (Lishman & Lee, 1973; Nashner & Berthoz, 1978; Worchel & Dallenbach, 1948). Each of these systems seems to contribute in important ways to the detection and correction of errors in the status of the body's equilibrium.

It is a rather universal observation that balance is more efficient with vision than without (e.g. Amblard & Cremieux, 1976; Travis, 1945); and that in general individuals find it more difficult to maintain control over balance when there is some distortion of or unusual variation in the visual information available to them from the environment in which they are balancing (e.g. Berthoz et al, 1975; Brandt et al, 1973; Brandt et al, 1975). DeWit (1972) has shown that adults who stood on a stabilometer in a dark room and faced a luminous rod which oscillated in the frontal plane tended to sway laterally in phase with the rod. Lee and Aronson (1974) have also shown a similar relationship between vision and antero-posterior sway in toddlers who swayed in concert with movement of the surrounding visual field, often to the extent that the child lost balance and fell over. Likewise if visual information is reduced, e.g. by providing the performer with only tunnel or central vision, balance performance deteriorates markedly. Overall evidence indicates that visual input often overrides other, more accurate sources of sensory information about the status of the body's equilibrium and contributes in significant ways to postural responses which may lead to inadequate or inappropriate balance control (e.g. Dichgans et al, 1976).

There seems to be at least four possible ways vision may play a role in balance control. First, there is reason to believe that in acquiring balance control the individual establishes an underlying pattern of vestibular-proprioceptive activity and then modulates or fine-tunes that pattern of activity by linking it through vision to pertinent information in the surrounding external environment (Butterworth, 1982; Forssberg & Nashner, 1982). Lee and Lishman (1975) have suggested that vision's most important role in balance is the 'tuning up' of proprioceptive information involved in balance, especially in situations where the individual is asked to maintain balance in less familiar, unpracticed positions or where, for some reason, proprioception is either impoverished or not well established. Begbie (1967) has shown that individuals who are deficient in vestibular function tend to have normal balance when vision is available but are very unstable in balancing in the dark on uneven or unfamiliar compliant surfaces.

Indirectly research has suggested that the visual system may act in part as a monitor of the external environment; that is, it may provide an objective means by which the performer can judge various aspects of the external environment (e.g. horizontals and verticals) and thereby maintain an appropriate body position (e.g. Llewellyn, 1971; Witkin & Wapner, 1950). Still others assert that the important role of vision in balance is to monitor the movement of the body itself and to verify the status of the body's equilibrium by directly assessing the nature and extent of the position and or movement of the body (e.g. Brown, 1981).

A final point of view (Wapner & Werner, 1950; Witkin, 1948, 1950) suggests that it is the 'visually apprehended relationship' between the body and the surrounding environment that is the most important contribution of vision to balance. In other words, this point of view suggests that vision acts to monitor body/environment relationships and to match-up body position and movement to environmental demands in an interactive way. A number of studies have shown that visual monitoring of the movement of the limbs and body is prerequisite to development of other aspects of motor control (e.g. refined eye-hand coordination and guided reaching behaviours) in young, developing organisms (Hein, 1974; Held & Bauer, 1974; Held & Hein, 1976).

Most work to date has been done on static balance and postural control. Little is known about how young children use vision to regulate balance in a dynamic movement situation. What visual information do young children use to establish and maintain control over balance? Is visual information used primarily to fine-tune underlying vestibular-proprioceptive activity, or is it used to monitor the environment? Is it used to monitor the movement of the body itself or to assess the relationship between the body and the environment in which it is moving? The purpose of the present series of studies was to investigate the role of vision in the regulation of dynamic balance control in young children.

EXPERIMENT 1

The purpose of Experiment I was to investigate the role of vision as a monitor of body/environment relationships in the development of dynamic balance control in young children. More specifically, Experiment I studied the effects of the type and amount of visual information available about body/environment relationships on the performance of a simple beam walking task in 6 and 8 year old children.

METHODS

Subjects. Participants were 52 six (n= 26) and eight (n= 26) year old boys and girls enrolled in selected elementary schools in the midwestern United States. There were equal numbers of boys and girls in each age group.

Task and Experimental Conditions. Each child was randomly assigned to walk a standard balance beam, 2" wide x 2" high x 8' long in one of five conditions.

> Condition 1: Full Visual Monitoring of Body/Environment Relationships. The child walked the beam in a full, normal visual environment (Control Condition);
>
> Condition 2: Visual Monitoring of the Environment Only. The child walked the balance beam in the dark with only the top surface of the beam illuminated by a piece of 2" luminescent tape placed across the full length of the beam (Beam Only Condition);
>
> Condition 3: Visual Monitoring of Upper Body/Environment Relationships. The child walked the beam in the dark with the beam illuminated as before and with a strip of 2" luminescent tape on each arm. This tape extended from the shoulder to the wrist (Beam-Arms Condition);
>
> Condition 4: Visual Monitoring of Lower Body/Environment Relationships. The child walked the balance beam in the dark with the beam illuminated as before and with 2" strips of luminescent tape on each leg. The tape extended from hip to knee (Beam Legs Condition);
>
> Condition 5: Visual Monitoring of Total Body/Environment Relationships. The child walked the beam in the dark with the beam illuminated and with 2" strips of luminescent tape on both arms and legs (Beam-Arms/Legs Conditions).

Procedures. Each child walked the balance beam in a heel-to-toe fashion. Initially each child was given four practice trials walking the beam in a normal, fully lighted room. Children then walked the beam under the task condition to which they had been randomly assigned. Four trials were given; the average of 4 trials was the dependent variable. Time to the nearest .01 second was recorded. If the child stepped off the beam as he/she walked, she/he stepped back on the beam and continued walking. Step-offs were reflected in performance scores by the arbitrary addition of one second per step-off to the total task completion time. A three-way ANOVA (5 Task Conditions x 2 Ages x 2 Sexes) was used to analyse the data.

RESULTS AND DISCUSSION

The main effect of task conditions was significant ($p= .01; F_{4,160}= 25.46$) and is shown in Figure 1. Scheffe's post hoc comparisons tests indicated that performances in the Beam-only condition were significantly different from (e.g. poorer than) performances in all other conditions. Thus when no visual information was available about body/environment relationships, performance deteriorated significantly. There were no significant differences

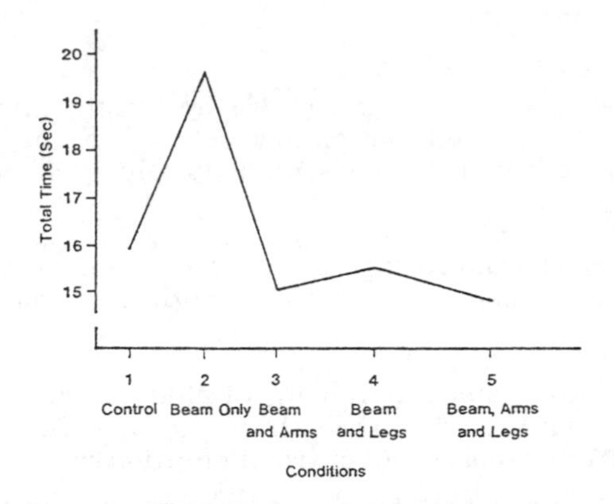

Fig. 1. Balance Performance: Main Effect of Task Condition.

among performances in any condition in which some form of visual information about the relationship of the body to the environment (beam) was present. These data suggest that monitoring of the external environment alone was not a sufficient condition for maintaining effective balance control in young children; rather effective balance seemed to require some form of visual information about the body's movement in relationship to the environment. Note that the form of the visual information needed to define such relationships was very flexible; it could be natural (e.g. full visual environment) or artificial (e.g. provided by luminescent tape), full (total body) or partial (legs or arms).

The interaction between age and task conditions was also significant (p= .01; F 4, 160= 18.80). See Figure 2. It is clear that task condition effects were almost entirely nested in the performance of six year old children. There were no significant differences in balance performances of 8 year olds under any task condition. Thus eight year old children performed as well under conditions where they could only monitor the environment as they did when they could monitor body/environment relationships. In contrast to this, six year olds performed significantly better when some form of visual information about the body's relationship to the environment was present. Overall, 6 year olds seemed to need to be able to visually monitor the body's movement in the environment to maintain effective control over balance. As before it did not seem to matter whether such information was full and natural (as in the control condition) or artificial and reduced (as in the various experimental conditions).

One might speculate that the motor control system of the six year old is at a point in development where it requires visual information to reaffirm the nature of the movement of the body in the environment to maintain effective balance control. Does this mean that the system of the older child can better integrate or use proprioceptive-vestibular information to effectively modulate and maintain control over balance?

Six year olds seem to be similar to a new or novice performers who need vision to maintain control over movement. Eight year olds are more like advanced or proficient performers who tend to need to rely less on vision to regulate movement behaviour. Although it is clear that a number of sensory and motor systems are integral to balance control, these data

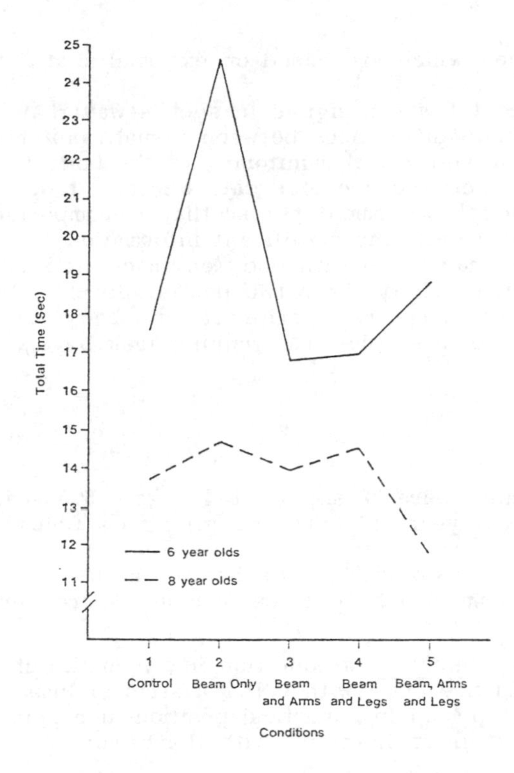

Fig. 2. Balance Performance: Age x Task Condition Interaction.

suggest that vision may play an important but changing role in the development of dynamic balance in young children.

EXPERIMENT II

One experiment of course does not tell it all. There were at least two major limiting factors in Experiment I. First, the external environment was defined solely in terms of the 'balance beam' itself. Clearly there are other aspects of the visual environment that are important in providing information about body/environment relationships that may be important to the development of adequate balance control in young children. For example, Lestienne et al (1977) reported that stimuli in the peripheral visual field play a significant role in producing the postural adjustments that are induced by moving visual scenes. Strelow and Brabyn (1981) have also presented data that indicate that a clearly defined and visible aiming point (e.g. a central visual field referent) markedly improves the accuracy with which adults walk a path in space; they also report that the presence of 'background' visual information in the peripheral visual field increases the accuracy with which individuals walk such a path. Wapner and Werner (1950) suggested some 30 years ago that vertical and horizontal referents were of utmost importance in maintaining appropriate spatial orientation. Recently Millar (1976, 1979, 1981) has proposed that one of the important by-products of visual experience for young children is the facilitation of use of strategies for coding spatial location which are based on external spatial referents.

Secondly, Experiment I was designed in such a way that it did not allow us to clearly evaluate differences between visual monitoring of body/environment relationships and visual monitoring of the body itself. In other words, it was not clear from the previous data whether it was visual information about the body's movement per se that was important to the process of balance control or if the significant information for such control was, in fact, that which had to do with body/environment relationships. Experiment II attempted to clarify these two points. Specifically, Experiment II investigated the effects of central, peripheral and body referent visual cues on the performance of a simple beam walking task by six and eight year old children.

METHODS

Subjects. Participants were 32 six (average age = 6.5 years) and eight (average age = 8.6 years) year old boys and girls from Columbia, S.C.

Task and Experimental Conditions. As before, each child was asked to walk a 2 inch balance beam in a heel-to-toe fashion. There were eight conditions:

> Central Visual Referent, a condition in which the child walked the balance beam with ONLY a strip of luminescent tape (2" x 6') placed in a vertical position at a point 4' beyond and in direct alignment with the beam;
>
> Peripheral Visual Referents, a condition in which two strips of luminescent tape were placed in a horizontal position 4' from the beam on either side of the beam and at approximately eye level of the child;
>
> Body Referents, a condition similar to the previous experiment in which strips of luminescent tape were placed on both the arms and legs;
>
> No Visual Referents, a condition in which the child walked the beam in total darkness.

The remaining conditions were combinations of the proceeding four conditions. In no condition was the beam illuminated, and an attempt was made to keep the room as dark and free of other light and miscellaneous background visual information as possible.

Procedure. We further screened the children for this experiment. Before entering the laboratory, all children walked a 2" beam identical to that used in the experiment proper in a heel-to-toe fashion and in the full visual environment. Any child who had difficulty walking the beam in the full visual environment did not participate in the experimental portion of the study.

Children in the study walked the balance beam three trials in each of the eight experimental conditions, a total of 24 trials. Total time to complete the task was recorded for each child.

Apparatus and Data Collection. Force transducers were placed under the supports of the beam at each end and were connected to a differential amplifer. The output of the differential amplifier was fed into an Apple-2E computer which was programmed to detect when the child was 'in' or 'out' of balance. Before beginning the experiment proper, each child's 'beam-weight' was determined. The child stood in the centre of the beam in a fully balanced position. A beam-weight 'value' for this fully balanced position was determined. The parameters for being 'in' balance were then set for that individual child. The general standard set for being 'in' balance for all children was 80%. This meant that if 80% of the child's weight was on the beam, the computer recorded this as time 'in' balance; if less than 80% of the child's weight was on the beam, the computer recorded this as time 'out' of balance.

Design. The design of the study was a 2 (6 and 8 year olds) x 8 (experimental conditions) x 8 (orders of presentation) factorial with repeated measures. Four children (two 6 and two 8 year olds were given one of eight randomised orders of the experimental conditions. An ANOVA with appropriate post hoc tests was used to analyse the data.

RESULTS AND DISCUSSION

Only the main effect of Central Visual Referent (P= .015; F1,211 = 5.93) and the three-way interaction between Age x Central x Body Referents (p= .05; F1,211 = 3.87) were significant. In general balance performance was better when there was a central visual cue available than when there was not.

Of importance to us is the three-way interaction effect shown in Figure 3. For both groups of children, without the central ('aiming') visual cue, balance performance was little affected by the presence or absence of 'body referent cues'. That is, when information about the position and/or movement of the body per se was present without some external environmental reference point to relate it to, there was little or no effect on balance performance in either 6 or 8 year old children. This suggested that in

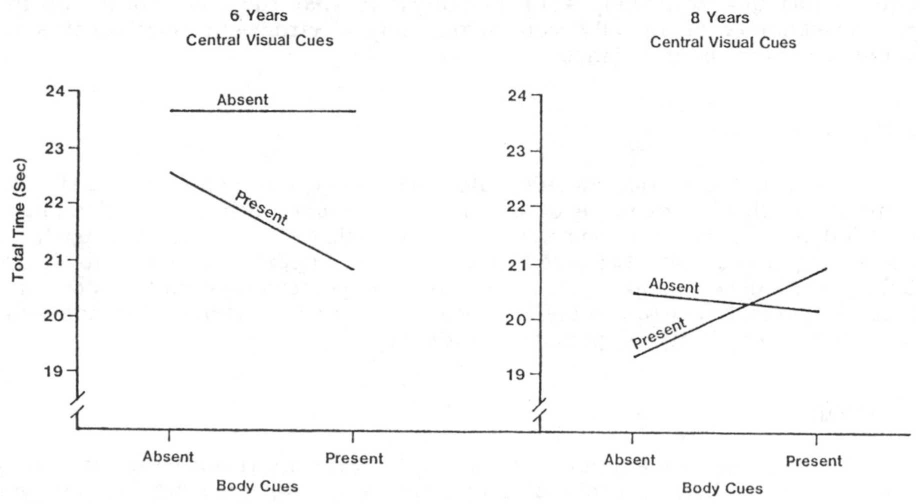

Fig. 3. Balance Performance: Central Cues x Body Cues x Age Interaction.

general visual monitoring of the movement and position of the body independent of the environment was not an important factor in the regulation of dynamic balance control in young children.

What happened when the central visual referent was present? Interestingly, the effect of pairing 'body referents' with 'environmental referents' was different for the two age groups. As before, for six year olds balance performance was significantly improved when visual information about body movement and visual information from the external environment (central visual cue) were combined. Under such conditions, the child could monitor, at least in a general way, the relationship between the body and the external environment in which it was moving. An unexpected effect was observed for 8 year olds. Time to complete the beam walking task was significantly poorer when both body referent cues and central visual cues were present simultaneously. That is, when 8 year olds performed under conditions where they could (or did) monitor body/environment relationships they performed more poorly than when they could (or did) monitor the external environment only. Is it possible that in some way, this unusual form of visual monitoring of body movement actually interfered with effective balance control? This could happen if the older child more spontaneously relies on vestibular-proprioceptive information for assessing the body's position and movement in space and selectively filters out direct visual information about the body. It is possible that one of the things that characterises dynamic balance development in normal children is a shift from monitoring body/environment relationships through vision to monitoring selected aspects of environment through vision and maintaining awareness of the body's position and movement through vestibular-proprioceptive information.

Overall data from Experiment II support the notion that visual monitoring of body/environment relationships may be important to effective balance control in younger children but may be less so for older children. If this is the case, perhaps one of the reasons that children with balance problems continue to have difficulty is that the mechanism(s) necessary for fine-tuning and using proprioceptive-vestibular information about the body's equilibrium fail to develop appropriately and that the child continues to rely on the strategy of visually monitoring body/environment relationships to achieve control over balance.

EXPERIMENT III

Because there was considerable concern on our parts that a single (and quite simple) measure of balance performance might be misleading, we decided to undertake Experiment III. The primary purpose of Experiment III was to investigate the questions posed in Experiment II but to do so by using multi-dimensional measures of balance performance and to describe balance performance by analysing beam traversal patterns. Our concern was with the replicability of previous findings.

METHODS

Methods were identical to those of Experiment II with the exception that total task time, number of step-offs, and total time 'in' balance were used as dependent variables. A MANOVA with appropriate post hoc tests

(Hotelling-Lawley Trace F Approximations) was used to analyse the data.

RESULTS AND DISCUSSION

What did we find when we looked at balance performance in this way? There were no age effects and no effects of 'body referents'. Only the main effect of Central Visual Referent ($p= .018$; $F_{ap,3,209} = 3.41$) and the interaction between central and peripheral visual referents ($p= .003$; $F_{ap,3,209} = 4.62$) were significant. Thus in contrast to the previous two experiments, age was not an important factor and body referent cues did not significantly affect performance singly or in combination with environmental cues. These data suggest that young children may not directly monitor the movement of the body or body/environment relationships in maintaining balance. Rather they seem primarily to use some combination of external central and peripheral (aiming and guiding) visual cues to modulate the processes involved in regulating dynamic balance control.

What external cues do children use? Data for total task time and number of step-offs for the Central/Peripheral Referents condition suggests that performance, in terms of both total task time and number of step-offs, was better when the central visual cue was present than when it was not. See Figure 4. Children stepped off the beam fewer times and traversed the beam more quickly when there was a referent or aiming cue in the central visual field than when there was not.

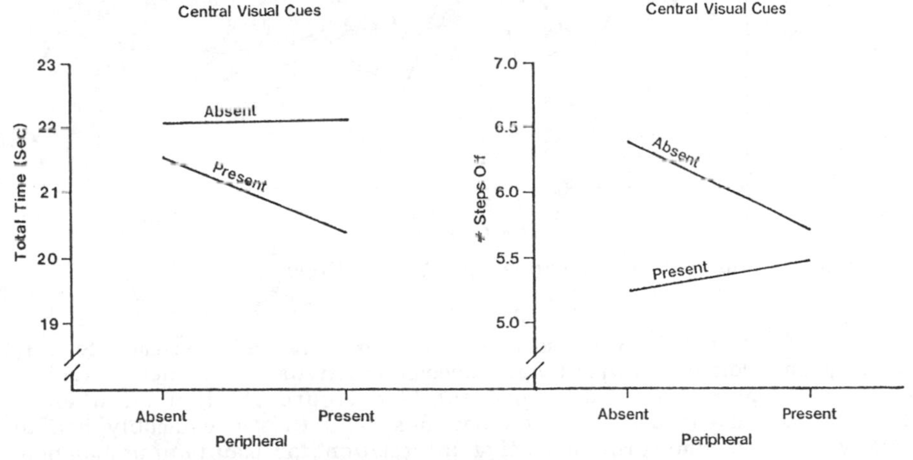

Fig. 4. Interaction Between Central/Peripheral Visual Cues: Total Task Time; Step-Offs.

In addition, total time to traverse the beam decreased significantly when the central referent cue was paired with peripheral visual cues. With regard to the number of step-offs, when a central visual referent was present, the peripheral cue was of little importance. In the absence of a central cue, the peripheral cue became very important. Under these conditions, the child tended to step off the beam significantly fewer times than when the peripheral visual cue was not available. In other words, in terms of number of step-offs, a peripheral visual referent was better than no referent at all. Overall the foregoing suggest that 6 and 8 year olds use both central and peripheral visual cues in maintaining control over balance. Of the two, the central visual referent (aiming cue) may be the more important.

Beam Traversal Patterns. We also looked at balance performance in terms of beam traversal patterns. We tried to describe or profile the pattern of the children's balance as they travelled across the beam under different task conditions. A 'beam traversal pattern' was defined as (a) the number of time periods used by the child to cross the beam (the time from when the child stepped onto the beam to his first step-off was defined as Period 1; the time from when the child stepped back onto the beam to the second step-off was defined as Period 2, etc.) and (b) the average duration of each time period. Two selected 'beam traversal patterns' are shown in Figures 5 and 6.

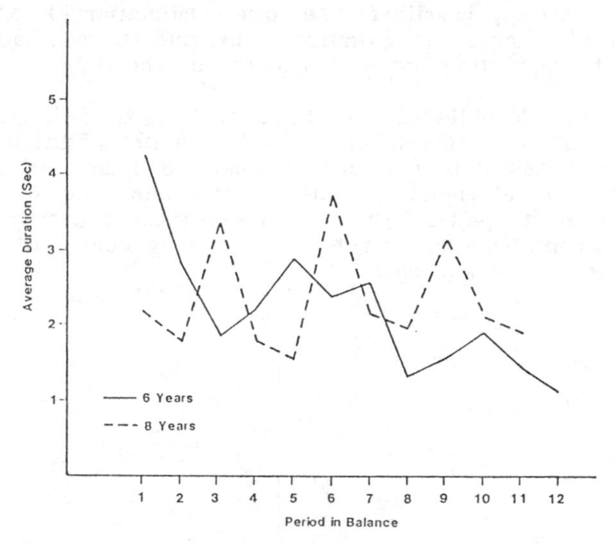

Fig. 5. Balance Performance: No Visual Cues.

Looked at in this way, some interesting differences seemed to exist in the way children of different ages accomplish dynamic balance control. When no visual referents were present (see Figure 5), that is, when children walked the beam in total darkness and thus presumably had to rely largely on vestibular-proprioceptive information for maintaining balance, both 6 and 8 year olds traversed the beam in approximately the same number of time periods (6 years= 13; 8 years = 12). Younger children, in contrast to older children however, tended to show an overall steady decline in the duration of the time periods spent 'in balance' on the beam. That is, the average duration of time actually spent 'in' balance for any given time period decreased as 6 year olds proceeded across the length of the beam. Does the sensitivity of the vestibular-proprioceptive system of the six year old decrease as time without opportunity for monitoring or fine-tuning such processes via visual information increases? Older children appeared to maintain a relatively constant level of time 'in' balance throughout beam traversal. That is, the time per period spent 'in' balance was relatively constant across the full length of the beam. Does the vestibular-proprioceptive

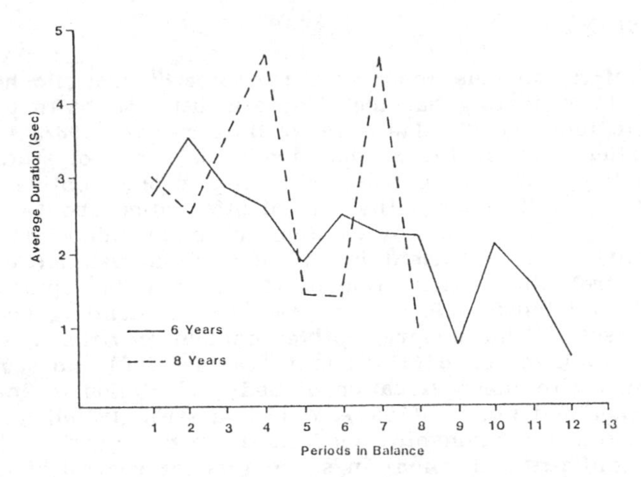

Fig. 6. Balance Performance: Central X Peripheral Cues.

system of the older child better maintain its sensitivity in the absence of visual cues typically available for monitoring or fine-tuning such information?

It should also be noted that characteristic of the beam traversal patterns of 8 year olds in the dark was rather regular or cyclical pattern of being 'in' balance for periods of short and long durations. In other words, eight year olds exhibited a pattern of dynamic balance in which a period of being 'in' balance for a longer duration was immediately followed by two periods of being 'in' balance for a shorter duration. This pattern did not change across time and was not characteristic of 6 year olds. What this means is at present not clear.

Patterns of beam traversal changed somewhat when children balanced with both central and peripheral visual referents present. See Figure 6. Under these conditions, older children crossed the beam in fewer time periods than when no external visual referents were available. The average duration of the periods of being 'in' balance was also longer. Thus eight year olds stayed 'in' balance for longer periods of time when external visual referents were present than when they were not. This of course suggests that the child had better control over his/her balance. As before, the cyclical pattern of two shorter 'in' balance periods followed by one longer 'in' balance period was observed.

In contrast, when central and peripheral visual cues were present, six year old children crossed the beam in approximately the same number of time periods as they did when they walked in the dark. In addition, the duration of the periods spent 'in' balance were only slightly greater than in the dark. Again, the average duration of time periods spent 'in' balance tended to decrease as the child traversed the beam. These observations suggest that older children may be more effective in using external visual vues to regulate dynamic balance than are younger children. Since integration of visual and knaesthetic information has been reported to undergo important changes during the period from 6 to 8 years (Birch & Lefford, 1963), these beam traversal patterns may be a reflection of more refined intersensory integration processes found in older children.

GENERAL DISCUSSION

What does all of this tell us about sensory-motor control and how children use vision in regulating balance? There is little doubt that vision has a proprioceptive function in balance (e.g. Butterworth, 1982; Lee & Lishman, 1975; Lestienne et al, 1977). Data from this series of studies point to some potentially interesting features of that proprioceptive function in dynamic balance. First it appears that visual information about body position or movement per se (e.g. movement of the body independent of the external environment) is not sufficient in and of itself to maintain effective dynamic balance control. Such information needs, at least in young children (6 year olds), to be related to information from the surrounding visual environment to be useful. This proprioceptive function of vision has been aptly described by Lestienne et al (1977) and Travis (1956) and seems to be directly concerned with the "evaluation of body orientation in space" (p. 364). Like Wapner and Werner (1950), our data strongly indicate that the 'visually apprehended relationship' between the body and the environment is a significant component in sensory-motor control of dynamic balance in young children. The type of visual information needed to evaluate body/environment relationships by the young child seems to be very general.

Although not totally clearcut, it would seem that developmentally there may be a trend away from the need to visually monitor body/environment relationships directly to maintain effective balance (e.g. at 6 years of age) to a shift toward greater reliance or use of vestibular-proprioceptive information for maintaining dynamic balance control at 8 years of age. Butterworth and Hicks (1978) have reported that the destabilising effects of vision on posture (in the form of movement of the visual environment) diminishes with growth and development in normal infants. Butterworth (1982) believes that this is in part a result of a gradual shift toward a more dominant role for vestibular-proprioceptive systems in balance as the nervous system matures.

Data from the present experiments also indicate that sensory-motor control in young children may be characterised by an increase in the capacity of the child with age to use or relie on external spatial referents to regulate balance. As Strelow and Brabyn (1981) have reported for adults, both peripheral and central visual field referents contribute to effective postural control, but in the case of young children, the central or aiming cue seems to be the more important of the two.

Beam traversal patterns suggest that even though 6 and 8 year old children both have better balance control with external visual referents than without, older children seem to be better than younger ones at using external visual referents to modify or adapt control over balance. Hay (1978, 1979) and McCracken (1983) report observations on the development of eye-hand coordination in children which may be pertinent here. Hay (1978) indicated that seven year old children were less able than older children 9-11 years) to reach accurately toward a stationary visual target when they could not observe the movement of the limbs. Hay (1979) suggested that this was in part due to the increased capacity of the older child to integrate visual and kinaesthetic information into motor control processes. It should be noted that the tasks used in Hay (1978), McCracken (1983) and the present series of studies took place in essentially 'closed' environments (e.g. reaching to or walking a stationary target). It may be that there is less need for the more mature sensory-motor system to visually monitory body or limb movements in closed environments where changes in such relationships are minimal. Under these circumstances, it may simply rely on external visual referents to guide bodily movements. It is possible that in 'open' environments monitoring of body/environment relationships may be much more important. More research is needed to verify such speculations.

References

Amblard, R. & Cremieux, J. (1976). Role of the visual motion information in the maintenance of postural equilibrium in man. *Agressologie, 17,* 25-36.

Begbie, G.H. (1967). Some problems of postural sway. In A.V.S. de Rueck and J. Knight (Eds.), *Myotatic, Kinesthetic and Vestibular Mechanisms.* London: J. and A. Churchill.

Berthoz, A., Pavard, B. & Young, L.R. (1975). Perception of linear horizontal self-motion induced by peripheral vision (linear vection). Basic characteristics and visual-vestibular interactions. *Experimental Brain Research, 23,* 471-489.

Birch, H.G. & Lefford, A. (1963). Intersensory development in children. *Monographs of the Society for Research in Child Development, 28,* 2-27.

Brandt, T., Dichgans, J. & Koenig, E. (1973). Differential effect of central versus peripheral vision on egocentric and execentric motion perception. *Experimental Brain Research, 16,* 476-491.

Brandt, T., Wist, E. & Dichgans, J. (1975). Foreground and background in dynamic spatial orientation. *Perception and Psychophysics, 17,* 497-503.

Brown, C.E. (1981). The Contribution of Visual Feedback from body Limb Position to Dynamic Balance Control. Unpublished Master's Thesis, The University of Toledo, Toledo, Oh.

Butterworth, G. (1982). The origins of auditory visual perception and visual proprioception in human development. In R. Walk and H. Pick (Eds.), *Intersensory Perception and Sensory Integration.* New York: Plenum Press.

Butterworth, g. & Hicks, L. (1977). Visual proprioception and postural stability in infancy: a developmental study. *Perception, 6,* 255-262.

Davis, W.J. & Ayers, J.L. (1972). Locomotion: control by positive-feedback optokinetic responses. *Science, 13,* 75-79.

DeWit, G. (1972). Optic versus vestibular and proprioceptive impulses measured by posturometry. *Agressologie, 13,* 75-79.

Dichgans, J., Mauritz, K.H., Allum, J.H.J. & Brandt, T. (1976). Postural sway in normals and atactic patients: analysis of the stabilizing and destabilizing effects of vision. *Agressologie, 17,* 15-24.

Forssberg, H. & Nashner, L. (1982). Ontogenetic development of posture control in man: adaptation to altered support and visual conditions during stance. *Journal of Neuroscience, 2,* 545-552.

Gibson, J.J. (1966). *The Senses Considered as Perceptual Systems.* Boston: Houghton Mifflin.

Hay, L. (1978). Accuracy of children on an open-loop pointing task. *Perceptual and Motor Skills, 47,* 1079-1082.

Hay, L. (1979). Spatial-temporal analysis of movements in children: motor programs versus feedback in the development of reaching. *Journal of Motor Behavior, 11,* 189-200.

Hein, A. (1974). Prerequisite for development of visually guided-reaching in the kitten. *Brain Research, 71,* 259-263.

Held, R. & Bauer, J. (1974). Development of sensorially guided reaching in infant monkeys. *Brain Research, 71,* 265-271.

Held, R. & Hein, A. (1976). Movement produced stimulation in the development of visually guided behavior. *Journal of Comparative Physiological Psychology, 37,* 87-95.

Lasky, R.E. (1977). The effect of visual feedback of the hand on the reaching and retrieval behavior of young infants. *Child Development, 48,* 112-117.

Lee, D.N. & Aronson, E. (1974). Visual proprioceptive control of standing in human infants. *Perception and Psychophysics, 15,* 529-532.

Lee, D.N. & Lishman, H.R. (1975). Visual proprioceptive control of stance. *Journal of Human Movement Studies, 1,* 87-95.

Lestienne, F., Soechting, J. & Berthoz, A. (1977). Postural readjustments induced by linear motion of visual scenes. *Experimental Brain Research, 28,* 363-384.

Lindberg, E. & Garling, T. (1982). Acquisition of locational information about reference points during locomotion: the role of central information processing. *Scandinavian Journal of Psychology, 23,* 207-218.

Lishman, J.R. & Lee, D.N. (1973). The autonomy of visual kinaesthesis. *Perception, 2,* 287-294.

Llewellyn, R.R. (1971). Visual guidance of locomotion. *Journal of Experimental Psychology, 95,* 245-261.

McCracken, H.D. (1983). Movement control in a reciprocal tapping task: a developmental study. *Journal of Motor Behavior, 15,* 262-279.

Millar, S. (1981). Self-referent and movement cues in coding spatial location by blind and sighted children. *Perception, 10,* 255-264.

Millar, S. (1976). Spatial representation by blind and sighted children. *Journal of Experimental Psychology, 21,* 460-479.

Millar, S. (1979). The utilization of external and movement cues in simple spatial tasks by blind and sighted children. *Perception, 8,* 11-20.

Mulder, T. & Hulstijn, W. (1985). Sensory feedback in the learning of a novel motor task. *Journal of Motor Behavior, 17,* 110-128.

Nashner, L.M. & Berthoz, A. (1978). Visual contribution to rapid motor responses during postural control. *Brain Research, 150,* 403-407.

Smyth, M.M. & Murray, A. (1982). Vision and proprioception in simple catching. *Journal of Motor Behavior, 2,* 143-152.

Strelow, E.R. & Brabyn, J.A. (1981). Use of foreground and background information in visually guided locomotion. *Perception, 10,* 191-198.

Travis, R.C. (1945). An experimental analysis of dynamic and static equilibrium. *Journal of Experimental Psychology, 35,* 216-234.

Wapner, S. & Witkin, H.A. (1950). The role of visual factors in the maintenance of body balance. *American Journal of Psychology, 63,* 385.

Williams, H.G. (1983). *Perceptual and Motor Development.* Englewood Cliffs, N.J.: Prentice, Hall.

Witkin, H.A. (1950). Perception of the upright when the direction of the force acting on the body is changed. *Journal of Experimental Psychology, 40,* 93-106.

Witkin, H.A. (1948). Studies in space orientation. I Perception of the upright with displaced visual field. *Journal of Experimental Psychology, 38,* 325-337.

Witkin, H.A. & Wapner, S. (1950). Visual factors in the maintenance of upright position. *American Journal of Psychology, 63,* 32.

Woollacott, M.H. (1983). Children's changing capacity to process information. AAHPERD Symposium, Minneapolis, MI.

Worchel, P. & Dallenbach, K.M. (1948). The vestibular sensitivity of deaf-blind subjects. *American Journal of Psychology, 61,* 94-99.

SECTION 5

POSTURE AND LOCOMOTION

FROM STEPPING TO ADAPTIVE WALKING: MODULATIONS OF AN AUTOMATISM

A.M. Ferrandez and J. Pailhous

1. INTRODUCTION

The fact that motor activity can greatly influence the development of intelligence was stated in particular by Piaget. Numerous studies have been conducted on motor activity but most of them have focused on the so-called sensorimotor stage, in infancy. During the subsequent stages of development, investigators seem to consider that verbal statements are more worthy of investigation than motor behaviour as a means of studying the underlying representational processes. Mounoud has nevertheless claimed that even in children who are old enough to express themselves perfectly well in words, the non-verbal, motor form of expression can be most informative as to how these processes develop. In children aged between 5 and 9, for instance, instead of using the subjects' verbal statements as is usually done in order to determine how the conservation and seriation of weights are acquired, it has been possible to efficiently deduce how children represented weights by analysing the motor behaviour they displayed when grasping and lifting objects (Mounoud & Hauert, 1982; Gachoud et al, 1983). By observing motor activity, it has also been possible to extend the study of concrete operations concepts to very young children. On the basis of non-verbal, motor data, Mounoud and Bower (1974) have shown that infants aged 15 months are to a certain extent able to perform items of conservation and seriation of weights. Various motor tasks have been used in studies of this type: the grasping and lifting of objects just mentioned, pointing towards a target under various conditions usually relating to the vision of the target and/or the pointing limb (Bard & Hay, 1983; Hay, 1979a, 1981; Hay & Bard, 1984; Sugden, 1980; see Hay, 1979b, for a review), and visuomanual tracking (Mounoud et al, 1983, 1985). These activities often involve the upper limbs, which are able to carry out a wide range of behavioural functions: tying shoe-laces, piano-playing, and knitting, for instance, are activities requiring a high degree of skill; threading a needle or hammering in a nail require each hand to fulfil a separate specialised function; pointing at somebody or describing a spiral staircase are activities which call upon the faculties of expression.

When a child is only just beginning to walk, he is also gradually learning to make use of the various registers of which the upper limbs are capable. At this age, he is also beginning to acquire a highly specialised automatic activity - that is, locomotion - with his lower limbs. These limbs are rarely used as means of expression except in dancing, an art which requires an extremely high degree of motor skill. The legs are not each highly specialised as the hands are (although one of them is the leader), and the skills which require training of the lower limbs (such as pedalling, skating running, or swimming) are often based on automatic locomotor habits. The main function of the legs is walking, and this is an automatic movement which shows a high degree of stability and regularity at all ages once it has been acquired. This stability is an asset to scientists, since it allows them, as Bernstein puts it, to distinguish "the random from the regular", so that by studying changes in locomotion due to special conditions, it is possible to establish what modulations are involved.

After outlining the development of the locomotor automatism, it is proposed to deal with various structural aspects and to discuss the modulations involved.

2. THE ONTOGENESIS OF THE LOCOMOTOR AUTOMATISM

> Johnny displayed far more stepping than Jimmy throughout the first year, but he did not walk alone sooner. (McGraw, 1935).

Most animals are able to move unaided only a few hours after birth, whereas human babies take about a year to be able to walk on their feet like adults. They go through several intermediate stages such as creeping and crawling (Benson et al, 1985). Learning to stand up and walk is an important achievement for children: it frees their hands so that they can reach and manipulate objects which were hitherto unattainable; they are able to diversify and develop their exploratory activities by combining manipulation with displacement (trajectories involving obstacles to be crossed become easier to master; objects that were out of reach become accessible). The multiplicity of possible displacements and the ease with which they can be made may facilitate the coding of spatial properties by means of an external frame of reference (Lepecq, 1985).

2.1. Posture and locomotion

Children all learn to stand and to walk at roughly the same time (Grillner, 1981). When they are about one year old (large variations), children are able to walk first when supported and then independently. Walking involves mastery of a series of states of equilibrium and disequilibriu Studies on the emergence of locomotion analysing the durations of the suppor and swing phases in the walking cycle have shown that the double-support phase is usually rather long in comparison with the duration of the cycle. Sutherland et al (1980) have described a rapid evolution of the decrease in the duration of the double-support phase up to 2 years of age approximately; but the characteristics of adult performance are not reached until several years later. Several reasons have been suggested for this: according to Sutherland et al (1980), this lack of stability can be explained by a lack of balance, the weakness of the plantar-flexor ankle muscles, and the lack of control of these muscles. Bril, Fontaine and Brenière (1985) have suggested that the reason why the double-support phase lasts so long may be that a resetting occurs between each step. This interpretation is not however in keeping with the results of Statham and Murray (1971), who, while reporting the same pattern of development as Bril et al, observed this event between the supported walking stage in which children require an adult hand to help them keep their balance, and the independent walking stage in which they eventually manage to keep their balance unaided. It is feasible that in these initial stages of walking, children may seek maximum stability and therefore this stability may be ontained by an over-flexion of hips and knees, as suggested by Statham and Murray (1971) and Forssberg (1985). Statham and Murray assume that this over-flexing serves to lower the centre of gravity with a view to achieving greater stability. In elderly people (over the age of 60), a similar attempt to ensure greater stability has been observed in the form of a greater degree of out-toeing than in younger subjects (Murray et al, 1964). This wider foot-angle can actually also be observed in young people, when they walk slowly: so that the above morphological characteristics of elderly people's gait may be simply attributable to the fact that they have a natural tendency to walk slowly (Murray et al, 1966). The processing of visual data moreover plays an important part in maintaining standing balance (Lee & Aronson, 1974), particularly in children under the age of 5 (Lee & Lishman, 1975; Shumway-Cook & Woollacott, 1985), where the function of vision is to provide proprioceptive information (Gibson, 1966). Vision has been found to have this function even before children are able to stand, when they are still beginning to maintain a sitting position (Butterworth & Hicks, 1977). Here it is peripheral vision which is involved in the processing of information, as shown by Pavard, Berthoz and Lestienne (1976) in adults and by Stoffregen et al (1985) in children. Stoffregen et al have furthermore shown that in walking, optical information is less necessary than in maintaining balance. These authors have attributed this finding to the fact that in walking optical information is less necessary than in maintaining balance. These authors have attributed this finding to the fact that in walking, the two feet "are spread apart along the line of motion, and this two point basis is more stable than when the feet are together (as in stance)".

2.2. Stepping and walking

Although children are only able to walk properly at the age of one, newborn infants show a stepping reflex which looks surprisingly like walking: when an infant is held in an erect position, his or her legs will perform rhythmic alternating movements, and if the child is gently moved forward, he can seem to be making several steps. This reflex usually disappears after 2 months or so, otherwise the maturation of the nervous system is said to be defective (Capute et al, 1976; Dekaban, 1959; DiLeo, 1967; Fiorentino, 1981; Illingworth, 1966; Menkes, 1980, Molnar, 1978; Peiper, 1963; Touwen, 1976; quoted by Thelen et al, 1982). Recent studies have shown that with training, this reflex can be maintained longer or even right up to the age when a child is able to walk (Zelazo, 1983; Zelazo et al, 1972). The debate as to why this reflex disappears has recently been revived (Prechtl, 1981): some authors claim that it is due to an inhibition resulting from the maturation of the cortex (Hofer, 1981; McGraw, 1940, 1943; Paulson & Gottlieb, 1968; quoted by Thelen et al, 1983); others attribute it simply to disuse (Zelazo, 1976; Zelazo et al, 1972). In a very elegant series of studies, Thelen and her collaborators have shown that the loss of the stepping reflex seems to be actually due to the dramatic increase in the mass of the legs, which can no longer be raised against the pull of gravity (Thelen & Fisher, 1982; Thelen et al, 1982). When children's legs are placed in water, they still perform stepping movements perfectly well (Thelen, 1983). Thelen's explanation is compatible with the fact that the stepping reflex disappears whereas kicking (rhythmic pattern observed in supine position) does not: the later reflex actually increases sharply between the age of 4 and 6 months, without any intervention (Thelen, 1979, 1981). Thelen and Fisher (1982) conclude that stepping and kicking might be "the same underlying movement, differently influenced by biomechanical demands". Thelen has underlined the similarities between the stepping and kicking pattern (synergic contraction of muscles in a single limb, and alternating movement) and locomotion and comes to the conclusion that "kicking is indeed a manifestation of the intrinsic neuromuscular programming later incorporated into erect locomotion" (Thelen et al, 1983).

Forssberg (1985), who has examined the development of the locomotor pattern from stepping in newborn infants to independent walking up to 18 months of age, expresses the opinion that "innate pattern generators in the spinal cord produce the infant stepping and also generate the basic locomotor rhythm in adults". He suggests that "neural circuits specific for humans develop late in ontogeny and transform the original, non-plantigrade motor activity to a plantigrade locomotor pattern".

3. STRUCTURE OF THE LOCOMOTOR AUTOMATISM

> The structural elements of the dynamics of a locomotor act may be certainly deciphered by means of more or less complex mathematical and physiological alphabets which permit the revealing through them of underlying central nervous processes (Bernstein, 1967).

Just as Bernstein proposed to identify the structure of locomotion as a means of understanding the underlying neurobiological mechanisms, we are proposing to investigate behavioural invariants from locomotor activity by investigating spontaneous and induced modifications in this activity. At a basic, elementary level, walking consists of putting one foot in front of the other and starting all over again; the automatism is expressed in both the morphology and the repetitive nature of walking. At a higher level, walking also consists of dividing up space with one's stride and time with one's cadence, and hence it is also the production of a velocity.

3.1. Morphological structure of walking

The bipedel locomotor pattern (found in humans as well as in birds when they are walking) is particularly simple and easy to describe. The body is displaced by means of an alternating series of extensions and flexions of the legs. Running and walking patterns have been described by Shapiro et al (1981) in terms of kinematic criteria. These authors studied the variations in the relative support and swing durations in walking and running (see also Grillner et al, 1979) and observed the duration of the flexion and extension phases. The relative durations of the stance, double-support and single-support phases composing the cycle have been investigated by Murray et al (1964). They also analysed the pattern of angle-rotation of the main joints involved in locomotion. Winter (1983) has found the joint angle patterns to be invariant, and the EMG profiles as well (consistent timing over the stride). Bernstein (1967) examined the pattern of forces and used it to analyse the structureal elements of which muscular activity is composed. He states that these structural elements "are of essential co-ordinational significance for the locomotor act and (that) to all appearences they must consequently have a peculiar genesis history and basis in the central nervous system or elsewhere" (Bernstein, 1967). This statement anticipates biological discoveries which were to be made much later in connection with the neural control mechanisms of the rhythmic aspects of locomotion (see in particular Delcomyn, 1980; Grillner, 1975, 1981; Shik & Orlovski, 1976).

3.2. The spatio-temporal structure of locomotion: the links between parameters

The links between the spatio-temporal parameters of locomotion have been mainly studied by varying the subjects' velocity, either using constraints (treadmill), or by requiring subjects to walk or run at different speeds. These studies have shown that a linear relationship exists between the duration of the stance or the swing phase, and the duration of the cycle. The slope of the regression line was found to differ between the two phases, which show that it is mainly the support phase which decreases when the duration of the cycle decreases. The duration of the swing phase decreases to a lesser extent (Herman et al, 1976; Murray et al, 1966). The same can be said of kicking in babies (Thelen et al, 1981) and in animal species such as cats and cockroaches (Pearson, 1976). Speed-related variations in the duration of the cycle have been observed in particular by Shapiro et al (1981) and by Grillner et al (1979), who reported a considerable decrease (in both walking and running subjects, at low speeds of 1 to 4 m/s) in the duration of the support phase, which was related to an increase in velocity. Similar results have been obtained on monkeys and cats (Vilensky & Gehlsen, 1984). It has been furthermore shown that the increase in velocity is accompanied by an increase in stride-length, both in young adults and in elderly subjects (Murray et al, 1966; Crowninshield et al, 1978). The spatio-temporal relationships between these parameters do not obey the same laws in adults as in small children (between the age of 1 and 2 years, the velocity is the reverse of that observed in adults), and the adult spatio-temporal pattern begins to emerge only around the age of 5 (Grieve & Gear, 1966).

Laurent and Pailhous (in preparation) decided to vary the stride-length or the cadence rather than the velocity: adult subjects instructed to walk to a set tempo given by audible signals showed a near-constant stride-length, which points to the existence of a strong link between velocity and cadence. When stride-lengths were constrained, both the cadence and the velocity were affected in the case of the shorter stride-lengths. With large stride-lengths, the velocity again reflected the imposed variation in stride-length and the cadence remained constant. Ferrandez and Pailhous (in preparation) have also found that strong links exist between velocity and cadence on the one hand, and velocity and stride-length on the other; whereas no significant relationship was observed between stride-length and cadence. This spatio-temporal gait pattern is set up by the age of 6 and becomes quite steady by the age of 8. It is found in children of both ages, both when walking normally and when performing some distracting task as they walk (such as counting their steps) which causes a decrease in the cadence.

3.3. The rhythmic structure of locomotion

There are many different forms of locomotion (limb alternation in walking in bipeds and quadrupeds, limb phase movement in galloping, wing phase movement in flying, natatorial and reptilian undulations), but they are all characterised by rhythmicity (Delcomyn, 1980; Grillner, 1981; Shik & Orlovski, 1976). This rhythmicity is what gives locomotor automatism its high degree of regularity. Bernstein has interestingly pointed out four particular aspects of locomotion: the fact that locomotion has a remarkably stable, typical structure "incorporating many dozens of characteristics for each normal subject"; locomotion is a movement which man has had time to master, both as a species (it is a "phylogenetically extremely ancient movement") and in terms of individual performance (it can be "mastered incomparably better and more completely than any individual professional skills"). Lastly, Bernstein stresses the automatic nature of locomotion, which set it apart from professional skills. He shows what a useful movement it can be to study, not only because of its repetitive nature but also because it allows us "to adopt constant criteria for the discrimination of the random from the regular". Actually, in any simple situation involving a single task - such as walking in a straight line over a normally lit, self-coloured, horizontal floor - locomotor activity involves a two-fold kinematic phenomenon: 1) it is very stable if one compares the length, cadence, and velocity of any stride in a sequence with the previous or subsequent stride; 2) and from one sequence of strides to another it is quite variable about a certain mean tendency. Any change in the condition (such as a slight change in the slope of the ground) tends to be simply reflected in a displacement of the mean tendency with large areas of overlap between distributions. Although all the strutural properties of locomotion have not yet been completely identified, it is reasonable on the basis of present knowledge to assume that the locomotor program parameters can be set but that they are not set in advance. In other words, one cannot speak about a basic stride in the way one speaks about a basic posture in the case of the erect position in man. The programmatic aspect of walking thus lies not in the duration or the length of the strides but for instance in the morphological consistency of the basic pattern, or in the fact that it is impossible to suddenly change the values of parameters from one step to another, or in the bonds of cadence and velocity... The program can also be manifested through an infinite number of kinematic and dynamic parameter values. The fact that the parameter values can be set in and not by the program is compatible with the fact that the parameters have variation ranges beyond which they no longer fit the program. for example because of biomechanical constraints, a certain stride length is impossible when a person is walking and forces him to break into a run (the double-support disappears). When speaking about modulations of locomotion (whether they are due to factors of cognitive origin such as the request to walk faster, or to environmental factors such as a change in the slope), we assume that the modulations in the parameters of walking come within the program's working limits. Lastly, it should be mentioned that proprioceptive reafferents are necessary for maintaining the locomotor program but they seem to play a decisive part in setting the parameter values (Wendler, 1974).

4. MODULATIONS OF THE LOCOMOTOR AUTOMATISM

> The overall picture is an intervention between subtle volitional corrections and basic central and peripheral elements all of which in a joint effort may produce movements ranging from a ballet dance to a tightrope walk (Grillner, 1981).

From the developmental point of view, studying an automatism is a good means of acquiring insights into the evolution of modulations because automatisms remain remarkably stable as an individual grows older. Once the adult pattern has been acquired (this has been said to occur at various ages dependeing on the authors' criteria: from 18 months according to Forssberg, 1985, to around 5 years according to Bernstein, 1967, or Grieve and Gear, 1966), the actual pattern will show no further changes until old age. By studying age-related changes in locomotion, information has been obtained about how modulations function. The first example we shall give concerns modulations induced by a simple rhythmic task (step-counting). The second concerns modulations affecting locomotion in high-level performances of a competitive sport (regulation of stride-length in long-jumping). The role of visual information and its implications for motor performance will be discussed.

4.1. Modulations of locomotion elicited by focusing attention on cadence

When children count their steps as they walk, the cadence at which they walk decreases. This has been observed at the age of 6 and 8, and neither affects the spatio-temporal structure nor the links between parameters (Ferrandez et al, 1985; Ferrandez & Pailhous, in preparation). The way in which this decrease in the cadence affects the walking parameters (velocity and stride-length) depends on the subject's age. At the age of 6, it was found that the above decrease in cadence led to an equivalent decrease in velocity, resulting in significant slowing down from normal walking to walking with a step counting constraint, although stride-length remained constant. At the age of 8, on the other hand, the change in cadence affected the velocity but also the stride-length to nearly the same extent. The strong links observed between the parameters "velocity plus cadence", and "velocity plus stride-length" show that the velocity is a key notion. These links seem to indicate that it might be the main parameter controlled. There are several possible ways of accounting for velocity control. The subject's knowledge of his own speed might result from a cognitive control in which the values of the stride-lengths (provided by bio-mechanical information) are multiplied by the values of the cadence (auditory information in particular informs a subject as to his tempo). These cognitive calculations seem rather too sophisticated to be plausible, however; and in addition this hypothesis is not consistent with our recent findings that there are no systematic links between stride-length and cadence (Ferrandez & Pailhous, in preparation). A more likely explanation might be one based on direct access to information concerning the velocity. Visual information provides a subject with a direct means of assessing his velocity. An individual's displacement gives rise to an optical flow in the opposite direction to that of the displacement. This proprioceptive function of vision, which consists of informing individuals about the characteristics of their own displacement, was brought to light by Gibson (1958). The experiment conducted by Ferrandez and Pailhous (in preparation) seems to show that the velocity is the main parameter to be controlled at both ages, and it is plausible to suggest that this control may be based on the use of visual information. The ontogenetic differences observed might be attributable to the differences in the amount of visual information available to subjects of different ages. The width of the visual field has been found, for instance, to increase with age, especially between the age of 6 and 8 (Whiteside, 1976; Lakowski & Aspinall, 1969). The ontogenetic differences observed in Ferrandez and Pailhous' experiment can thus possibly be interpreted as follows: the differences in the amount of visual information available to 6 and 8 year-olds in the peripheral field may account for the fact that in 6 year-old subjects, the decrease in the cadence leads to a roughly equivalent decrease in velocity (and the stride-length remains constant), whereas in subjects aged 8, the decrease in velocity caused by the decrease in the cadence is partly compensated for by an increase in stride-length.

4.2. Stride-length regulation in locomotor pointing

A person crossing the street will place his or her preferred foot on the pavement without having to make any very consipicuous readjustment to the last step (Pailhous & Clarac, 1984). In fact, the adjustment begins several steps before that, and consists of either shortening or lengthening the last few steps. A small spatial change can thus lead to a relatively large adjustment, since the change is repeated at each step. People are thus capable 1) of anticipating what the future position of their foot on the pavement would be if they went on walking without any change in step; and 2) of changing their step slightly so as to reach to other side safely. These cognitive operations take place without the subject being aware of them. Studies have been made on long-jumpers' approach run up to the take-off board in order to determine what adjustments are made to their stride-length in order to ensure 1) that their pushing foot lands on the board, 2) that it is placed as accurately as possible (near the edge, but without overlapping), and 3) that they achieve maximum speed. Lee et al (1982) have shown that stride adjustment does not occur throughout the approach run, but that it is applied at a particular moment, 5 or 6 strides before the board. The question arises as to how the distance (or the time) to be run is encoded at that point. Visual information certainly plays a large part, both in assessing the distance between the athlete and the take-off board and in the form of visual flow indicating the speed at which the athlete is running. In the opinion of Lee and collaborators (Lee et al, 1982; Lee, 1976; Lee & Reddish, 1981), the distance remaining to be covered to the take-off board may be encoded not in spatial but temporal terms (time to contact). The results obtained by Lee et al (1982) seem to corroborate this hypothesis: they show that stride-length is controlled by adjusting the suspension time (temporal parameter). It has not yet been exactly established, however, how this temporal coding takes place. Since visual information provides the contact point and the speed of displacement, it can be processed to give the time to contact whenever this is required. Laurent (1981) has put forward a different interpretation: he suggests that the characteristics of strides may be used to calculate the position of the imaginary target which would be reached if the subject's stride-length remained unchanged. This virtual target might then be compared at regular intervals with the real target and the stride-length increased or shortened as required to reduce the difference between the two targets as far as possible. The latter interpretation is based on the assumption that athletes are extremely well acquainted with their own stride characteristics. Laurent (1981) has shown that this is so in the case of highly trained athletes but not in that of those with less experience. This particular sporting event differs from others such as sprinting in that it requires a particularly high degree of skill to encode the distance, process this information, and establish what modulations are required. Sprinting does not involve any such amplitude accuracy component, nor does locomotion in general (apart from tasks such as the road-crossing one mentioned above).

5. CONCLUSIONS

As we have seen, locomotion, because of its automatic nature, is an activity which, once properly acquired, offers the advantage of being stable from one age to another, which is rarely the case with acquired skills: we are taught to write, but not to walk. Whatever children's social and cultural background, and even their previous motor experience (apart from a few very extreme cases involving special training, cf. Zelazo for example), they all begin to walk roughly at the same age and in the same way. The first stage in movement development (stepping) unquestionably foreshadows mature walking: the rhythmic pattern and the synergy of the muscles in the limbs are suggestive of the locomotion that will be mastered later on. Other motor activities such as manual pointing are not so easy to distinguish and investigate. For one thing, this movement in babies involves temporal characteristics (slowness, step-by-step, cf. von Hofsten, 1982) which are quite different from the ballistic characteristics of the fully mature movement; for another, the hand position which is typical at an early age - the hand open, the forefinger half extended and the other fingers bent inwards - can be taken to be an early form of either grasping or pointing, depending on which characteristic is thought to be the main one. The upper limbs are able to carry out a wide range of different functions and can use a large variety of repertoires of possible movements. This wider range of possibilities can be explained in biomechanical terms, for example (the shoulder joint has more degrees of freedom than the hip), but basically it is the locomotor function which causes the difference: walking frees the upper limbs so that they can perform numerous activities and this in turn restricts the lower limbs to one main activity: performing locomotor automatism.

One of the main advantages of locomotion as a subject of investigation is the fact that it is susceptible of modulation. Far from being a rigid type of movement, locomotion, because of the many modulations of which it is capable, can adapt to complex tasks requiring a high degree of accuracy. The long-jumper's adjustment of stride-length demands a high degree of skill as well as involving distance-coding and a knowledge by the athlete of his own stride characteristics. Since locomotion is a rhythmic activity, continuous data can be coded in discrete terms (distance in terms of stride-length and time in terms of cadence). The particular moment at which the information is discretised might be that at which the foot strikes the ground. Muzzi et al (1984) have studied the co-ordination between clap and walk and observed "the particular saliency of heel strike within the step cycle as the anchor point around which the modulated clap cycle was focused". In the co-ordination between breathing and running, it has also been reported that the respiratory cycle was synchronised to the footfall cycle (Bramble & Carrier, 1983). The velocity, which is a continuous parameter, is thought to be deducted from the continuous visual input provided by the optical flow. This information may however be discretised in certain cases. An extreme example of the discretisation of visual information during walking is provided by bipedal locomotion in pigeons: Frost (1978) has observed that pigeons apparently make forward and backward movements and show that the purpose of these movements is to stabilise the visual scene: the head-bobbing disappears when the visual scene is fixed by making the pigeons walk on a treadmill. The role played by vision in locomotion has not yet been fully elucidated. Visual information is certainly known to play an important part in maintaining posture, but little is known about how visual information (concerning speed as well as changes of directions for example) brings about modulations of stride-length and cadence during locomotion. In ongoing experiments by Pailhous, Ferrandez, Fluckiger and Baumberger, adult subjects are requested to walk straight ahead under various visual optical flow conditions (sets of luminous points moving forwards or backwards and at various speeds). The duration and length of subjects' strides are being analysed. Any modulations in these two parameters will show whether the optical flow is related to the spatio-temporal parameters of locomotion (stride-length and cadence). It is not always easy to establish the role of cognitive processes in observed modulations. In the case of the vision-induced modulations of locomotion, there is no need to refer to high processes: the flocculus, a structure located in the cerebellum, seems to play an important part in adaptive changes in the vestibulo-occular reflex observed in monkeys (Lisberger et al, 1984). In modulations induced by rhythmic tasks, determining the involvement of cognitive processes is equally complex: co-ordinated running and breathing rhythms have been observed in several mammalian species, which seems to indicate that processing occurs at a quite elementary level. When this type of co-ordination was investigated in humans, however, it was reported that inexperienced ones were found to have clock-work precision of locomotor-respiratory coupling (Bramble & Carrier, 1983). Muzii et al have studied another type of co-ordination between the upper and lower extremities: clapping and walking. These authors report that "the temporal structure of the step cycle appeared to determine the timing of arm movements" (in clapping). They link this result to those obtained by Ballesteros et al (1965) and Craik et al (1976) on arm swing during stepping. On the basis of these findings concerning the relationships between locomotor rhythm and arm swing rhythm in normal walking, Muzzi et al have concluded that their results are compatible with the coupled oscillator concept put forward in particular by Grillner (1981) in connection with co-ordinated rhythmic patterns. Forssberg suggests that there exists "a hierarchical system for human locomotor control similar to that of quadrupeds, but with additional neural mechanisms that transform the original pattern" (Forssberg, 1985).

In short, an automatism such as locomotion can be a worthwile tool for studying the cognitive processes underlying motor activity. One should naturally be cautious in assuming that the modulations involved are necessarily of cognitive origin, since locomotion can be modulated both at very elementary levels and by highly complex cognitive constraints.

ACKNOWLEDGEMENTS

This work was undertaken thanks to a grant from the scientific association Naturalia et Biologia.

References

Ballesteros, M.L.F., Buchthal, F., Rosenfalck, P. (1965). The pattern of muscular activity during the arm swing of natural walking. *Acta Psychologica Scandinavica, 63,* 296-390.

Bard, C. & Hay, L. (1983). Etude ontogénétique de la coordination visuo-manuelle. *Revue Canadienne de Psychologie, 37(3),* 390-413.

Benson, J., Welch, L., Campos, J.J. & Haith, M.M. (1985). The development of crawling in infancy (poster abstract). *Cahiers de Psychologie Cognitive, 5(3-4),* 238.

Bernstein, N. (1967). *The co-ordination and regulation of movements.* Oxford: Pergamon.

Bramble, D.M. & Carrier, D.R. (1983). Running and breathing in mammals. *Science, 219,* 251-256.

Bril, B., Fontaine, R. & Brenière, Y. (1985). Analytical study of walking development (poster abstract). *Cahiers de Psychologie Cognitive, 5(3-4),* 239-240.

Butterworth, G. & Hicks, L. (1977). Visual proprioception and postural stability in infancy. A developmental study. *Perception, 6,* 255-262.

Capute, A.J., Accardo, P.J., Vining, E.P.G., Rubenstein, J.E. & Harryman, S. (1978). *Primitive reflex profile.* Baltimore: University Park Press.

Craik, R., Herman, R. & Finley, F.R. (1976). Human solutions for locomotion II. Interlimb coordination. In R.M. Herman, S. Grillner, P.S.G. Stein and D.G. Stuart (Eds.), *Neural control of locomotion.* New York: Plenum Press.

Crowninshield, R.D., Brand, R.A. & Johnston, R.G. (1978). The effects of walking velocity and age on hip kinematics and kinetics. *Clinical Orthopaedics, 132,* 140-144.

Dekaban, A. (1959). *Neurology of infancy.* Baltimore: Williams and Wilkins.

Delcomyn, F. (1980). Neural basis of rhythmic behavior in animals. *Science, 210,* 492-498.

Di Leo, J.H. (1967). Developmental evaluation of very young infants. In J. Hellmuth (Ed.), *Exceptional infant. Vol. 1. The normal infant.* Seattle: Special Child Publications.

Ferrandez, A.M., Loarer, E. & Pailhous, J. (1985). Modulation of locomotion in 6 and 8 year-old children induced by focusing attention on frequency (poster abstract). *Cahiers de Psychologie Cognitive, 5(3-4),* 297-298.

Fiorentino, M.R. (1981). *A basis for sensorimotor development. Normal and abnormal: The influence of primitive, postural reflexes on the development and distribution of tone.* Springfield, Ill: Charles C. Thomas.

Forssberg, H. (1985). Ontogeny of human locomotor control: I. Infant stepping, supported locomotion and transition to independent locomotion. *Experimental Brain Research, 57(3),* 480-492.

Frost, B.J. (1978). The optokinetic basis of head-bobbing in the pigeon. *Journal of Experimental Biology, 74,* 187-195.

Gachoud, J.P., Mounoud, P., Hauert, C.A. & Viviani, P. (1983). Motor strategies in lifting movements: a comparison of adult and child performance. *Journal of Motor Behavior, 15(3),* 202-216.

Gibson, J.J. (1958). Visually controlled locomotion and visual orientation in animals. *British Journal of Psychology, 49,* 182-194.

Gibson, J.J. (1966). *The senses considered as perceptual systems.* Boston: Houghton Mifflin.

Grieve, D.W. & Gear, R.J. (1966). The relationships between length of stride, step frequency, time of swing and speed of walking for children and adults. *Ergonomics, 5(9),* 379-399.

Grillner, S. (1975). Locomotion in vertebrates: central mechanisms and reflex interaction. *Psychological Review, 55(2),* 247-304.
Grillner, S. (1981). Control of locomotion in bipeds, tetrapods, and fish. In V.B. Brooks (Ed.), *Handbook of Physiology. Section I: The nervous system, vol. II.*
Grillner, S., Halbertsma, J., Nilsson, J. & Thorsteinsson, A. (1979). The adaptation to speed in human locomotion. *Brain Research, 165,* 177-182.
Hay, L. (1979a). Spatial-temporal analysis of movements in children: motor programs versus feedback in the development of reaching. *Journal of Motor Behavior, 11(3),* 189-200.
Hay, L. (1979b). Le mouvement dirigé vers un objectif visual chez l'adulte et chez l'enfant. *L'Annéé Psychologique, 79,* 559-588.
Hay, L. (1981). The effects of amplitude and accuracy requirements on movement time in children. *Journal of Motor Behavior, 13(3),* 177-186.
Hay, L. & Bard, C. (1984). The role of movement speed in learning a visuo-manual coordination in children. *Psychological Research, 46,* 177-186.
Herman, R.M., Wirta, R., Bampton, S. & Finley, F.R. (1976). Human solutions for locomotion. I: Single limb analysis. In R.M. Herman, S. Grillner, P.S.G. Stein and D.G. Stuart (Eds.), *Neural control of locomotion.* New York: Plenum.
Hofer, M.A. (1981). *The roots of human behavior: an introduction to the psychobiology of early development.* San Francisco: W.H. Freeman.
Hofsten, C. von. (1982). Eye-hand coordination in the newborn. *Developmental Psychology, 18(3),* 450-461.
Illingworth, R.A. (1966). *The development of the infant and young children, normal and abnormal.* London: E & S Livingstone (3rd. Ed.).
Lakowski, R. & Aspinall, P. (1969). Static perimetry in young children. *Vision Research, 9,* 305-312.
Laurent, M. (1981). Problèmes posés par l'étude du pointage locomoteur d'une cible visuelle. *Cahiers de Psychologie Cognitive, 1,* 173-197.
Lee, D.N. (1976). A theory of visual control of braking based on information about time to collision. *Perception, 5,* 437-459.
Lee, D.N. & Aronson, E. (1974). Visual proprioceptive control of standing in human infants. *Perception and Psychophysics, 15,* 529-532.
Lee, D.N. & Lishman, J.R. (1975). Visual proprioceptive control of stance. *Journal of Human Movement Studies, 1,* 87-95.
Lee, D.N., Lishman, J.R. & Thomson, J.A. (1982). Regulation of gait in long jumping. *Journal of Experimental Psychology, Human Perception and Performance, 8(3),* 448-459.
Lee, D.N. & Reddish, P.E. (1981). Plummeting gannots: A paradigm of ecological optics. *Nature, 293,* 293-294.
Lepecq, J.C. (1985). Object location and distance estimation during passive movements in infants (poster abstract). *Cahiers de Psychologie Cognitive, 5(3-4),* 241-242.
Lisberger, S.G., Miles, F.A. & Zee, D.S. (1984). Signals used to compute errors in monkey vestibulo-ocular reflex: possible role of flocculus. *Journal of Neurophysiology, 52(6),*
McGraw, M.B. (1935). *Growth: A study of Johnny and Jimmy.* New York: Appleton Century.
McGraw, M.B. (1940). Neuromuscular development of the human infant as exemplified in the achievement in erect locomotion. *J. Pediatr., 17,* 747-771.
McGraw, M.B. (1943). *The neuro-muscular maturation of the human infant.* New York: Columbia University Press.

Menkes, J.H. (1980). *Textbook of child neurology.* Philadelphia: Lea & Febiger.
Molnar, G.E. (1978). Analysis of motor disorder in retarded infants and young children. *Am. J. ment. def., 83,* 213-222.
Mounoud, P. & Bower, T.G.R. Conservation of weight in infants. *Cognition, 3(1),* 29-40.
Mounoud, P. & Hauert, C.A. (1982). Development of sensorimotor organisation in young children. In G. Forman (Ed.), *Action and thought: from sensori-motor schemes to symbolic operations.* New York: Academic Press.
Mounoud, P., Hauert, C.A., Mayer, E., Gachoud, J.P., Guyon, J. & Gottret, G. (1983). Visuo-manual tracking strategies in the three to five year-old children. *Archives de Psychologie, 51,* 23-33.
Mounoud, P., Viviani, P., Hauert, C.A. & Guyon, J. (1985). Development of visuo-manual tracking in 5 to 9 year-old children. *Journal of Experimental Child Psychology, 40,* 115-132.
Murray, M.P., Drought, A.B. & Kory, R.C. (1964). Walking patterns of normal men. *Journal of Bone and Joint Surgery, 46(2),* 335-360.
Murray, M.P., Kory, R.C., Clarksson, B.H. & Sepic, S.B. (1966). Comparison of free and fast speed walking patterns of normal men. *American Journal of Physical Medicine, 45(1),* 8-24.
Muzii, R.A., Lamm Warburg, C. & Gentile, A.M. (1984). Coordination of the upper and lower extremities. *Human Movement Science, 3,* 337-354.
Pailhous, J. & Clarac, F. (1984). Approche comportementale de la locomotion: éléments d'analyse chez l'homme et chez l'animal. In J. Paillard (Ed.), *La lecture sensorimotrice et cognitive de l'expérience spatiale: direction et distance.* Paris: Editions du CNRS, collection Comportements.
Paulson, G. & Gottlieb, G. (1968). Developmental reflexes: the reappearence of foetal and neonatal reflexes in aged patients. *Brain, 91,* 37-52.
Pavard, B., Berthoz, A. & Lestienne, F. (1976). Rôle de la vision périphérique dans l'évaluation du mouvement linéaire. Interaction visuo-vestibulaire et effects posturaux. *Le Travail Humain, 39(1),* 115-138.
Pearson, K. (1976). The control of walking. *Scientific American, 235,* 72-86.
Peiper, A. (1963). *Cerebral function in infancy and early childhood.* New York: Consultants Bureau.
Prechtl, H.F.R. (1981). The study of neural development as a perspective of clinical problems. In K.J. Connolly and H.F.R. Prechtl (Eds.), *Maturation and development: Biological and psychological perspectives.* London: SIMP and Heinemann.
Shapiro, D.C., Zernicke, R.F., Gregor, R.J. & Diestel, J.D. (1981). Evidence for generalized motor programs using gait pattern analysis. *Journal of Motor Behavior, 13(1),* 33-47.
Shik, M.L. & Orlovski, G.N. (1976). Neurophysiology of locomotor automatism. *Physiological Reviews, 56(3),* 465-501.
Shumway-Cook, A. & Woollacott, M.H. (1985). The growth of stability: postural control from a developmental perspective. *Journal of Motor Behavior, 17(2),* 131-147.
Statham, L. & Murray, M.P. (1971). Early walking patterns of normal children. *Clinical Orthopaedics, 79,* 8-24.
Stoffregen, T., Schmuckler, M. & Gibson, E. (1985). Development of use of optical flow in the control of stance and locomotion (poster abstract). *Cahiers de Psychologie Cognitive, 5(3-4),* 246-247.
Sugden, D. (1980). Movement speed in children. *Journal of Motor Behavior, 12(2),* 125-132.
Sutherland, D.H., Olshen, R., Cooper, L. & Woo, S.L. (1980). The development of nature gait. *Journal of Bone and Joint Surgery, 62(3),* 336-353.

Thelen, E. (1979). Rhythmical stereotypies in normal human infants. *Animal Behavior, 27,* 699-715.

Thelen, E. (1981). Kicking, rocking and waving: contextual analysis of rhythmical stereotypies in normal human infants. *Animal Behavior, 29,* 3-11.

Thelen, E. (1983). Learning to walk is still an "old" problem: a reply to Zelazo (1983). *Journal of Motor Behavior, 15(2),* 139-161.

Thelen, E., Bradshaw, G. & Ward, J.A. (1981). Spontaneous kicking in month-old infants: manifestations of a human central locomotor program. *Behavioral and Neural Biology, 32,* 45-53.

Thelen, E. & Fisher, D.M. (1982). Newborn stepping: an explanation for a "disappearing" reflex. *Developmental Psychology, 18(5),* 760-775.

Thelen, E., Fisher, D.M., Ridley-Johnson, R. & Griffin, N.J. (1982). Effects of body build and arousal on newborn infant stepping. *Developmental Psychobiology, 15(5),* 447-453.

Thelen, E., Ridley-Johnson, R. & Fisher, D.M. (1983). Shifting patterns of bilateral coordination and lateral dominance in the leg movements of young infants. *Developmental Psychobiology, 16(1),* 29-46.

Touwen, B. (1976). *Neurological development in infancy.* London: SIMP and William Heinemann Medical Books.

Vilensky, J.A. & Gehlsen, G. (1984). Temporal gait parameters in humans and quadrupeds: how do they change with speed? *Journal of Human Movement Studies, 10,* 175-188.

Wendler, G. (1974). The influence of proprioceptive feedback on locust flight coordination. *Journal of Comparative Physiology, 88,* 173-200.

Whiteside, J.A. (1976). Peripheral vision in children and adults. *Child Development, 47,* 290-293.

Winter, D. (1983). Biomechanical motor patterns in normal walking. *Journal of Motor Behavior, 15(4),* 302-330.

Zelazo, P.R. (1976). From reflexive to instrumental behavior. In L.P. Lipsitt (Ed.), *Developmental Psychobiology: the significance of infancy.* Hillsdale, N.J.: Lawrence Erlbaum.

Zelazo, P.R. (1983). The development of walking: new findings and old assumptions. *Journal of Motor Behavior, 15(2),* 99-137.

Zelazo, P.R., Zelazo, N.A. & Kolb, S. (1972). Walking in the newborn. *Science, 176,* 314-315.

DEVELOPMENTAL CHANGES IN THE RELATIVE TIMING OF LOCOMOTION

M.A. Roberton

A simple way to describe the study of motor development is to say that it focuses on the changing motor coordination(s) which occur across an organism's lifespan. Most laypeople would understand that definition, and most specialists would accept it as a rough approximation of what they do. Yet, few, contemporary motor development researchers take the opportunity to study *age change* (as opposed to *age differences*), and few actually study either the *act* or the *process* of "becoming coordinated": that evolving concatenation in space and time of the movements of body parts to accomplish a given task.

Traditionally, however, describing the actions involved in becoming coordinated has been the province of motor development research. Frequently, these descriptions have been cast in the form of developmental sequences, chronicling the qualitative changes that occur with time in the organisation of body parts to accomplish a task, such as walking. Yet, when one examines the last 100 years of work in this area (using the publication of Darwin's, 1877, observations on his son as a marker), the number of carefully-described sequences, validated with longitudinal data, are pitifully small. Of these, the number concerned with the processes underlying the changes described are fewer yet. Recently, however, several developmentalists have returned to the study of locomotion in an effort to understand the developing control structures underlying sequential change in the patterns of coordination. Their initial work will be the focus of this paper.

TIMING RELATIONSHIPS IN ADULT LOCOMOTION

A basic concept associated with the notion of coordinated, skillful movement is the precise ordering of spatial-temporal motor events; skilled movers have their body parts in the right place at the right time; and the order in which the body levers move to that position seems precisely timed in terms of successive accelerations and decelerations. Recently, motor control specialists have begun studying these timing relationships in adults. Spurred by the evidence of Grillner (1975), Pearson (1976), and Wetzel and Stuart (1976) for spinal, limb "pattern generators" in animals, investigators have been studying temporal relationships in human adult handwriting (Gentner, 1982; Terzuolo & Viviani, 1979, 1982), walking and running (Shapiro, Zernicke, Gregor & Diestal, 1981), speech (Kelso & Tuller, in press), and various laboratory tasks (see Schmidt, 1985). The guiding hypothesis for this research is that timing relationships which remain invariant over modifications of the skill (by speed changes, for instance) may be external manifestations of control mechanisms, such as spinal generators.

While not without controversy (see Gentner, 1982), the overwhelming, current opinion seems to be that certain, invariant timing relationships do exist between at least some constituent lever actions (or EMG patterns) within the tasks studied. These relationships are not seen clearly in the absolute timing of actions, but are revealed when the timing relationships are normalised by setting some referent, such as the total time for the complete movement, to 100%. Constituent parts of the movement, when seen relative to the total cycle, do not seem to change as the cycle is "scaled up" by increasing the over-all velocity of the movement. These invariants in the face of scaling are thought to represent the "deep structure" of the system as opposed to the changeable, "surface" structures (Schmidt, 1985).

Findings on adult locomotion illustrate these points. Grieve (1968) was among the first to suggest that study of the mechanisms underlying walking needed a "whole-range" approach in which invariant relationships would be sought across a variety of walking speeds. He demonstrated a linear relationship between the duration of the time taken for leg swing and the speed of the walk, suggesting a relative timing mechanism generalising across speeds. In 1981 Shapiro, Zernicke, Gregor, and Diestal investigated this phenomenon further. They filmed five persons walking on a treadmill at a variety of speeds from 3-6 km/hr and running at various speeds from 8-12 km/hr. Although these subjects doubled their walking speed during the filming and increased their running speed by 1.5 times, the relative timing of the four phases of the Phillippson (1905) step cycle stayed statistically the same within the walk and within the run. At the same time, however, the absolute times consumed by these portions of the cycle increased dramatically (especially for walking) as speed increased. Thus, only when timing was examined relative to the total duration of a cycle were invariant relationships easily determined. In addition, these relative times were reliably different between walking and running, a finding which corroborated the technique's ability to distinguish between qualitatively-different gaits.

IS THERE A "TIMER"?

Two basic views of motor control have been used to explain these findings of relative timing invariance in locomotion and other skills. Shapiro et al (1981) adopted the more prevalent view, represented by Schmidt's (1980, 1985) generalised motor program theory. Schmidt has hypothesised that invariants are unchangeable aspects of a motor program, which is "called up" by the performer prior to the execution of a skill. Other characteristics in the program are changeable parameters. For instance, Schmidt (1985) feels speed of execution is a changeable feature; relative timing of constituent parts and, perhaps relative forces, are unchangeable aspects.

Kelso (1981) and his colleagues (Kelso & Tuller, in press) have posed an alternative view. They see relative timing invariance as a consequence of the motor system's dynamics and as a signature of a "coordinative structure". They argue against an external timer, such as a motor program, feeling that time "evolves from the 'playing out' of the dynamics" of the system (Kelso & Tuller, in press). The coordinative structure, whose presence may be signalled by the invariant timing, is a "temporary marshalling of many degrees of freedom into a task-specific functional unit" (Kelso, Tuller, Vatikiotis-Bateson & Fowler, 1984, p. 828). That becomes, in most cases, a collective of muscles, "often spanning several joints, that is constrained to act as a unit" (Turvey, Shaw & Mace, 1978, p. 563).

At this point in the study of adult motor control, the relative timing issue needs further, convincing evidence of invariances in a variety of motor skills, especially invariances which would show "during-movement" relationships between limbs or muscles groupings, rather than simply "start-stop" relationships. In particular, study of inter-limb coordination has been rare, especially of arm-leg relationships (Muzii, Warburg & Gentile, 1984). Statistical analyses also need to be more convincingly presented, since the finding of an "invariance" may simply be the result of too little statistical power. Finally, the area also needs resolution to the issue of whether timing invariances are extrinsic or intrinsic to the muscular system, i.e., of whether they exist prior to the movement or are a consequence of the movement.

"DEVELOPMENTAL INVARIANCES"

In contrast to the area of adult motor control, the motor development field has not studied relational invariances to any great degree. As Wade (1982) has pointed out, the entire issue of spatial-temporal relationships across body parts within a task has received surprisingly little developmental interest other than as a peripheral part of developmental sequence research. Obviously, for those who study change, the notion of no change or invariance is the opposite side of the coin, and a very interesting side, at that. In a very real sense, the most convincing tests of the meaningfulness of the search for invariants should come out of motor development. If certain features of the timing of motor skills are "really" invariant, then that invariance should be retained over relatively long portions of the lifespan, rather than simply over speed changes at one point in time. Yet, developmentalists would also not be surprised to find that invariants could be emergent, that is, developing at a certain point in the lifespan, but not before. Indeed, such events might be expected to accompany the so-called qualitative changes noted in developmental sequence research. Even so, after their emergence, such invariants should then be retained for relatively long periods of time.

WALKING

Notable exceptions to the dearth of developmental work on intra or inter-limb timing relationships are the pioneering studies by Thelen and her co-workers and Clark and her co-workers. Thelen (Thelen, Bradshaw & Ward, 1981) studied videotapes of the supine kicking behaviours of 8 infants. Focusing on one leg, she counted the videoframes at which movement began, stopped, or changed direction. She found that the relationships of the interkick interval and the kick time to the total kick cycle were similar to the ratios for adult stance and swing to total step cycle in walking. In a subsequent paper (Thelen & Fisher, 1982), kinematics and EMGs of the infant kick appeared related to the kinematics and EMGs of reflex stepping. These results, taken with work on adult locomotion, led Thelen to argue for a common, spinal pattern generator responsible for the spatial-temporal patterns of walking and infant kicking. Moreover, she felt these invariances were established at least by 1 month of age. Thelen (Thelen, Ridley-Johnson & Fisher, 1983) has also looked at inter-leg coordination patterns within kicking. The ability to alternate kicks was quite high even in 2 week olds, suggesting that inter-limb coordination "is a very fundamental property of human leg movements" (Thelen et al, 1983, p. 38).

Clark, (Clark, Phillips & Bower, 1983; Clark, Phillips & Whitall, 1984) has been building on the Thelen work by examining toddler locomotion. She and her colleagues have filmed beginning walkers from the onset of walking through the first year. They found that swing to stance ratios in the single leg began to approximate that of the adult walker as early as two weeks after walking onset. They further found that at approximately three months of walking age the infants began to exhibit a temporal organisation between the two legs that had many similarities to adult walkers. The period prior to this time was characterised by variable and asymmetrical interlimb phasing. In a third study (Whitall, Clark & Phillips, 1985) they demonstrated that new walkers, who were supported to ease the postural demands of the skill, showed more mature, inter-leg coordination than, in some cases, unaided, 4-week walkers. Their conclusions were that intra-leg coordination precedes inter-leg coordination and that the tuning of the coordinative structures to gravitational demands and reactive forces takes about 3 to 6 months of unaided walking. Both the Thelen et al and the Clark et al studies strongly suggest that the basic patterns of intra- and inter-leg coordination for walking are available quite early, but that context-demands, such as postural system control or leg mass, may mask the functioning of these structures at these early ages.

HOPPING

These pioneering, creative, developmental efforts encouraged me to examine relative timing relationships in a quite-different locomotor skill, the hop over distance (as opposed to hopping in place) (Roberton & Halverson, in preparation). Available to me were 15 years of longitudinal, cinematographic data on the same youngsters working to master this task. Specific questions of interest were whether timings could be detected, which remained invariant for a substantial number of years; whether these invariants would be present from initial attempts at the skill or whether they would emerge over time; and conversely, whether some timings were, indeed, developmental, showing change with the passage of time.

Hopping is an interesting locomotor skill for several reasons. First of all, it has phyletic origins. The rudimentary hop (or "limping reaction", as Peiper, 1963, called it) is present as a reflex in a number of species: displacement of the body away from the supporting limb and base of support will elicit a flexion, and then, extension response of that limb to lift it off the ground and replace it under the animal's body. Lateral, forward, and backward hopping responses can be elicited in intact animals, including man Peiper, 1963). Bard (1933) concluded that the hopping response was cortically controlled since ablation of specific cortical areas depressed the response. Herdman et al (1983) have recently challenged this view, finding that the response was slowed but not extinguished after complete spinal cord transection in the cat. They suggested that the basic neural circuitry for the response lies in the cord, but that supraspinal influences are definitely necessary to tune the response. Thus, hopping is yet another skill where developmentalists can speculate about the relationship between the "reflex" and its analogue in voluntary behaviour.

Secondly, the hop over distance has an interesting, evolving coordination between the two arms and the two legs. As the illustrations at the top of Figure 1 indicate, in the advanced hop the non-support leg swings forward to accompany support leg extension, then backward during the flight phase of the hop. The arm opposite the non-support leg also pumps forward and

and back, and the remaining arm works in opposition to that movement. As usual, what is thought of as a simple, childhood skill is really a set of complex coordinations.

TIMING IN THE ADVANCED HOP

The hopping data I examined were a collection of longitudinal films on 7 children, followed for approximately 15 years by Lolas Halverson at the University of Wisconsin-Madison, U.S.A. (Halverson, Roberton & Harper, 1973). Each child was filmed 4 times a year from ages 3-4, every six months from years 5-7, and yearly, thereafter, until their 16th to 18th year. The children were filmed using one, later two 16mm cameras running at 64 fps. Side and front views were taken serially when one camera was used; simultaneously after a second camera was introduced in 1971.

To obtain relative timing information, the frames for onset/cessation of potentially key actions of the four limbs were identified in the films of the children. Every useable hop across the 15 years was included for each child. From the key frames the duration of any event of interest could be calculated using the known frame time. These absolute times were, then, converted to percentages of the total time used for a particular hop cycle. The resulting relative data were averaged across all the children at each age. Inter-observer agreement was within 1 frame. Across occasionally-differing camera speeds, this error could cause, at most, a 4% miscalculation in the relative times.

Figure 1 depicts the averages of normalised data on 13 trials of the hop in which the 7 children studied were categorised as having reached advanced levels in both their arm action and their leg action (Halverson, 1985). The children were 15-18 years of age at the time. The bottom bar represents the phases of the hopping leg during the hop cycle, which is portrayed from foot touch, the first detectable contact of the foot with the surface in the act of landing, to foot touch of the next landing.

I have divided the hopping leg action into three discernible phases: Support Phase I, from foot touch to the point of deepest knee flexion; Support Phase II, from deepest knee flexion until take-off; and the Flight Phase. In the advanced hop, approximately 47% of the hop cycle is taken up in flight, and 54% (with rounding error) in support. The greatest amount of support time is used in Phase II, which is the time of force generation. Phase II ends in take-off, which is also the time of fullest knee extension.

Superimposed on the cyclic action of the hopping leg is the movement of the non-hopping leg, which Roberton and Halverson (1984) called the "swing leg". As the illustrations at the top of Figure 1 show, the swing leg moves through a range of close to 90° both forward and upward, and then down and back in the course of one hop. As the second bar from the bottom of Figure 1 indicates, the swing forward begins about 7% into the hop cycle and ends roughly 10% before take-off. The backward swing starts about 6% into the flight phase and ends simultaneously with the end of the cycle, foot touch.

Superimposed on both actions of the legs are the swinging or pumping actions of the arms (Figure 1). Working in opposition to each other, the arm contralateral to the swing leg pumps forward at the same time as the swing

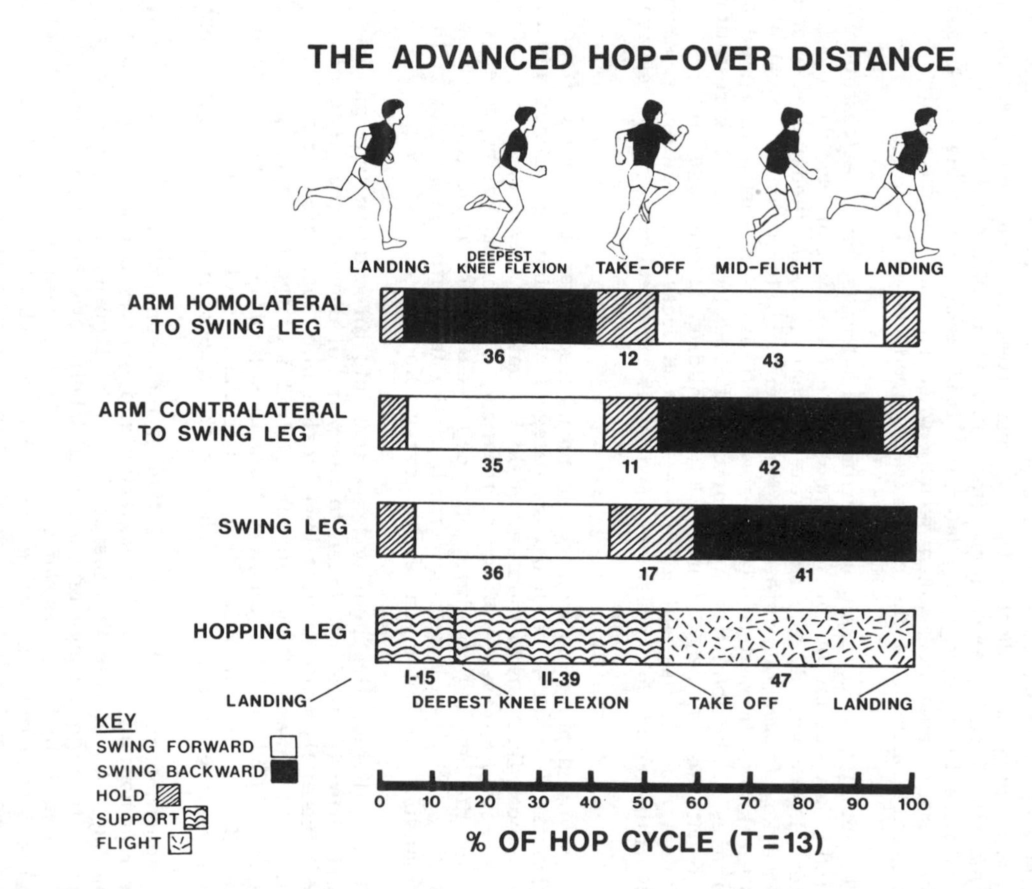

Fig. 1. Relative timing (normalised) across 13 trials of the advanced hop when the 7 children in the longitudinal sample were 15-18 years old.

leg and for the same duration. Meanwhile, the arm on the same side as the swing begins backward movement, again for approximately the same duration: 36% of the cycle. The reverse swings of the arms and the leg are again tied, having similar durations of about 42%. It is interesting that the "hold" periods of the arms (when they are not moving) are similar at the end of each movement, but slightly different from the hold periods of the swing leg. The temporal coordination of the arms and swing leg seems to be most close in the duration of the movement. The two arms, however, are closely tied, both in terms of duration and in terms of initiation and cessation of movement.

Orlovskii and Shik (1965) noted that during treadmill walking or trotting, duration of the swing phase was the most impervious to deformation in the dog. The tightest limb relationships were between contralateral limbs, then hind to forelimbs (Shik & Orlovskii, 1965). These relationships seem to hold also for the human hop, even though the arms are not weight-bearing. This latter observation favors neuro-muscular, oscillator mechanisms over strictly mechanical explanations, although certain biomechanical factors cannot be totally ruled out.

TIMING RELATIONSHIPS WITHIN THE HOPPING LEG

As indicated earlier, the hop can be divided into a support phase and a flight phase. Figure 2 charts the change in absolute flight time for the children from age 3-18. The actual time-in-flight at age 18 is double the time-in-flight at age 4.25, yielding the customary developmental curve motor development specialists love to see. When these data are converted to percentages relative to total hop time, however, the resulting graph (Figure 3)

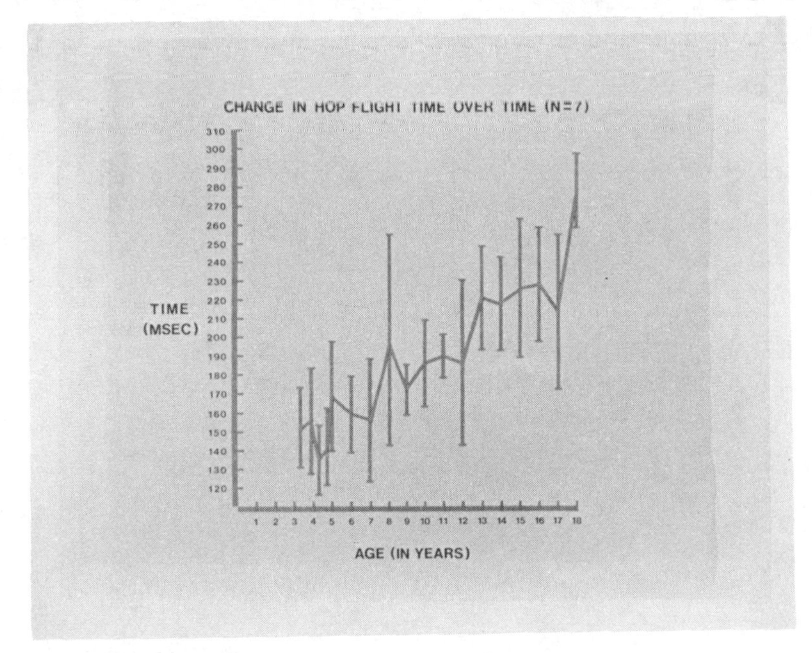

Fig. 2. Longitudinal change in means and standard deviations for absolute flight time.

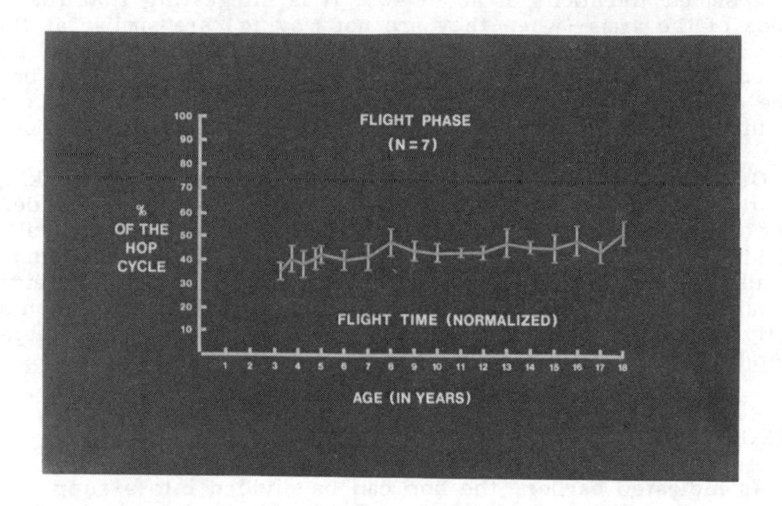

Fig. 3. Longitudinal change in means and standard deviations for normalised flight time.

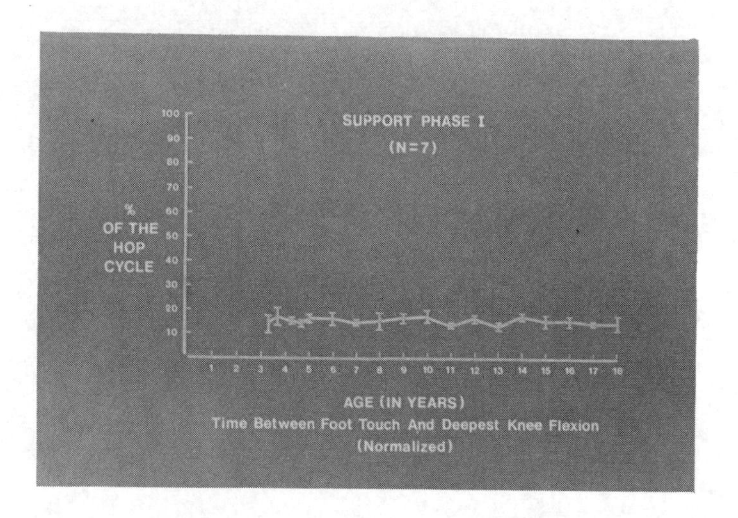

Fig. 4. A relative timing invariance present for 15 years. Normalised means and standard deviations are plotted by age.

is startling. The almost 200% increase in absolute flight time is reduced to a 16% increase in relative flight time. Note also the reduction in the standard deviations. Relative to the greater time needed for the total hop, the flight time actually increased only 16% in 15 years. Relative times for the support phase of the hop, in turn, decreased by the same amount. Since measurement error could account for only a 4% change, 16% is still "meaningful" in terms of change. The difference between 200% and 16%, however, is a dramatic illustration of why relative relationships are important dependent variables for developmentalists to study.

When the hopping leg was further examined for changes in relative timing, the first invariance in timing was discovered. Figure 4 illustrates the relative time used for Support Phase I across the 15 years. These normalised data indicate no change in that portion of the hop which takes place from the time of landing to deepest knee flexion in the landing leg. There is no trend in the data and the range of values was only 3.5%: the children were "the same" at age 3 as they were at age 18. To my knowledge, this is the first timing invariance demonstrated over such a long period of the lifespan.

In addition, Support Phase 1 is analogous to that portion of the walk known as the E_2 phase of the Phillippson step cycle. Shapiro et al (1981) found that the E_2 phase, normalised to the total cycle, was the only phase that did not change across all speeds of *both* walking and running. It would appear that the time needed for the landing to dissipate downward force in the locomotor skills of walking, running, and hopping is under the control of an invariant system that is in operation from the earliest attempts at these skills.

When Support Phase II of the hop (the time from deepest knee flexion to take-off) was examined, two more timing invariances were discovered. The time between deepest knee flexion and the beginning of knee extension (Support Phase IIa) and the duration of knee extension (Support Phase IIb) also showed no trend across the 15 years. Indeed, Support Phase IIc was completely responsible for the 17% decline in the relative timing of the support phase in relation to the total hop cycle (see Figure 5). This period is the time occurring between full knee extension and toe-off. The shortening of this time represents a lessening of the flexion response used by primitive hoppers to leave the ground (Roberton & Halverson, 1984). By age 18 flexion of the hopping leg occurs only 5% ahead of take-off rather than 22%. The advanced hop is primarily an extensor response with flexion used only to clear the toe from the ground.

TIMING OF OTHER BODY PARTS

The developmental paths for the timing relationships of the arms and swing leg to the hopping leg and to each other are all either emergent and then invariant or emergent and then developmental. Their emergent characteristic is due to the qualitative changes which occur between the beginning hop and the advanced hop. These changes have been ordered into developmental sequences by Roberton and Halverson (1984) and partially validated by Halverson and Williams (1985) and Halverson (1985). Briefly, in early hopping the child holds the swing leg immobile, thus *avoiding* having to time the movement of this segment. Only later in development does that leg begin to swing up and down. The arms show dramatic changes as well.

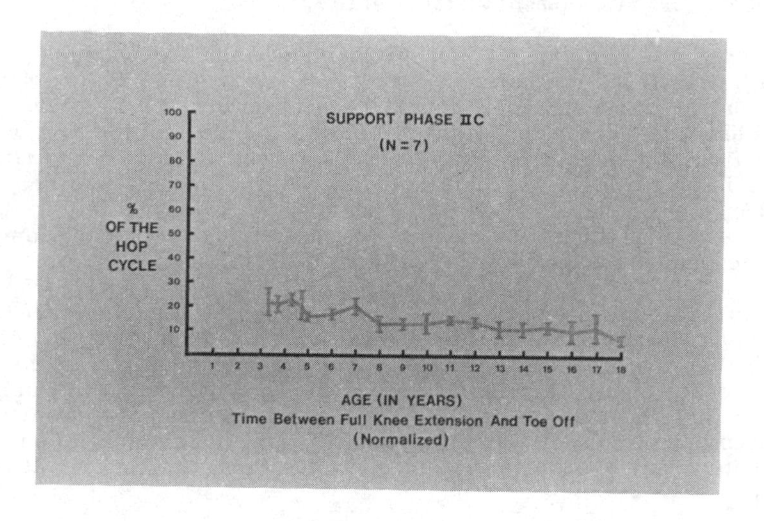

Fig. 5. The only portion of the support phase of the hopping leg to show developmental change over a 15 year period. Normalised means and standard deviations are plotted by age.

At first, they also do not move or move only in reaction to postural disturbances. When movement begins, it is bilateral - both arms pumping up and down synchronously instead of moving in opposite directions. Only in the final level of the hop are the arms synchronised to the swing leg and in opposition to each other.

Figure 6 illustrates the emergence of the timing of the swing leg and its gradual linkage to the beginning of knee extension in the hopping leg. Although the swing leg began swinging in some of the children at 4 years of age, the timing relationship was not worked out until approximately 9 years of age. From then on, the relationship between the two events was invariant, with the swing leg beginning forward movement 20% of the hop cycle ahead of the beginning of knee extension in the hopping leg. Similarly, the timing relationship between the arm contralateral to the swing leg and swing leg showed a period of growing entrainment from age 5-9, with invariance thereafter.

A final example from the findings is Figure 7, showing the two arms as they worked over a number of years to coordinate the timing relationships

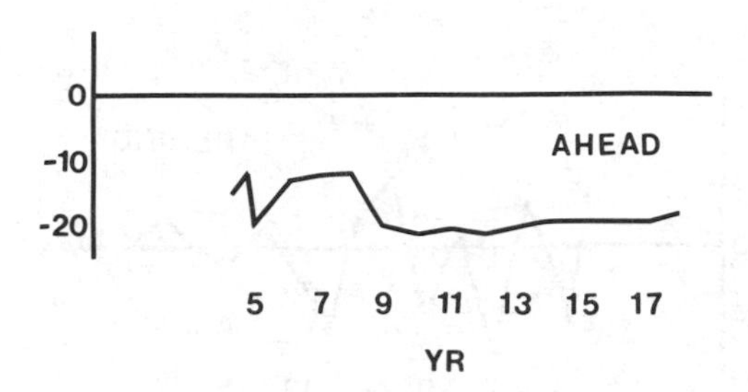

Fig. 6. The emergence of swinging action in the non-support leg and its gradual linkage to a time point 20% ahead of the beginning of knee extension in the support leg (represented by zero on the graph). The negative percentages mean that the swing leg begins forward/upward movement ahead of the beginning of knee extension.

of "opposition". Not until 14 years of age did the end of the backswing of the contralateral arm begin to coincide with the end of the forward swing of the homolateral arm. This graph is an example of an emergent timing followed by a more gradual working out of the relative timing relationship.

These hopping data, then, contain examples of relative timing invariants, which were present from the initial attempts at the skill and remained to adulthood; of emergent invariants, which were absent at first, appeared, took some time to develop but were then constant for a long period of time; and of emergent timings which were absent at first, appeared, and then showed "classic" development, taking years to coalesce. In the first case, the coordination appeared to be functioning as soon as the system was functioning. It appears to be part of an innate or very-early-to-appear coordinative structure incorporated into several locomotor forms. In the second case, the coordination appeared to require some degree of practice or physiological change before it was acquired. In the last case, practice would seem the likely requirement in such a slowly-developing coordination.

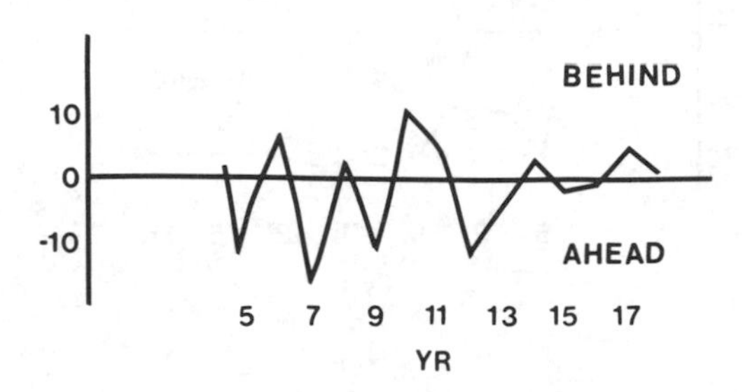

Fig. 7. The emergence of arm action in the hop and the gradual development of a simultaneous stop at the end of both arm swings. The plotted line is the stopping time of the arm contralateral to the swing leg. Negative values indicate stops before the stop of the homolateral arm (the zero line); positive values are stops after the stop of the homolateral arm. These longitudinal data are normalised for 7 children.

BUT, IS RELATIVE TIMING SUFFICIENT?

As a group, the developmental data on relative timing in locomotion are quite fascinating, especially the growing evidence for potentially innate or very-early-appearing invariances in the weight-bearing legs. Yet, as interesting as these data are, a caveat seems in order. Even if instances of invariant relative timing turn out to be plentiful, both in developmental and in adult transfer studies, it may be a mistake to assume that one can extrapolate "time" directly backward to the nervous system or to a "motor program" Movement does not occur in space alone nor in time alone; it is a spatial-temporal phenomenon. Before automatically assuming that time is the parameter being metered out by a motor program, additional research into where the body parts have traveled in the time under study needs to occur. While initial emphasis has been on relative timing, that timing may be the signature of more interesting phenomena detectable at other levels of analysis. For instance, Kelso and Tuller (in press) suggested phase portrait analysis as a second step to pursue in the study of invariance. By comparing the relative positions and simultaneous velocities of body segments during the time elements of interest, they suggest that time may fall out as a resultant of the relative motions rather than as a cause. The key invariant relationships in movement may be position-velocity *states* rather than time. The appealing aspect of their argument is that physiological evidence exists for position and velocity receptors (muscle spindles and tendon organs), but none exists for "time" receptors.

In addition, Winter (1984) has warned that what appears to be invariant at one level of analysis may be variable at another level of analysis. For instance, he found that very different (flexor one time, extensor another) moments of force at the knee and hip could produce the same kinematic configuration of the lower leg in walking. On the other hand, Winter's data imply that the hip and knee moments co-vary, suggestive of a coordinative structure whose function is to get the lower leg to a certain spatial-temporal location in whatever way it can.

In conclusion, the field of motor development appears to be the most proper testing place for the question of (spatial) temporal invariance in motor skills. The long periods of time over which developmentalists view their subjects provide the ideal situation in which to look for the complement of change: no change. That relative timing invariances present from initial attempts at a skill can remain present as long as 15 years later has now been established. The search for the meaning of these "developmental invariances", however, is just beginning.

References

Bard, P. (1933). Studies on the cerebral cortex: localized control of placing and hopping reactions in the cat and their management by small cortical remnants. *Archives of Neurological Psychiatry, 30,* 40-74.

Clark, J., Phillips, S. & Boyer, J. (1983). Temporal characteristics of infant gait across speeds. *Psychology of motor behavior and sport - 1983.* Abstracts of the Annual Meeting of the North American Society for the Psychology of Sport and Physical Activity, East Lansing, MI.

Clark, J., Phillips, S. & Whitall, J. (1984). The development of interlimb coordination in upright locomotion. *Abstracts* of the 1984 Olympic Scientific Congress, Eugene, OR.

Darwin, C. (1877). A biographical sketch of an infant. *Mind, 2,* 285-294.

Gentner, D. (1982). Evidence against a central control model of timing in typing. *Journal of Experimental Psychology: Human Perception and Performance, 8,* 793-810.

Grieve, D. (1968). Gait patterns and the speed of walking. *Biomedical Engineering, 3,* 119-122.

Grillner, S. (1975). Locomotion in vertebrates: Central mechanisms and reflex interaction. *Physiological Reviews, 55,* 247-303.

Halverson, L. (1985). Longitudinal changes in hopping over distance. *Psychology of motor behavior and sport-1985.* Abstracts of the Annual Meeting of the North American Society for the Psychology of Sport and Physical Activity, Gulf Park, MS.

Halverson, L., Roberton, M.A. & Harper, C. (1973). Current research in motor development. *Journal of Research and Development in Education, 6,* 56-70.

Halverson, L. & Williams, K. (1985). Developmental sequences for hopping over distance: A prelongitudinal screening. *Research Quarterly for Exercise and Sport, 56,* 37-44.

Herdman, S., Douglas, M., Shell, D., Volz, D., Yancey, S., Chambers, W. & Liu, C. (1983). Recovery of the hopping response after complete spinal cord transection in the cat. *Experimental Neurology, 81,* 776-780.

Kelso, J.A.S. (1981). Contrasting perspectives on order and regulation in movement. In J. Long and A. Baddeley (Eds.), *Attention and Performance IX.* Hillsdale, N.J.: Erlbaum.

Kelso, J.A.S. & Tuller, B. (in press). Intrinsic time in speech production: Theory, methodology, and preliminary observations. In E. Keller and M. Gopnik (Eds.), *Sensory and motor processes in language.* Hillsdale, N.J.: Erlbaum.

Kelso, J.A.S., Tuller, B. Vatikiotis-Bateson, E. & Fowler, C. (1984). Functionally specific articulatory cooperation following jaw perturbations during speech: Evidence for coordinative structures. *Journal of Experimental Psychology: Human Perception and Performance, 10,* 812-832.

Muzii, R.A., Warburg, C.L. & Gentile, A.M. (1984). Coordination of the upper and lower extremities. *Human Movement Science, 3,* 337-354.

Orlovskii, G. & Shik, M. (1965). Standard elements of cyclic movement. *Biofizika, 10,* 935-944.

Pearson, K. (1976). The control of walking. *Scientific American, 235,* 72-86.

Peiper, A. (1963). *Cerebral function in infancy and childhood.* New York: Consultants Bureau Enterprises.

Phillippson, M. (1905). L'autonomie et la centralisation dans le system des animaux. *Trav. Lab. Physiol. Inst. Solvay (Bruxelles), 7,* 1-208.

Roberton, M.A. & Halverson, L.E. (1984). *Developing children: Their changing movement.* Philadelphia: Lea & Febiger.

Schmidt, R. (1980). On the theoretical status of time in motor-program representations. In G. Stelmach and J. Requin (Eds.), *Tutorials in motor behavior*. Amsterdam: North-Holland.

Schmidt, R. (1985). The search for invariance in skilled movement behavior. *Research Quarterly for Exercise and Sport, 56,* 188-200.

Shapiro, D., Zernicke, R., Gregor, R. & Diestal, J. (1981). Evidence for generalized motor programs using gait pattern analysis. *Journal of Motor Behavior, 13,* 33-47.

Shik, M. & Orlovskii, G. (1965). Coordination of the limbs during running of the dog. *Biofizika, 10,* 1037-1047.

Terzuolo, C. & Viviani, P. (1979). The central representation of learned motor patterns. In R. Talbott and D. Humphrey (Eds.), *Posture and movement*. New York: Raven.

Terzuolo, C. & Viviani, P. (1982). On the relation between word-specific patterns and the central control of typing: A reply to Gentner. *Journal of Experimental Psychology: Human Perception and Performance, 8,* 811-813.

Thelen, E., Bradshaw, G. & Ward, J.A. (1981). Spontaneous kicking in month-old infants: Manifestation of a human central locomotor program. *Behavioral and Neural Biology, 32,* 45-53.

Thelen, E. & Fisher, D. (1982). Newborn stepping: An explanation for a "disappearing reflex". *Developmental Psychology, 18,* 760-775.

Thelen, E., Ridley-Johnson, R. & Fisher, D. (1983). Shifting patterns of bilateral coordination and lateral dominance in the leg movements of young infants. *Developmental Psychobiology, 16,* 29-46.

Turvey, M., Shaw, R. & Mace, W. (1978). Issues in the theory of action: Degrees of freedom, coordinative structures, and coalitions. In J. Requin (Ed.), *Attention and Performance VII*. Hillsdale, N.J.: Erlbaum.

Wade, M. (1982). Timing behavior in children. In J.A.S. Kelso and J. Clark (Eds.), *The development of movement control and co-ordination*. New York: Wiley.

Wetzel, M. & Stuart, D. (1976). Ensemble characteristics of cat locomotion and its neural control. *Progress in Neurobiology, 7,* 1-98.

Whitall, J., Clark, J. & Phillips, S. (1985). Interaction of postural and oscillatory mechanisms in the development of interlimb coordination of upright bipedal walking. *Psychology of motor behavior and sport-1985.* Abstracts of the Annual Meeting of the North American Society for the Psychology of Sport and Physical Activity, Gulf Park, MS.

Winter, D. (1984). Kinematic and kinetic patterns in human gait: Variability and compensating effects. *Human Movement Science, 3,* 51-76.

SECTION 6

CULTURAL INFLUENCES

MOTOR DEVELOPMENT AND CULTURAL ATTITUDES*

B. Bril

1. INTRODUCTION

Is motor development influenced by cultural environment? Are there "motor styles" common to members of a given cultural group?

In an experimental study, Marisi (1977) analysed genetic and environmental contributions to motor performance and concluded that "initially extragenetic factors appears to account for existing individual differences in motor performance...The strength of this genetic control, however, systematically diminishes throughout the course of practice obeying a monotonic trend over trials" (p. 203).

This statement suggests that important differences in environment leading to very different practices will have a non-negligeable effect on motor performance.

This paper is devoted to the idea that the influence of cultural attitudes should be studied through two main directions:
1. Child rearing and training practices since birth, and especially postural and vestibular stimulation and deliberate training will give rise to different "motor styles" during the first year of life and will influence rates of motor development. The literature on this topic will be discussed. Examples taken from the Bambara culture will illustrate the discussion.
2. If differences in motor behaviour do exist in different cultures, of what nature are they and what accounts for them? One way of studying this problem is to work on conditions of transmission and learning.

The comparative study of motor development in a wide enough range of cultural variations reveals the importance of environmental effects on motor development. This type of research is essential as it is impossible, for ethical reasons, to experience drastic variations in the child environment for quite long periods (one may refer to the experiment of Dennis (1938), which we consider as unjustifiable).

* The field research for this study was supported by the Direction de la Coopération Scientifique et Technique du Ministère des Relations Exterieures (France). The Institut des Sciences Humaines (Bamako) is thanked for its assistance during my stay in Mali. I wish to thank also Mamadou Bengali who assisted me during field work in 1984, Catherine Marlot for great help with manuscript preparation, and Emanuelle Bril for drawings of Figure 1. I am grateful to the inhabitants of Dugurakoro and especially mothers and infants who participated in the study.

How to investigate the notion of cultural milieu? Kroeber (1948, cited by Mundinger, 1980) gives the following definition: "...the mass of learned and transmitted motor reactions, habits, techniques, ideas and values and the behaviour they induce, is what constitutes culture". This way of defining culture is commonly accepted but may appear not very pertinent for psychological studies. As we are dealing currently not with "what" is "culture" but how cultural attitudes may influence motor behaviour, we shall refer to Segall's view (1984), the problem being to identify "whatever ecological, sociological and cultural variables might link with established variation in human Behaviour" (p. 154). Another interesting view is proposed by Super and Harkness (1982). They define what they call the "developmental niche" which focuses on culture as it is experienced by any individual.

The concept of culture still gives rise to very controversial issues. The reader should easily be convinced by referring to the recent debate devoted to differing views on "culture" (Rohner, 1984; Jahoda, 1984; Segall, 1984).

2. MOTOR DEVELOPMENT AND CULTURAL ATTITUDES

In the thirties, a few authors argued that to achieve normal development, a child did not need social or motor stimulation. Dennis (1938, 1940) stated that "the infant within the first year will "grow up" of his own accord" (p. 157). Buhler (1935) concluded from ethnographic work on Albanian children that the characteristic trend of normal development is "irrespective of specific environmental influences" (p. 85). These ideas, which seem to have been accepted for some time, have been very much challenged since then.

Many studies have emphasised differences in the rate of motor development across cultures (age of onset of head control, sitting, walking, etc.). A very controversial issue is whether or not there are differences in physical maturity at birth. In 1957, Geber and Dean reported that Baganda babies (in Uganda, Africa) were at birth at "a more advanced state of development than newborn European children". Three characteristics of this advance were noted: muscle tone, head-control, absence of certain neonatal reflexes. These findings have not been corroborated in subsequent studies (Warren & Parkin, 1974; Brueton, Palit & Possner, 1973; Konner, 1972). For a detailed discussion of this problem, see the recent work of Super (1981).

2.1. Motor development during the perinatal period

A more interesting issue for our purpose is the study of newborn behaviour during the first days after birth, and of motor development after this period up to 18-24 months. There, again, different reviews (Super, 1980, 1981; Lester & Brazelton, 1982) discuss this topic. Brazelton's studies are probably the most strikingly relevant with regard to neonatal behaviour: they focus on the idea that one should view infant behaviour in its cultural context, "both as a shaper of and as shaped by cultural expectations". The theoretical purpose of the research was to "highlight the complex interaction between genetic and environmental influences on neonatal behaviour" (Lester & Brazelton, 1982). Their major claims are that there exists a twofold influence: not only environmental conditions may influence child rearing practice, but also the kinds of babies that are "produced" by the society will in turn influence these practices. Different studies with newborn African babies (Keefer, Dixon, Tronik & Brazelton, 1978 cited by Lester & Brazelton, 1982; Brazelton, Koslowski & Tronick, 1976), in Kenya and Zambia respectively, show that environment and especially maternal responsiveness to babies reinforce capacities in the neonate. The ten Zambian infants who have been compared to 10 US infants on days 1, 5 and 10 after birth showed poorer scores on almost all items* on day 1 but were higher in half of them on day 10. For the authors, this astonishing recovery was due to cultural expectation for early motor development, very different from that of US mothers. In the case of Gussii children, not only their motor activity was higher than that of the US group, but they maintained an excellent motor coordination while handled or when excited, a situation interpreted by the authors as very rewarding to the adult and therefore encouraging pursuit of the interaction. In contrast, a study of Zinecanteco Indian infants (Brazelton, Robey & Collier, 1969) showed that passive caretaking practices (for example, cradling or breastfeeding the baby rather than allowing him to cry, and a quiet pattern of maternal interaction), will reinforce certain aspects of motor behaviour, viz. moderate vigor, free and fluent motor activity, no intense crying, quiet, alert states for long periods. The authors suggest that these characteristics of motor activities are reinforced by subsequent handling practices.

One conclusion that can be drawn from the studies cited above is that it is very difficult to investigate the reasons for the differences or similarities in behaviour and development between groups. Prenatal history, intra-uterine environment have an influence on infant behaviour at birth (Lester & Brazelton, 1982) and are very hard to analyse.

2.2. Motor development during the first two years

A pioneering work undertaken by Geber and Dean (1957) on the psycho-motor development of Ugandan children, concludes that there is an overall precocity of several weeks (compared to American natives) during the first year, a precocity which diminishes during the second year. Since then, many studies have challenged this finding. Reviewing 50 cross-cultural studies of psychomotor development, Werner (1972) concludes that there is an acceleration of psychomotor development among samples of infants reared in traditional communities, the African groups showing the greatest acceleration, followed by Latin Americans and Indians, with White Euro-Americans coming last. At the same time, Warren (1972) discussed the so-called African infant precocity and concludes that it has not been satisfactorily demonstrated. His arguments against these findings are based on the difficulty in comparing scores obtained by different methods**, the comparison between results in different cultures, and the lack of attention devoted to

---

* The items were the following: motor activity, tempo at height, rapidity of buildup, irritability, consolability, social interest, alertness, follow up with eyes, reactivity to stimulation, defensive movements, cuddliness. For further details, see Brazelton, T.B. Neonatal Behavioral Assessment Scale, *Clinics in Developmental Medicine, 50*. London: William Heinemann Medical Books, Philadelphia: J.P. Lippincott, 1979.

** The testing procedures used the most often are selected from the following: Gesell, Terman-Merrill, Brunet-Lézine, Bayley motor-scale, Griffith, Brazelton neonatal behavioural assessment scale.

identifying independent variables that account for differences in development. Another criticism that may be addressed to many of the studies cited is the use of an overall index of development, such as the Developmental Quotient (DQ) of the Gesell developmental schedule for gross motor behaviour (Moreover the yardstick of 100 DQ is considered as the norm for American children). Then this overall index very often masks specific differences in motor development.

Various arguments, including genetic ones, have been put forward as an explanation of these influences in motor development during the first years: variations in prenatal care and maternal nutrition (such as protein intake) (Brazelton et al, 1969, 1976), type of ecological setting (e.g. altitude: Brazelton et al, 1969; Saco-Sollitt, 1981), permissive v.s restrictive home surroundings, various handling practices after birth (Brazelton et al, 1969, 1976; Geber, 1973; Ainsworth, 1977), and especially backcarrying (Goldberg, 1977; Kilbride et al, 1970).

2.3. The search for independent variables: the role of specific cultural practices on sensori-motor development

More recent studies have focused less on the overall evolution of motor development than on the identification of specific experimental variables related to specific behavioural items. An analysis of the different items of the diverse testing procedures in previous studies yields the conclusion that there is no overall precocity for African children. Only for some items can a real precocity be shown (head control, sitting or standing alone, walking, ...) while for others (such as crawling, turning over) African babies were often behind their European counterparts. These observations lead to the hypothesis that specific environmental experiences affect specific behaviours. This view has been explicitely formulated only recently, giving rise to a new research trend.

The work of Kilbride (1980) is a very good example of this evolution. First, comparison with Euro-American norms have been abandoned. Second, two African cultural settings have been chosen because of specific differences in their socio-cultural system and, consequently, in adult values. Those two cultures are very similar (horticulturalist with important fishing, disperse settlement, extended family and multiple caretakers, almost similar prenatal and caretaking practices), except on the following point. In Baganda, adult values emphasise social skills, particularly of a manipulatory bent, which serve as a means for upward mobility in the sociopolitical order. Samia values, on the other hand, emphasise clan cooperation, harmony and individual responsibility, with comparatively little preoccupation given to active social manipulation. The Baganda seem to emphasise "social" labor, while the Samia train for "productive" labor (p. 137). In both societies, the infant gets a great deal of physical stimulation; motor skills such as early sitting are encouraged, although crawling is not.

In Kilbride's research, the rate of development of three sensori-motor behaviours was assessed: smiling, sitting, crawling. The items used were selected from the Bayley scale (a scale with six items was used for smiling and sitting). The results showed that whereas the first items are passed at about the same age, a divergence appears gradually for both smiling and sitting. Samia babies passed item 6 on the smiling scale at 4.9 months while Baganda babies passed it at 3 months. The results were inverted for sitting: 5.6 months for Samia babies, 6.0 months for Baganda babies. In both cases mean differences in smiling and sitting score were statistically significant. Concerning pre-walking progression, no difference between the two samples was found. A comparison with the American norms provided by Bayley shows a significant advance of both Baganda and Samia babies; on the pre-walking progression no global difference was exhibited.

For Kilbride, these findings argue in favor of acquired social (here sensori-motor) skills, "through culturally constituted experience" (p. 145). The results are in accordance with his hypothesis: Baganda emphasise more infant sociability (defined here for the child as smiling skill), the Samia favoring situations that free them for work (sitting skill).

A suggestion given here is that Baganda and Samia caregivers both train their children for sitting, the training being more intensive for Samia infants. Samia mothers report that they systematically train their infants to sit from about two months of age. Unfortunately, the author confesses that no observable data on the time devoted to training are available.

Here we come to a very important point, which constitutes in our opinion an open research field that could yield an essential source of data for future research.

2.4. Deliberate teaching and incidental practices

Kilbride (1980) and some other researchers (Super, 1976; Konner, 1972, 1977) focus on the distinction between what is generally called deliberate teaching (for example babies are trained to sit, being put on the lap, in a hole in the ground or in a basin) and incidental practices (being held on the back or the hip while the mother is working or walking). In fact, except in very few cases, it is certainly difficult to draw a boundary line between these two situations.

Unfortunately, as far as we know, there exist very few data on this topic. Super (1976) and Konner (1977) give some statistical data, only for a few items. Physical contact with mothers and other caretakers are estimated for Kung children under 4 years (a Bushman population of South Africa), and compared with data for US or European babies. While Kung children under 18 weeks are in bodily passive contact for more than 70% of time, US and European children are in a similar situation less than 25% of time (Konner, 1977). In the same study, Konner describes the "typical infant positions" during the early weeks of life, but does not give any estimation of the time spent in such positions. In the Kipsigis population (Kenya), Super (1976) gives for one-month olds the figure of 60% for the time spent sitting during waking hours vs. 40% for an American sample. But here again, we lack more precise information: is it sitting with a vertical trunk position, or, as it seems to be, a semi-sitting position as in a European sitting chair?

Further on, Super (1976) discusses deliberate teaching of walking, but here, again, he does not investigate how often and how long this teaching takes place.

Referring to more experimental studies such as those of Korner and Thoman (1970, 1972) and as a conclusion from his study, Konner (1977) emphasises the importance of vertical posture, vestibular stimulation, physical contact and conscious training effort. For Super (1976), for example, the game that consists of holding the infant under the arms and bouncing him on one's lap, that Kipsigis adults play with the child from one month on, prompts the child to respond with the standing or stepping reflex. This would be an everyday life version of Zelazo et al experiment on walking in the newborn (1972). With these authors we postulate that the amout and quality of stimulation produced by everyday child care may affect motor development.

2.5. Experimental studies on the influence of postural and vestibular stimulations on motor development

Since the reviews of Warren (1972) and Werner (1972), a few experiments have demonstrated the importance of certain types of postural and vestibular stimulation.

Vestibular dysfunction may lead to delay in acquisition of head control, slow motor development and postural difficulties (Eviatar & Eviatar, 1982). Not only is vestibular stimulation used in therapy programmes, but everyone knows that rocking a child does quiet him. A study of Clark et al (1977) supports the claim that vestibular stimulation improves gross motor skills significantly. Preambulatory infants from 3 to 13 months participated in the experiment. There were 16 sessions of semi-circular canal stimulation during four weeks. Two sessions took place two days a week. A session consisted of 10 spins in a rotating chair. Reflex tests and motor skill tests were administered prior to and after the treatment. Comparison with a control group supported the hypothesis that exposure to vestibular stimulation accelerates motor development in infants. A recent study with developmentally delayed children (MacLean & Baumeister, 1982) confirms these results.

Thelen (1980) argues that specific caregiving practices, and especially vestibular stimulation provided by the caregiver, are associated with a decrease of stereotyped behaviours in the infant. Korner and Thoman's studies (1970) test the efficacy of contact, upright position and vestibular stimulation on visual alertness in neonates. Vestibular stimulation and upright position have a significant effect on alertness. Contact alone has no effect. The same results are reported in their study on soothing neonates (1972); contact alone has no effect, while vestibular stimulation has patent effects. These results on visual alertness are very important for our purpose. For Clark et al (1977) "vestibular stimulation of the infants (in their study) may have facilitated maturation of the vestibulo-ocular reflex and, in turn, provided the visual system a more stable retinal image against which motor involvement with the environment developed more rapidly...The stimulation (in their study) may also affect motor behaviour through vestibulospinal reflex facilitation" (p. 1229).

To test these hypotheses according to cultural variations, very detailed estimations of the kinds of stimulation offered to the infant during the first year of life are needed.

2.6. "Postural time table" of Bambara infants

In order to carry out further investigations such as those of Kilbride, or to test hypotheses on the role of handling practices on sensori-motor development, we need to refer to precise statistical data. The available data generally concern duration of contact or sitting posture. To our knowledge, no data are available on the amount and nature of vestibular stimulation provided to infants during the first year of life. In addition, more precise data are needed on the conditions of elicitation of certain types of stimulation.

That is why we have undertaken a study concerning what we call the "postural time-table" of the infant, from birth to the onset of walking. We give here preliminary results of a study which is being carried out in a Bambara community in Mali (Africa)*. The purpose of the study is to evaluate, through daily observation, the different kinds of postural and vestibular stimulation (active and passive) the child is exposed to during day-time. Moreover we study how these stimulations evolve with motor development during the first year. Two levels of information are recorded. First we noted (with pencil and paper) the postural activity of the child, from about 7.30 a.m. (that is, starting just after the first meal), to 6.30 p.m. (that is, just before the evening meal).

The following items were coded: state of alertness (awake or asleep), position (lying, semivertical sitting on one's lap, sitting, standing), holding (on the lap, on the hip, on the back, etc.), person interacting with the child, mother's activity (working at home or in the fields, resting time, playing with the child, etc.).

Concurrently, that is the second level of information, we video-recorded 10 to 15 minutes of each of these situations, so that we could estimate more precisely the different postures of the child and the nature of the vestibular stimulations (frequency and amplitude).

We give here some results concerning 4 children of respectively 4,8, 11, 23 weeks; this represents about one hundred hours of observation. Days of observation have been chosen according to mother activities.

2.6.1. Carrying on the back

Being carried in a sling involves consequences that have been subject to different interpretations. Some authors emphasised the beneficial effect of such a practice (Geber, 1958; Konner, 1972; Ainsworth, 1977). This posture strengthens neck and trunk musculature. S. Goldberg carried on further her investigation (1977) although she did not have indication on how long infants are carried on the back, at an early age; she inferred it from data reported by mothers, assuming that a child who has been very much carried at 12 months had a good chance of having been carried a great deal at 4 or 6 months. Her findings show that long sling carrying is correlated with advanced motor behaviour at 6 months, no correlation at 4 months, while at 12 months the infants who were the least carried had the highest motor development (on Bayley motor scale).

These results suggest that the relationship between postural stimulation such as sling carrying, and motor performance is very dependent on the

---

* The Bambara people live in West Africa, mostly in Mali. They are concerned almost exclusively with agriculture; they grow cereals and vegetables for their subsistence, a great part of which is sold on local markets. Most families are partriarchal extended families, and polygamy is still very often present. This situation has two main implications: first a child has multiple caregivers; second a woman who has one or two co-wives shares domestic work (which represents a great amount of work) with others; she then benefits by more free time for gardening (the money she earns by selling her production belongs to her) or nursing her children.

level of development of the child; while the effect is positive on a 6 month-old infant, it is negative on a 12 month-old, and this for completely different reasons: sling carrying restrains a 12-month old from motor activity, whereas it favors certain aspects of motor stimulation in the youngest. If one can easily imagine why it restrains the child's activity after 12 months, it is more difficult to estimate what elicits postural and motor stimulation.

In fact, it is important to examine this practice more carefully, and I shall take here examples from the Bambara culture. First, there are different ways of putting the child in the sling, depending on his/her age and degree of alertness at the precise moment he/she is carried: a child under 4 months is always tied "arm in" the sling (Fig. 1a and b, see next page), the very small ones (up to two months) having an extra sling maintaining the nape of the neck; after 4 months the two solutions are offered to the child: when he/she is sleeping, the former solution is adopted; when he/she is awake, his/her arms are freed (Fig. 1d). Concerning the impact of the type of carrying on motor development, we find it important to look for the different constituents of postural motor or vestibular stimulations this situation implies for the child.

As a Bambara mother traditionally stays at home during 40 days after a birth, the infant is rarely held on the back during that period, or at least during the first two weeks. This is especially true in large families with the presence of multi-caretakers. At the time the child is to months old, the mother has already resumed her activities. From that time on, up to the time the baby is able to sit, he/she will be carried quite a lot: at two months, a child spends about 40 to 45% of day-time in the sling. When he/she is in the sling, a child is asleep approximately 70 to 80% of the time; this represents 75 to 80% of day sleeping time.

As soon as the child is able to sit (at about five months), the time spent in the sling decreases to about 25% of day time; the child is asleep, when on the back, the same amount of time as at two months, which still represents 75 to 80% of day sleeping time.

Though our data are not sufficient to make any generalisation, they were confirmed by "spot observation". It is important to know that for children under six months, back carrying is used most of the time when the child is sleeping. This result contrasts with studies concluding that sling carrying restrains manual and visual exploration (Rakowska-Jaillard, 1983). Another way of carrying children gradually develops (as the child progresses with sitting): that is hip carrying. Whereas we do not find it at four weeks, at two months, it appears several times a day, but each time for very short periods from a few seconds to 3-4 minutes. At five months it becomes a significant way of carrying children, representing a little less than 10% of observation time, that is about 25% of carrying time.

2.6.2. Postural stimulation

Postural stimulations refer to all incitements to control and monitor the head and the whole body. When a child is lying in a crib, or on a mat, there is no external stimulation. But when a child is held for more than 90% of day time, which is the case for the two children observed at two months, he/she has to adjust constantly to the movements of the person who is holding him/her. Besides this, the structure of the extended family and of social life favors the holding by many different people. Our data suggest that the child

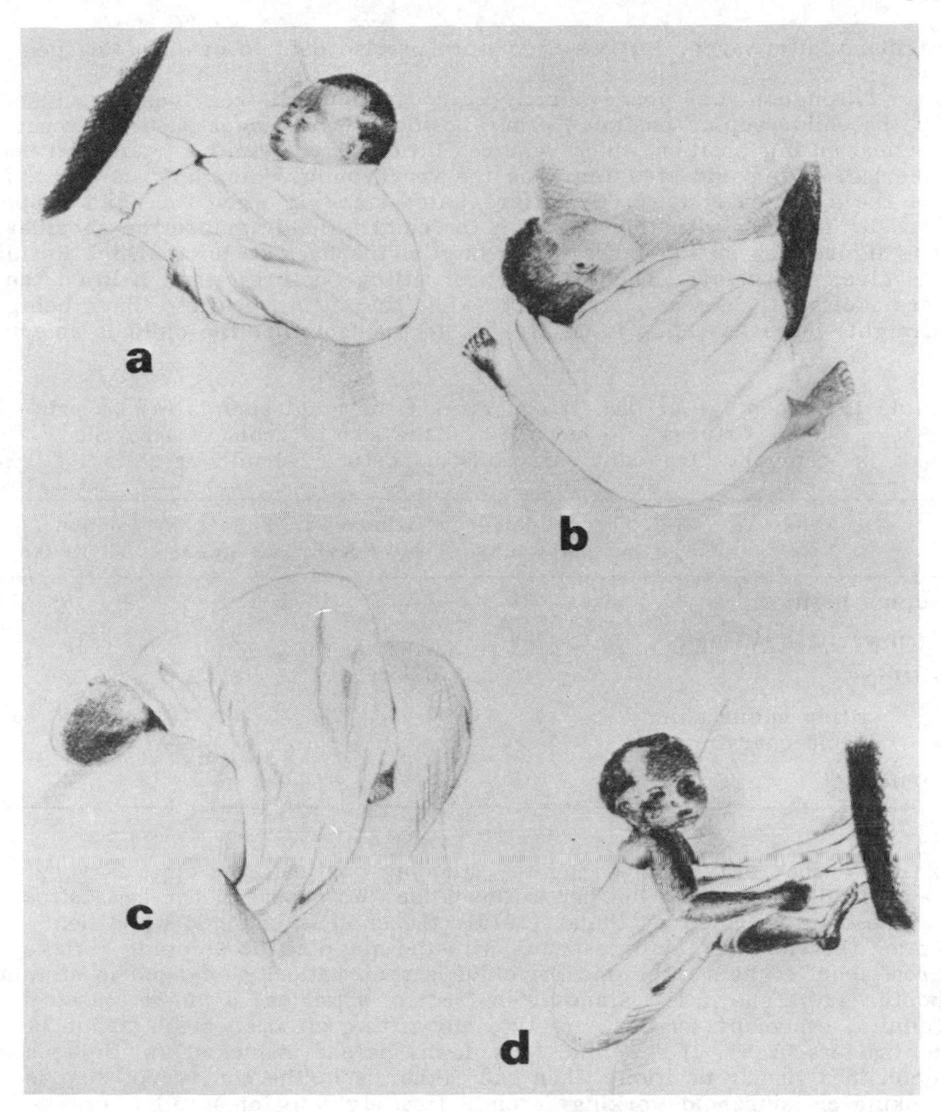

Fig. 1. Different positions of a child in sling back carrying. a, b, c: a child of two months sleeping "arms in"; c gives the position of the child when the mother is doing dish or cloth washing, a posture which is very frequent during domestic work. d: a child of eight months, "arms freed" from the sling.

changes holding partner three to five times an hour. Here again, he/she has to readjust to various handling styles! It seems that it is from five weeks (when the mother resumes work) to four or five months that the child is the most often in contact (that is "held") with somebody. During the first weeks, the figures are about 70% of time of observation; at two months we find 95%, and 85% at 5.5 months. These figures seem to drop regularly afterwards. But we need more precise data to confirm this point.

Throughout our observations, we coded four different postures taken by the child: supine position (prone position almost never occurs), semi-vertical sitting position which requires little exercise of the trunk and neck muscles, sitting and standing. For the very young, "standing" is probably not the appropriate term: we differentiated standing when the child supports himself, from the situation in which the child is held against the shoulder. The figures for sitting include carrying on the back or on the hip. Results are given in Table 1. The semi-vertical sitting posture, when held on the caretaker's lap decreases gradually, while the sitting posture (back being straight) increases; this is mainly due to the fact that the child is able to

Table 1. Percentage of time of observation the child spends in the main four postures. To have 100 as the sum of each column, the category "frequent variations of posture" should be added.

	Abdou 4 weeks	Bakaro 8 weeks	Yaya 11 weeks	Madou 23 weeks
Supine position	33	5	5	6
Semi-vertical sitting	39	21	22	15
Sitting	19	64	52	72
sitting minus sling or hip carrying	19	22	7	39
Standing	0	2	2	4

sit on his/her own. Concerning the standing posture, the child is very early held standing on his/her mother's lap. We observed the same situation as the one described by Super (1976): the child is bounced while held under the shoulder, and responds with the standing or stepping reflex. From about eight months on, the child is systematically engaged in standing postures: he/she is left standing in front of a mortar, a bucket, a stool (adults, especially females, are typically sitting on small stools about 20 centimeters high). If the child falls down, he/she is picked up, and placed again in a similar position. When the mother is in the courtyard, that is, cooking or household working, a child from eight to ten months remains in this position about 25% of the time*.

2.6.3. Vestibular stimulation

Vestibular stimulations are categorised into two main classes:

- *Deliberate stimulation* from the adult; two main situations are differentiated: "bouncing game" corresponds to the situation previously described; it really aims at pleasing the child. Each up and down bouncing lasts about 600 ms, the amplitude of the vertical movement being about 40 cm.

* These figures have been estimated from six hours of video-recording made by the author in 1981, and concerning a 8-month-child. These films concerned the child when she was in the courtyard exclusively.

The number of consecutive bouncings may be over 60! It ranges usually from 10 to 20, followed by a few second pause, and the game may go on for more than 5 minutes! This bouncing game is very stereotypes throughout Bambara people. The rhythm appears to be independent of the person. "Swaying" seems to quiet the child. It can be a quite slow lateral rotation (a backward and forward motion lasts about 750 ms): the child is held in the arms and the caretaker rotates his/her trunk in a backward and forward motion. The other way of quieting a child is to make a very rapid "vibration" (of a period of 200 ms) with the child in the arms or on the back.

- *Incidental stimulation:* when the child is on the back, on the hip or even on the lap of his/her caretaker, he/she is rarely left motionless. Women are used to work with their child on their lap or on their back. Consequently, the child is constantly stimulated. Here again, three classes of vestibular stimulation are distinguished: steady stimulations either of small amplitude, due to walking or work such as bolting of flour (duration of the movement: 280 ms), or with high amplitude such as the pounding. The third category includes all irregular stimulations, e.g. when the caretaker comes and goes in the courtyard to prepare the food or the fire; we estimated that, in this case, a woman bends down about 1.5 time per minute. When the child is on her back, this means for him/her a rotation in the sagittal plane of about 110° counterclockwise, and then clockwise. Another situation occurs when the child is with older children that successively hold him/her.

As can be seen, lots of different situations are encountered. It seems that vestibular stimulations are maximal at about two or three months. They represent respectively 15%, 46% and 39% of the time of observation at 1 month 2 months and 5.5 months. The interesting fact is that deliberate stimulation decreases at 5.5 months. They represent about 26% of vestibular stimulations at 2 months and drop to 6% at 5.5 months. Irregular stimulation represents more than 50% of vestibular stimulation at two months, and drop to 40% at 5.5 months. The evolution of the number and type of vestibular stimulation is easily explanable by the evolution of children/adults or eldest interaction.

These data on postural and vestibular stimulation need to be completed and extended to other cultural contexts, including European ones. Experimental work (Clark et al, 1977; MacLean & Baumeister, 1982; Korner, 1972) gives strong evidence that vestibular and postural stimulation have demonstrable effects on muscular tonicity, gross and fine motor skills and even more cognitive skills (Pomerleau et al, 1982). Hypotheses that attribute differences in motor development to various experiences in postural and vestibular stimulation offered by catetaking practices, are highly plausible, but more extensive field observations are needed. Controlled comparisons including quantitative analyses are necessary to investigate more fully the relationship between environmental factors and various aspects of motor and cognitive development.

3. ACQUISITION OF COMPLEX MOTOR SKILLS AND CULTURAL ATTITUDES

Are there specific motor skills culturally speaking? If the answer is positive, how are they transmitted and learned? This question seems to be less popular than the previous one, and has been far less explored.

A few anthropologists have focused on the cultural form of gestuality. Most often through written description, the authors have listed various motor habits, such as eating, sleeping, pointing, spitting, sitting postures etc. or emblematic gestures (Bailey, 1942; Brewer, 1951). The problem is that these descriptions are often ambiguous. Very few attempts have been made to undertake comparative studies of postures or motor habits. In 1936, M. Mauss encouraged such a programme of research, but with no real success. A good example of comparative work is Hewes' paper (1955) on "world distribution of certain postural habits". Hewes recorded information on about one hundred of the commonest postures such as sitting, kneeling, crouching and squatting.

Two chapters of the book edited by Brooke and Whiting (1973) *Human Movement, a Field Study,* are devoted to comparative studies and especially to cross-cultural aspects of motor behaviour (Carroll, 1973; Hendry, 1973). But all these studies emphasise those differences in motor activities that are most directly related to the technical and socio-economic characteristics of cultural groups (an African woman will pound, bolt, carry on her head, activities that a French woman will never perform).

More analytic work has been done by Lomax et al on variations in movement features. Working on "expressive behaviour", and especially on dances, Lomax et al (1969) delineate "motor styles" according to three main features: a) body attitude (that is the dynamic postural base line for all activity); b) the parts, or areas of the body most frequently articulated; c) the geometry of dimensionality of the movement that results (that is linear, curved, looped). Unfortunately, their data are mainly qualitative: for example, stance is classified as narrow, wide and very wide; or acceleration is coded along a seven point rating scale, which registers strong tendencies and not numerical frequencies.

Despite the scale of this comparative study (the sample covers over 250 dances for 400 cultures), it is an anthropological work, that may provide ideas for more psychological work, but is hardly of direct use for studies on motor behaviour and development.

In recent literature on motor behaviour, the role of socio-cultural factors has been acknowledged by different authors. Smoll (1982) notes that "various aspects of the cultural milieu are known to condition or modify the expression of underlying motor processes" (p. 340). Higgins (1985) goes further and says that "psychological and socio-cultural factors may affect both behavioural outcomes and the structure of the movement" (p. 140), even if she does not say clearly what is meant by "structure".

Ethnographic data show clearly that morphological and biomechanical factors are not the only ones to influence the way a motor task is solved: see for example the different ways of sitting, or the different solutions to the problem of carrying loads (on the head, the shoulders, the back, etc.).

What could be interesting for theories on the development of motor skills is the assumption that cultural factors could affect the structure of the movement. Concerning the implications of postural behaviours, Hewes (1955) noted that research on metabolic efficiency of various postures has been restricted, because it does not take into account cultural data (see for instance Bouisset, 1981 for standing or chair-sitting). Unfortunately, as noted by Smoll (1982) "because investigators (in cross-cultural studies) have rarely focused on motor variables, we are essentially limited to speculative interpretations..." (p. 340). As far as we know, there are almost no experimental studies in that domain. The major problem is to determine which aspects of the structure of the movement remain invariant across cultural differences.

Walking is a domain that is worth exploring. Supported by ethnographic data, Mauss stated in 1936 that there were no natural ways of walking. He pointed out that such a motor skill was "learned" through cultural transmission and education. Here again there are very few available data. Bernstein (1967) assumed that normal walking may not differ in its structure but "only in the rhythms and amplitudes of the ratios" (p. 61) between parameters.

The only comparative study on walking we found concerns spontaneous cadence in urban setting (Pélosse, 1959). The results of Pélosse's study shows that singificant differences exist in spontaneous cadence for male in Paris (2.45 step/s), Hamburg (1.94 step/s), Copenhague (1.75 step/s). Data from China (Basler, 1929, cited by Pélosse) give 2.06 step/s. No hypotheses are proposed to explain these differences. The only conclusion is that the cadence found in Copenhagen is nearer to an "optimal cadence", that is with maximal energetic economy (1.45 to 1.50 step/s; data from Atzler (1927) and Magne (1920) cited by Pélosse).

Our data concerning female walking in a Bambara rural community show a slower cadence than what is generally admitted in studies on human gait. For instance, Larsson et al (1980) give for women a cadence of 2.2 step/s for ordinary walking. We found for a sample of five women an average of 1.82 step/s with a range of 1.52 to 2.03 step/s. We videotaped 16 females from 4 years to 12 years. Here again, we found cadence systematically inferior to those given by Sutherland et al (1980) (see Table 2).

Table 2. Comparison of data on female cadence (step/sec) from a Bambara rural community and from the US. Subjects were asked to walk at a spontaneous cadence. (Figures in parentheses give the range of cadence for each group).

	Adult	Children			
		4/5 years	6 years	7/8 years	9/12 years
	n= 5	n= 5	n= 4	n= 4	n= 3
Bambara	1.82	2.36	2.16	2.10	2.06
	(1.52-2.03)	(2.16-2.47)	(2.07-2.34)	(2.06-2.24)	(1.96-2.12)
US (published data)	2.2*	2.62**	2.50	2.37	

* From Larsson et al (1980) (females)
**From Sutherland et al (1980) (boys and girls)

These data are essentially descriptive, and corroborate Bernstein's statement: only rhythm has been investigated. Pélosse (1959) argues that biomechanical factors are not the only ones to account for the differences of cadence. If these differences are confirmed in different cultural settings, how is spontaneous cadence modulated by cultural environment?

In a recent study on the development of gait in African children, Hennessy et al (1984) emphasised the remarkable consistency of gait pattern. They interpreted the decline of walking cadence at a younger age for African children as compared with American children (Sutherland et al, 1980) as due to motor precocity. Even if motor precocity is a factor, Hennessy et al's study does not consider the possible cultural variation in cadence among these people as compared to American norms. We think that if these variations are confirmed, it is important to take them into account for further exploration.

4. CONCLUSION

This paper is mainly a plea for collecting more comparative data, so that it will be possible to formulate precise hypotheses on the factors that may affect motor development and the structure of movement.

In view of the scarcity of data concerning cultural variation of motor activity, only very cautious hypotheses may be advanced. Cross-cultural comparisons, with identical experimental techniques, are needed to explore further the universal as well as the culture-specific aspects of motor development, and to confirm (or invalidate) Higgins' (1985) statement that socio-cultural factors may affect the "structure of movement".

References

Ainsworth, M.D.S. (1977). Infant Development and Mother-Infant Interaction among Ganda and American families. In P.H. Leiderman et al (Eds.), *Culture and Infancy*. New York: Academic Press.

Bailey, F.L. (1942). Navaho motor habits. *American Anthropologist, 44,* 210-234.

Bernstein, N. (1967). *The Coordination and Regulation of Movement.* Oxford: Pergamon Press.

Bouisset, S. (1981). *Postures and Movements.* In Scherer (Ed.), Paris: Masson.

Brazelton, T.B., Robey, J.S. & Collier, G.A. (1969). Infant Development in the Zinacanteco Indians of Southern Mexico. *Pediatrics, 44,* 274-290.

Brazelton, T.B., Koslowski, B. & Tronick, E. (1976). Neonatal Behavior among Urban Zambians and Americans. *Journal of the American Academy of Child Psychiatry, 15,* 97-107.

Brewer, W.D. (1951). Patterns of Gesture among the Levantine Arabs. *American Anthropologist, 53,* 232-237.

Brueton, M.J., Palit, A. & Prosser, R. (1973). Gestational Age Assessment in Nigerian Newborn Infants. *Archives of Disease in Childhood, 48,* 318-320.

Buhler, C. (1935). *From Birth to Maturity.* London: Kegan Paul, Trenen, Trubner & Co Ltd.

Carroll, J. (1973). Topic Areas-developed: Comparative Studies. In J.D. Brooke and H.T.A. Whiting (Eds.), *Human Movement: a Field Study.* London: Henry Kimpton Publishers.

Clark, D.L., Kerutzberg, J.R. & Chee, F.K.W. (1977). Vestibular Stimulation Influence on Motor Development in Infants. *Science, 196,* 1228-1229.

Dennis, W. (1938). Infant Development under Conditions of Restricted Practice of Minimum Social Stimulation: a Preliminary Report. *The Journal of Genetic Psychology, 53,* 149-158.

Dennis, W. (1940). The Effect of Cradling Practices upon the Onset of Walking in Hopi Children. *The Journal of Genetic Psychology, 56,* 77-86.

Eviatar, L. & Eviatar, A. (1982). Development of Head Control and Vestibular Responses in Infants Treated with Aminoglycosides. *Developmental Medicine and Child Neurology, 24,* 372-379.

Geber, M. (1958). The Psychomotor Development of African Children in their First Year and the Influence of Mother Behavior. *Journal of Social Psychology, 47,* 185-195.

Geber, M. (1973). L'environnement et le Développement des Enfants Africains. *Enfance, 3-4,* 145-174.

Geber, M. & Dean, R.F. (1957). The State of Development of Newborn African Children. *Lancet, 272,* 1216-1219.

Goldberg, S. (1977). Infant Development and Mother-Infant Interaction in Urban Zambia. In P.H. Leiderman et al (Ed.), *Culture and Infancy.* New York: Academic Press.

Hendry, L.B. (1973). Topic Areas-Developed: Human Movement, a Societal Study. In J.D. Brooke and H.T.A. Whiting (Eds.), *Human Movement: a Field Study.* London: Henry Kimpton Publishers.

Hennessy, M.J. & Dixon, S.D. (1984). The Development of Gait: a Study of African Children Aged One to Five. *Child Development, 55,* 844-853.

Hewes, G.W. (1955). World Distribution of Certain Postural Habits. *American Anthropologist, 57,* 231-244.

Higgins, S. (1985). Movement as an Emergent Form: its Structural Limits. *Human Movement Science, 4,* 119-148.

Jahoda, G. (1984). Do We Need a Concept of Culture? *Journal of Cross-Cultural Psychology, 15,* 139-151.
Kilbride, J., Robbins, M.C., Kilbride, P.L. (1970). The Comparative Motor Development of Baganda. American White and American Black Infants. *American Anthropologist, 72,* 1422-1428.
Kilbride, P.L. (1980). Sensorimotor Behavior of Baganda and Samia Infants: a Controlled Comparison. *Journal of Cross-Cultural Psychology, 11,* 131-152.
Konner, M.J. (1972). Aspects of the Developmental Ethology of a Foraging People. In N. Blurton-Jones (Ed.), *Ethological Studies of Child Behavior.* Cambridge: Cambridge University Press.
Konner, M.J. (1977). Infancy among the Kalahari Desert San. In P.H. Leiderman, S.R. Tulmin and A. Rosenfeld (Eds.), *Culture and Infancy: Variation in Human Experience.* New York: Academic Press Inc.
Korner, A.F. & Thoman, E.B. (1970). Visual Alertness in Neonates as Evoked by Maternal Care. *Journal of Experimental Child Psychology, 10,* 67-78.
Korner, A.F. & Thoman, E.B. (1972). The Relative Efficacity of Contact and vestibular-Proprioceptive Stimulation in Soothing Neonates. *Child Development, 43,* 443-453.
Larsson, L.E., Odenrick, P., Sandlund, B., Weitz, P. & Oberg, P.A. (1980). The Phases of the Stride and their Interaction in Human Gait. *Scan. Rehab. Med., 12,* 107-112.
Lester, B.M. & Brazelton, T.B. (1982). Cross-Cultural Assessment of Neonatal Behavior. In D.A. Wagner and H.W. Stevenson (Eds.), *Cultural Perspective on Child Development.* San Francisco: W.H. Freeman and Co.
Lomax, A., Bartenieff, I. & Paulay, F. (1969). Choreometrics: a method for the study of cross-cultural pattern in film. *Sonderdruck aus Research Film, 6(6).*
MacLean, W.E. & Baumeister, A.A. (1982). Effect of Vestibular Stimulation on Motor Development and Stereotyped Behavior of Developmentally Delayed Children. *Journal of Abnormal Child Psychology, 10(2),* 229-245.
Marisi, Dan.Q. (1977). Genetic and Extragenetic Variance in Motor Performance. *Acta Genet. Med. Gemellol., 26,* 197-204.
Mauss, M. (1936). Les Techniques du Corps. *Journal de Psychologie, 32* (3-4), paru in: *Sociologie et Anthropologie.* Paris: PUF, 1973.
Mundinger, P.C. (1980). Animal Cultures and a General Theory of Cultural Evolution. *Ethology and Sociobiology, 1,* 183-223.
Pélosse, J.L. (1959). Cadence Spontanée de la Marche en Milieu Urbain: étude comparative. *Biotypologie, 20,* 72-77.
Pomerleau, A., Courchesne, M. & Malcuit, G. (1982). Relation entre les stimulations vestibulo-kinesthésiques fournies par la mère et les comportements exploratoires du nourrisson de 9 mois. *Psychologica Belgica, 22(1),* 25-37.
Rakowska-Jaillard, C. (1983). L'Enfant Africain: Géométrie et Portage au dos. In E. Herbine et M.C. Busnel (Eds.), *Aube des Sens.* Paris: Stock.
Rohner, R.P. (1984). Toward a Conception of Culture for Cross-Cultural Psychology. *Journal of Cross-Cultural Psychology, 15,* 111-138.
Sacco-Pollitt, C. (1981). Birth in the Peruvian Andes: Physical and Behavioral Consequences in the Neonate. *Child Development, 52,* 839-846.
Segall, M.H. (1984). More than we Need to Know about Culture, but are Afraid not to Ask. *Journal of Cross-Cultural Psychology, 15,* 153-162.
Smoll, F.L. (1982). Developmental Kinesiology. Toward a Subdiscipline Focusing on Motor Development. In J.A.S. Kelso and J.E. Clark (Eds.), *The Development of Movement control and Coordination.* John Wiley & Sons Ltd.

Super, C.M. (1976). Environmental Effects on Motor Development: The Case of "African Infant Precocity". *Developmental Medicine and Child Neurology, 18,* 561-567.
Super, C.M. (1980). Cross-Cultural Research on Infancy. In H.C. Triandis et al (Eds.), *Handbook of Cross-Cultural Psychology: Developmental Psychology, vol. 4.* Allyn and Bacon Inc.
Super, C.M. (1981). Behavioral Development in Infancy. In R.H. Munroe, R.L. Munroe and B.B. Whiting (Eds.), *Handbook of Cross-Cultural Human Development.* New York: Garland STPM Press.
Super, C.M. & Harkness, S. (1982). The Infant's Niche in Rural Kenya and Metropolitan America. In L.L. Adler (Ed.), *Crosscultural Research at Issue.* New York: Academic Press.
Sutherland, D.H., Olshen, R., Cooper, L. & Savio, L.Y. Woo (1980). The Development of Mature Gait. *Journal of Bone and Joint Surgery, 62-A,* 336-353.
Thelen, E. (1980). Determinants of Amounts of Stereotyped Behavior in Normal Human Infants. *Ethology and Sociobiology, 1,* 141-150.
Warren, N. (1972). African Precocity. *Psychological Bulletin, 78(5),* 353-367.
Warren, N. & Barkin, J.M. (1974). A Neurological and Behavioral Comparison of African and European Newborns in Uganda. *Child Development, 45,* 966-971.
Werner, E.E. (1972). Infants around the World: Cross-cultural Studies of Psychomotor Development from Birth to two Years. *Journal of Cross-Cultural Psychology, 3(2),* 111-134.
Zelazo, P.R., Zelazo, N.A. & Kolb, S. (1972). "Walking" in the Newborn. *Science, 176,* 314.

THE ACQUISITION OF AN EVERYDAY TECHNICAL MOTOR SKILL: THE POUNDING OF CEREALS IN MALI (AFRICA)*

B. Bril

1. INTRODUCTION

This article focuses on the acquisition of everyday technical motor skills. Most of the studies on the development of motor skills deal with fundamental motor skills such as prehension, walking, throwing, kicking, running, jumping, catching, etc. (see for example Wickstrom, 1983). Very little attention has been paid to more cultural motor skills and especially to those "technical" skills, shared by most of the members of a community: the pounding of cereals in West Africa is one of those skills every woman has to perform almost everyday.

Pounding may be veiwed as a complex motor skill, culturally specific, and will be learnt by any female child through imitative activities beginning as free play copied on adult models.

Free imitative activities will be defined as activities in which the adult does not interfere (i.e. no verbal instruction, no correction) implying that:
1. the child discovers *gestural properties* by himself;
2. the *difference* from adult gestuality is *gradually reduced;*
3. the distance between child and adult gestuality *is not arbitrary,* but constitutes an *adjustment* of a smaller and weaker body to a tool (mortar and pestle) made for adults.

What is interesting to note is that there is no explicit teaching of such a skill**: the adult does not interfere directly on movement learning. This means that:
1. the child has free access to the working place and ustensils of the

---

* The data used for this study have been selected during two stays in the village of Dugurakoro, 20 miles from Bamako (Mali). The author wishes to thank all the women and children who participated in the study. This study has been supported by a grant n°97 703 19 from the D.G.R.S.T. A first version of this paper was presented at the 7th biennal Meeting of the ISSBD in August 1983 (Munich) under the title: Acquisition and transmission of culture: children learning of everyday technical gestuality - the pounding of millet.

** Almost all everyday motor skills are learnt by children in the same way. The study reported here is part of a larger project, concerned with the cultural transmission of motor skills acquired by children without any explicit instruction from adults.

adult; she can play with damaged pestles and mortars, and even with objects in good working order when the adult is not using them;

2. from three years on, the child is asked to accomplish a goal-oriented task that presents greater and greater difficulties: first bruising of condiments, then crushing and finally pounding.

In this paper, which is partly descriptive, we show how the child masters different aspects of the adult movement. Four main aspects of the development of the movement will be discussed: postural stability, temporal components of the movement and relative timing of the different phases of the movement, coordination of the body segments. The last point deals with synchronisation with a partner; this issue is interesting because the child is confronted with an additional environmental variable to take into account.

2. THE POUNDING ACTIVITY

Pounding is an important part of daily work of any Bambara female. All three meals are based on cereals that have first been ground more or less finely. Three main cereals are ground: mostly millet and some corn and rice. Even if it is difficult to estimate precisely how long a woman is pounding every day, it may vary from one to two hours a day.

Men will never pound, and young boys are teased when seen pounding.

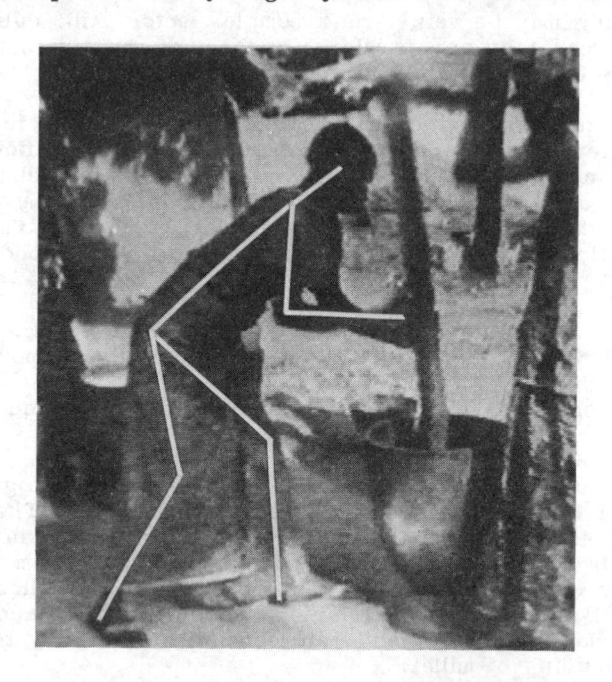

Fig. 1. Woman pounding: body segments taken into account for movement analysis. Seven critical points have been chosen (head, shoulder, elbow, wrist, hip, knee and heel) for the definition of the four following joint angles: shoulder, elbow, hip, knee. (This picture is a video frame reproduction).

Pounding is a technique that can be performed either individually or by two or three persons together, sometimes more.

The tools used are highly standardised and are composed of (Fig. 1)
- a mortar, the size of which depends on the ingredients to be pounded;
- a pestle that may be of two kinds:
  . a condiment pestle, light and about 80 cm long
  . a heavy pestle, weighting 6 to 8 pounds, and 90 to 120 cm long.

Adults always use the heavy pestle to pound cereals; owing to its weight, children of three and four years usually use a condiment pestle, either for play or for more functional work.

3. ADULT POUNDING SKILL: THE MATURE PATTERN OF MOVEMENT

Before discussing developmental data, it is important to consider the mature pattern of pounding skills; this issue is developed more fully elsewhere (Bril, 1983).

Pounding consists of the repetition of a basic elementary movement, lasting 1000 to 1250 msec, depending on the activity of the woman and on the ingredients being pounded. The basic elementary movement has been analysed as a three-phase gesture, based on the movement of the pestle:

1. the pestle is in contact with the contents of the mortar (phase a)
2. the pestle is moved up (phase b1) and positioned correctly (phase b2)
3. the pestle is moved down (phase c).

Diagrams of the movement is shown in Figure 2.

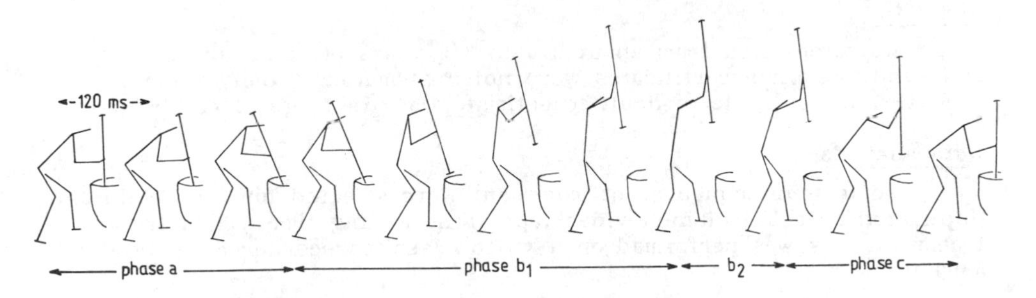

Fig. 2. Adult "basic elementary movement": the body segments given are those of Figure 1. Duration between two diagrams is 120 ms.

The duration of the three phases is very stable (see Table 1), if we consider relative values. Phase a is the shortest one and represents from 19% to 21.5% of the movement duration. Phase b, the longest, represents 53,5% to 56%, and phase c 24.5% to 26.5%. Pounding alone or with a partner does not modify the relative duration of the movement.

Table 1. Temporal structure of the elementary movement in five adult women. Mean duration of the elementary movement and relative duration of the three phases of the movement (n= number of successive elementary movements in the sequence taken into account to calculate the mean; values in parenthesis represent standard deviation.

		Ss_1	Ss_2	Ss_3	Ss_4	Ss_5
Mean duration of movement (in msec)		1000 (24) n= 10	1101 (13) n= 10	1193 (21) n= 9	1134 (29) n= 28	1230 (21) n= 14
relative duration of the phases	a	.203 (.015)	.190 (.014)	.213 (.044)	.219 (.025)	.202 (.032)
	b	.535 (.020)	.558 (.024)	.542 (.043)	.535 (.031)	.537 (.023)
	c	.262 (.021)	.251 (.017)	.244 (.018)	.245 (.018)	.261 (.016)

4. METHODS AND DATA

Video-recorded observations were collected in 1980, 1981 and 1984 in a Malian Bambara village, Dugurakoro. Adults and children were filmed by the author in a "natural" setting during their everyday activities. The video recorder was a JVC connected to a camera JVC GX-775, using batteries as there is no electricity available.

Subjects

Twelve children from about 2.6 to 8/9 years old and adults were observed. As birth certificates were not systematically delivered until recently, it was quite difficult to estimate the exact age of children.

Data analysis

Two to four sequences of movement were selected for each child and duplicated on a 3/4 of inch video-tape while adding time. Then frame by frame analysis was performed on a video cassette recorder Sony Umatic Vo 5850 P.

The displacement of head, shoulder, elbow, wrist, hip, knee and heel was measured during the execution of each movement, in the sagittal plane (see Figure 1). A pointer developed for laboratory measurement gave the coordinates of each point. These data were then processed on a micro-computer IMS 5000. Trajectories of the different points and values of joint angles during the movement were calculated.

5. CHILDREN ACQUISITION OF POUNDING SKILL: developmental data

For Fowler and Turvey (1978), learning a motor skill consists of discovering an optimal organisation of the movement. In fact, it is very difficult, if not impossible, in a situation of imitative learning to define what aspects of the movement are mastered through imitation or discovery or both.

However, it is important to note that the adult woman never interfers directly in the movement process itself: she will never make any comments on the movement itself; her only remarks are relative to the result of action. In addition she never refers to herself as a model (Bril, 1984) that is she never says to a child: "look at me" or "do as I do", etc.

5.1. Stability of basic postural features

Any motor activity may take two forms of movements, that may be referred to as "posture-preserving system" and "transport system" (Fitch, Tuller & Turvey, 1982). Postural movements are concerned with keeping the body upright. On those movements are surimposed movements of parts of the body or transport movements. Performing a movement disturbs the upright posture and may even put off the balance of the body; then the subject has to make a movement to restore the balance.

In the adult, transport movements are usually anticipated by postural adjustment of the rest of the body (Gahery & Massion, 1981), so that balance will not be disturbed. That is the case when a woman is pounding: she maintains equilibrium while the pestle is moving. Most of the women held their left foot in front of the other (see Figure 1): out of 13 women we observed while pounding, 10 put the left foot ahead. During the elementary movement the weight of the body shifts from the front leg (usually the left one) to the rear leg while the pestle starts moving up (phase b1), shifting back on the front leg at the end of phase b1 and while positioning the pestle (phase b2) for the moving down phase. As in field situation we were unable to use either E.M.G. data or force data, therefore we measured postural stability only through displacement of the feet. In adults the feet are fixed in a sequence of movement.

In children this stability is absent: the child, up to 7 or 8 years, moves her feet very frequently. Two indices have been computed:

1. frequency of shifts, which is the ratio:
   total number of shifts
   number of elementary movements in a sequence.
2. frequency of shifts of the rear foot, which is the ratio (for a sequence of n movements):
   number of shifts of rear foot
   total number of shifts (both feet).

The weight of the pestle seems to be here of great importance when the pestle is light (that is under two pounds). The number of shifts decreases very rapidly with age (Fig. 3). The child is able to master the kinetic energy produced by the movement of the pestle. The situation is very different with a heavy pestle (between 6 and 8 pounds). From our data, no evolution concerning postural stability is observed. Figure 3 shows that the number of shifts remains very high throughout the period of acquisition: even at 7-8 years, a child moves her feet more than once every three movements. The back foot moves much more often than the front one which is the supporting limb during more than 75% of movement time.

5.2. Temporal component of the movement

Stability of relative timing of the different phases of movement is often considered as an invariant feature of mature pattern of movement (Schmidt, 1975, 1980; Summers, 1981). This invariant property has been shown for

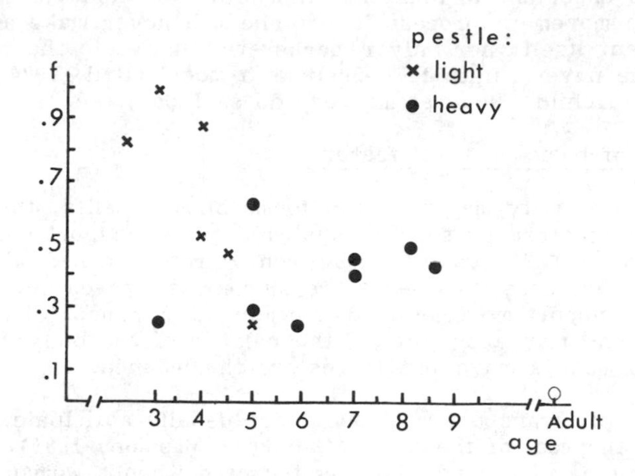

Fig. 3. Stability of basic postural features as a function of age of the child and weight of the pestle. Stability is define as the frequency of feet shifting during a sequence of n elementary movements. A shift correspond to a displacement of a foot. (Each point corresponds to the frequency of foot shifting for one child).

"learned" movement such as handwriting (Viviani & McCollum, in press), finger-tapping (Summers, 1975), or "innate" movement such as walking (Shapiro et al, 1981).

This invariance in relative duration of the different phases has been shown for pounding, within one woman and across the sample of woman in the study. Table 1 gives results concerning five different women. In a sequence of successive movements, the duration of the movement is almost constant for each woman, as well as the relative timing of the different phases. An inter-woman comparison shows that the timing is constant even if the total duration of the movement varies.

As Roberton points it out in a developmental study of "hopping" (1985, this volume), "little developmental information exists on to whether relative timing is an emergent or invariant feature of ontogeny".

We shall consider successively the timing of the basic elementary movement, then the phasing (relative timing of the three phases) of the movement.

5.2.1. Mean duration of the basic elementary movement

A comparison of five women across the sample shows that when pounding under usual condition, the duration of elementary movement ranges between 1000 ms and 1300 ms. Within a sequence of movements, there is almost no variation in the timing of movement (see Table 1).

In children, the duration of the basic movement becomes steady, 1050 to 1200 ms, shortly after the beginning of acquisition, at about 3 to 3.5 years. The regularity in duration of movement increases with age, but also depends on the weight of the pestle (see Figure 4).

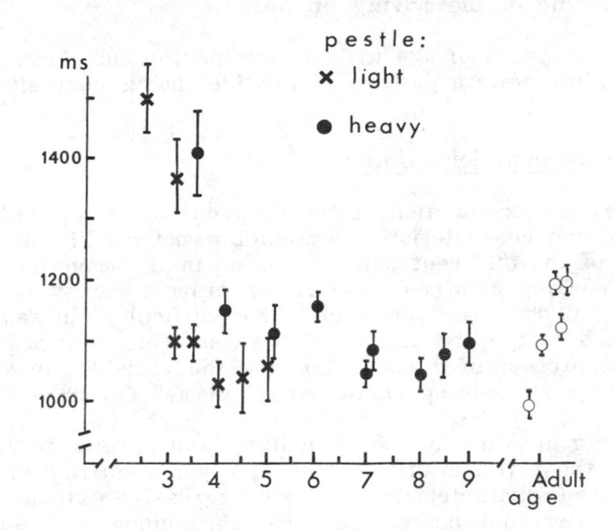

Fig. 4. Evolution of mean duration of basic elementary movement according to the child's age and the weight of the pestle. (Each point corresponds to the mean duration for one child during a sequence of movements).

5.2.2. Relative duration of three phases

In the youngest children (3 to 4 years) the relative duration of the different phases of the movement are very different from the one of the adult. Here again the weight of the pestle has a strong influence on the relative timing. The main characteristic of phasing in children is the longer duration of phase a (see Figure 5), which may represent more than 40% of the duration of the movement when the pestle is a heavy one, compare with

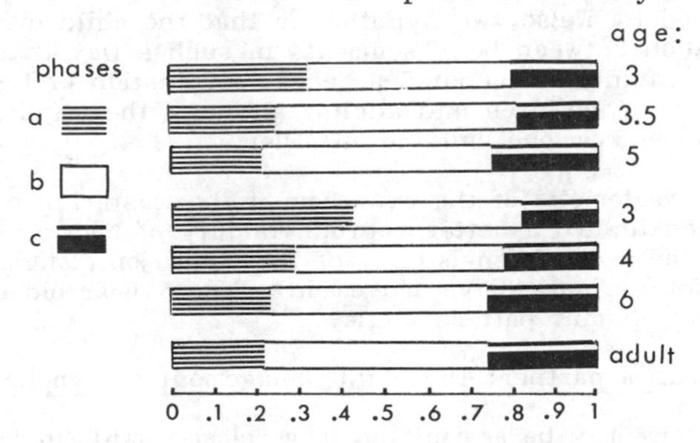

Fig. 5. Relative duration of the three phases of the elementary movement: evolution according to the child's age and the weight of the pestle.

20 to 22% for an adult.

It seems that the child has to readjust the holding of the pestle just before the beginning of the moving up phase.

As early as 5 years of age with a light pestle, and 6 years with a heavy one, a child shows a pattern of relative timing very similar to the adult pattern.

5.3. Motor coordination: joint motion

The pattern of coordination of the different body segments appears to be very stable, and characteristic of pounding motor skill. The regulation of the activity of the different joints involved in the movement may be viewed as the working of a coordinative structure (Turvey et al, 1982). As Kelso points out (1982), the yound child has difficulty "in sequencing the participating limbs". For the individual the mastering of coordination may be seen as "the process of *discovering* how the variables in a very complex system are related for solving particular problems" (p. 28).

When looking at adult joint coordination, the pattern is very clear: Figure 6 shows the patterns of variation of 4 joints during an elementary movement; the main characteristics are the successive extension of hip joint, then shoulder (after an important flexion), then elbow. In addition, the knee joint shows first a strong flexion, then an extension starting simultaneously with the elbow extension. Although we have no further analysis of the phenomenon, we may say that such coordination of body segments minimises the forces necessary to move the pestle up by keeping the centre of gravity of the pestle as near as possible to the body. This pattern of coordination is quite stable (see Fig. 7).

The pattern of coordination observed in adults is not found in very young children. The main characteristics of children coordination is the synchrony found in shoulder and elbow joints, with no flexion of the elbow during phase a. This synchrony may be a constraint of the same nature than the temporal invariance between limbs studied by Kelso et al (1979). With practice the child will break it down, giving independence to the two joints.

As suggested by Kelso, we hypothesise that the child discovers an optimal coordination between body segments in such a way that minimises weariness. Very rapidly, at about 5-6 years coordination of the body segments is similar in children and adults, although the amplitude of the movement may vary from one child to an other.

Another characteristic of the evolution of the mastering of the movement is the progression toward a better reproductability of limb coordination. Figure 7 shows the lack of consistency of the elbow joint angle pattern for the 3-year-old for the successive movements. The 5-year-old child shows a smaller variability of joint pattern angle.

5.4. Pounding with a partner: the child management of synchronisation

Pounding alone may be assimilated to a "closed skill" in Poulton's (1958) sense, while pounding with a partner will appear as an "open skill". Pounding with a partner (in the same mortar) implies to synchronise one's

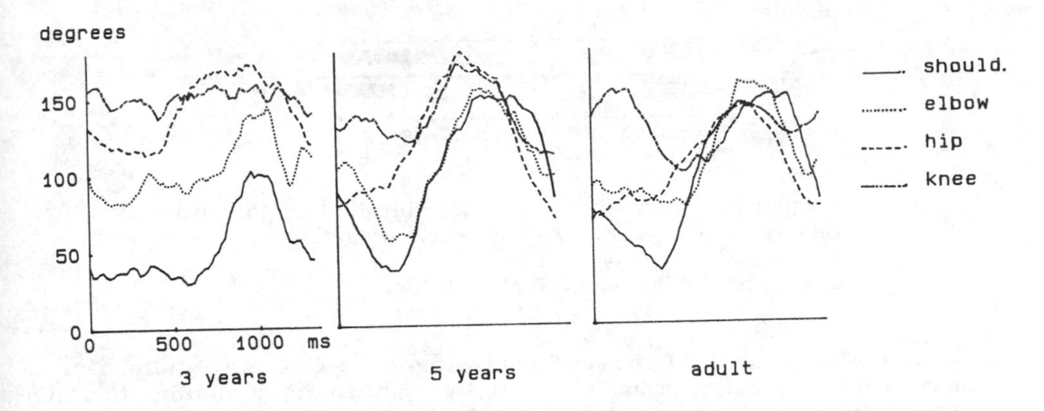

Fig. 6. Relation between angular position of hip, shoulder, elbow and knee: comparison between an adult and two children aged, respectively, 3 years and 5 years.

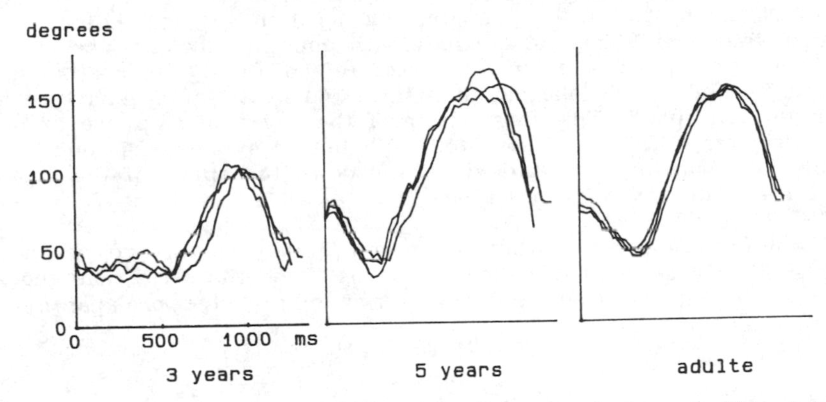

Fig. 7. Reproductibility of the movement: variation of elbow joint during three consecutive movements for an adult and two children (the same as in Figure 6).

movement with the other person's. For an adult woman, this synchronisation does not seem to have any impact on the timing of the movement. The phasing stays exactly unchanged.

On the contrary, the necessity to synchronise leads the child to modify her rhythm, with respect to the relative duration of the three phases. This results in:

- a complete stop after the moving-up phase, between b1 and b2 for the 3 and 4-year-olds;
- instead of a stop, a lengthening of the duration of phase b2 for children from 4 to 6-years of age. This amplification then decreases with age (see Fig. 8).

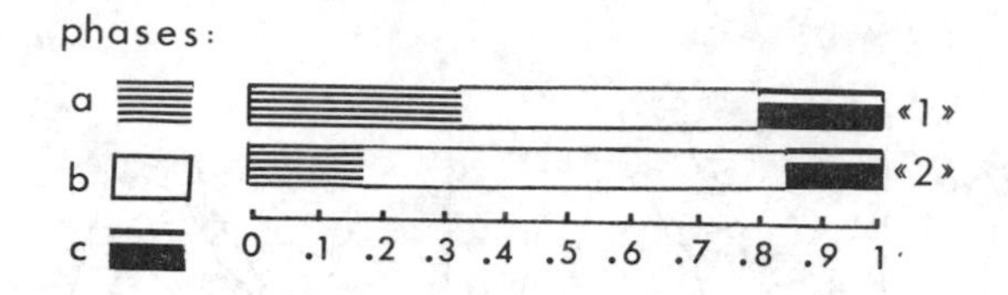

Fig. 8. Comparison between the relative duration of the three phases in a 3 year-old child when pounding:
1 - alone
2 - with a child partner of 4 years.

In fact, if we look at the figures of the younger ones more carefully, it appears that the relative timing is not really modified: once the duration of the stop is taken out, the relative timing is very much comparable to the timing in the adult.

While the child is pounding alone, she does not have to master any external element, except the mortar and pestle size, location, etc. which are constant throughout a sequence of movement. The major problem encountered when pounding with a partner is the necessity to anticipate the "location" of the pestle of the partner, this location varying with time. It seems then that a child cannot evaluate with enough precision the location of her partner's pestle, she ten overcomes this difficulty by positioning her pestle up, in such a way she can wait until the pestle of her partner has left enough free space. The lengthening of the duration of phase b2 instead of a complete stop, may be a step toward a better synchronisation. The child does not have to stop, but she slows down the speed of the pestle during the end of phase b1 and phase b2.

It is interesting to note that, even at 5 or 6 years of age, when the phasing and body segment coordination seems to be the same than the adult one, any change in environmental events may disturb temporal parameters of the movement.

6. DISCUSSION

We analysed the learning of pounding skill through the study of three types of factors: postural stability, temporal characteristics of the movement and patterns of displacement of body segments.

Two characteristics of the learning of pounding skill emerged:
1. On the one hand, there is a similar evolution of phasing and coordination of body segments: the child shows a temporal pattern and coordination pattern similar to that of the adult at about the same age, that is around 5 years of age; this evolution depends on the weight of the pestle, that is on the force necessary to move the pestle up.
2. On the other hand, postural stability, although increasing with age, is still not completely mastered at 7 or 8 years.

From these data, we may put forward the hypothesis that there is a correlation between phasing and body segment coordination. Is it the discovery of an optimal coordination that allows the phasing to stabilise or the reverse? At present we cannot answer this question.

The stabilisation of the "basic posture" does not seem necessary to master the temporal and coordination parameters of the movement. Therefore two questions arise: is this absence of postural stability due to lack of anticipation on the part of the child, or are these frequent shifts in any case necessary to compensate her weaker strength, thus permitting a good coordination of body segments? The great variability we found across the sample of children using the heavy pestle may indicate that children use postural stability as a degree of liberty necessary to master the kinematic properties of the movement.

In this study we analyse the evolution of the movement execution, but no information is given on how the process of control evolves. In a more experimental study (manuscript in preparation) we analyse the role of visual and auditory feedback in pounding skill. The first results show that visual and auditory feedback decrease with practice, thus corroborating what is usually accepted (Johnson, 1984). But it is only in case of suppression of both visual and auditory feedback that the movement is really perturbed.

A last word should be said on the conditions of learning. This study shows that without any explicit teaching, children master different gestural techniques when they are very young. The fact that there is no explicit teaching does not mean that adults take no part in the acquisition process. We observed for example in an adult-child pair that the adult adapted her performance to that of her child partner by making longer phase b, and shorter phase a (see Fig. 9) thus facilitating synchronisation on the part of the child. In the sequence of 14 successive movements analysed, phase a had a relative duration of .16, which was smaller than all the data analysed for adult (see Table 1).

This leads us to the problem of how cultural transmission of domains such as gestuality proceeds. Very often, imitation, imprinting, conditioning, teaching are called upon. The problem to debate is the type of transmission process involved for different domains, movement being one particular domain.

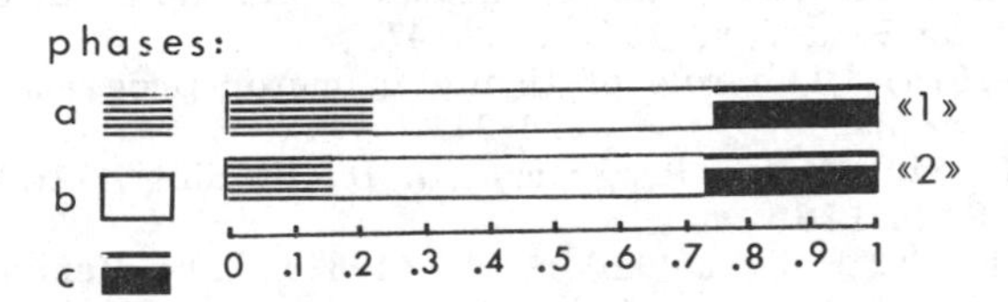

Fig. 9. Comparison of the relative duration of the 3 phases of movement in an adult when pounding:
1 - with an adult partner
2 - with a child partner of 3.5 years of age.

References

Bril, B. (1983). Analyse d'un geste de percussion perpendiculaire lancée: la mouture du mil dans un village bambara. *Bulletin Geste et Image, 3,* 97-118.

Bril, B. (1984). Acquisition et transmission du geste quotidien: le cas des techniques domestiques dans une communauté Bambara du Mali. Paper presented at the UNICEF-UNESCO Conference *Maîtrise du geste et pouvoir de la main chez l'enfant.* Paris: November.

Fitch, H.L., Tuller, B. & Turvey, M.T. (1982). The Bernstein Perspective: Tuning of Coordinative Structures with Special Reference to Perception. In J.A.C. Kelso (Ed.), *Human Motor Behavior: An Introduction.* London: L.E.A.

Fowler, C.A. & Turvey, M.T. (1978). Skill Acquisition: An Event Approach with Special Reference to Searching for the Optimum of a Function of Several Variables. In G.E. Stelmach (Ed.), *Information Processing in Motor Control and Learning.* New York: Academic Press.

Gahery, Y. & Massion, J. (1981). Coordination Between Posture and Movement. *Trends in Neuroscience,* 199-202.

Johnson, P. (1984). The acquisition of skill. In M.M. Smyth and A.M. Wing (Eds.), *The Psychology of Human Movement.* Academic Press Inc.

Kelso, J.A.S. (1982). Concepts and issues in human motor behavior: coming to grips with the jargon. In J.A.S. Kelso (Ed.), *Human Motor Behavior.* London: L.E.A.

Kelso, J.A.S., Southard, D. & Goodman, D. (1979). On the nature of human interlimb coordination. *Science, 203,* 1029-1031.

Poulton, E.C. (1957). On prediction in skilled movements. *Psychological Bulletin, 80,* 113-121.

Roberton, M.A. The Development of Arm-Leg Timing in Hopping over 13-14 Years, this volume.

Schmidt, R.A. (1975). A schema theory of discrete motor skill learning. *Psychological Review, 82,* 225-260.

Schmidt, R.A. (1980). On the Theoretical Status of Time in Motor-Program Representations. In G.E. Stelmach and J. Requin (Eds.), *Tutorial in Motor Behavior.* North-Holland Publishing Company.

Shapiro, D.C., Zernicke, R.F., Gregor, R.J. & Diestel, J.D. (1981). Evidence for Generalised Motor Programs Using Gait Pattern Analysis. *Journal of Motor Behavior, 13(1),* 33-47.

Summers, J.J. (1975). The role of timing in motor program representation. *Journal of Motor Behavior, 7,* 229-242.

Summers, J.J. (1981). Motor Programs. In D. Holding (Ed.), *Human Skills.* John Wiley & Sons Ltd.

Turvey, M.T., Fitch, H.L. & Tuller, B. (1982). The Bernstein perspective. I. The problems of degrees of freedom and context-conditioned variability. In J.A.S. Kelso (Ed.), *Human Motor Behavior.* London: L.E.A.

Viviani, P.Z. & McCollum, G. (in press). The relation between linear extent and velocity in drawing movements. *Neuroscience.*

Wickstrom, R.L. (1983). *Fundamental motor patterns.* Philadelphia: Lea & Febiger.

SECTION 7

SPEECH & LANGUAGE

PARALLELS BETWEEN MOTOR AND LANGUAGE DEVELOPMENT

V.J. Molfese and J.C. Betz

1. INTRODUCTION

Issues pertaining to the development of biological and behavioural processes have sparked a flood of research in recent years. Our interests in this area have been focused on the development of cognitive skills and brain processing mechanisms in samples of infants tested longitudinally from birth to approximately 36 months of age (Molfese & Molfese, 1985, 1985a,b). With our involvement in the behavioural assessments of these infants there has been a chance to observe repeatedly how specific skills develop relative to other skills. Of particular interest to this paper are the parallels that seem to exist between motor skills developments and language skills developments. That there should be parallels seems to be controversial.

Eric Lenneberg's "Biological Foundations of Language" (1967) represents an attempt to focus attention on what he believed to be the primary source of language. With the biological basis of language as his core assumption, Lenneberg sketches his concept of the emergence of language as an "unfolding of capacities" (p. 127); "a series of generally well-circumscribed events which take place between the second and third year of life" (p. 127). From Lenneberg's viewpoint, "the central and most interesting problem is whether the emergence of language is due to very general capabilities that mature to a critical minimum at about 18 months to make language, and many other skills, possible or whether there might be some factors specific to speech and language that come to maturation and that are somewhat independent from other, more general processes" (p. 126).

In developing this theme, Lenneberg generates two testable hypotheses. First, although Lenneberg takes note of "the remarkable synchronisation of speech milestones with motor-developmental milestones" he nevertheless claims that "the language-maturational process is independent of motor-skeletal maturation" (p. 131). Not only does he separate language development from motor development, but he calls attention to the "maturational histories" of motor skills and motor coordinations. He states that "the specific history for speech control stands apart dramatically from histories of finger and hand control" (p. 131). He further argues that although both language onset and the onset of gait are both regulated by maturational processes, they are nevertheless independent of one another (p. 131). As evidence he cites instances where "speech and language emerge at their usual time while motor development lags behind" (p. 132). Conversely, there exist children with "normal" motor development who through no congenital nor traumatic cause exhibit delayed speech development. Our interest in this issue of the independence of language development and motor development is not that there are children that show such dissynchronies but, rather, are such dissynchronies the norm?

Second, Lenneberg's view of the emergence of language development also produces a testable hypothesis. Lenneberg assumes that the general rate of development in children may not be constant in the formative years: "there may be transient slowing in the rate of maturation, with subsequent hastening" (p. 133). However, he adds that this alternation does not apply to the narrower rate of language development. More specifically, although general development is characterised by irregularity, "there is a remarkable degree of regularity in the emergence of language" (p. 133). From this it might be hypothesised that the emergence of language is more regular than that of motor development.

This paper uses data from a longitudinal study to address two hypotheses generated from basic points Lenneberg contends are valid for language and motor skills:

1. language-maturation is independent of motor-skeletal maturation.
2. the emergence of language is more regular than motor development: motor development history stands apart from language development history.

2. PROCEDURES

2.1. Subjects

The data used to evaluate the two hypotheses generated from Lenneberg's theory were obtained from a longitudinal study. The data set is composed of scores obtained from infants who were part of a study on brain-language relations. This data set is composed of infants who were either tested from birth to age 36 months at 6 month intervals or were tested from 12 months to 36 months at 6 month intervals. These infants had birth weights ranging from 1401 to 2270 gm (X= 3258.97), and gestational ages ranging from 35 to 43 weeks (X= 38.8). The Bayley Scales of Infant Development were used to assess development at each six month testing. Scores on the Bayley were obtained from 67 six-month olds, 31 12-month olds, 24 18-month olds and 16 24-month olds.

These infants are primarily white, from the middle class with parents who were married, husbands employed and with both parents obtaining at least 8 years of schooling. These infants were ideal subjects to use with the infant tests, described below, since such tests were normed on middle-class, primarily white infants.

2.2. Measures

The two measures to be discussed here are the Bayley Scales of Infant Development (Bayley, 1969) - mental scale and the Denver Developmental Screening Scale. The Bayley Scales are designed for the evaluation of a child's developmental status in the first two and a half years of life. The Scales are composed of two subscales: a mental scale and a motor scale. The mental scale, which is used in the research we are reporting, assesses sensory-perceptual acuities, object constancy, memory, learning and problem solving, socialisation, verbal communication, and abstract thinking. The 163 items can be identified as separately taping verbal (production and comprehension) and motor (fine and gross) skills. Examples of verbal and motor items are shown in Tables 1-4 below.

Table 1.

BAYLEY SCALES OF INFANT DEVELOPMENT

MENTAL SCALE

Verbal Production Items

Age (range)	Item
0.9 (.5 - 9)	Vocalizes once or twice
1.6 (.5 - 5)	Vocalizes at least 4 times
2.1 (1 - 6)	Vocalizes to E's social smile and talk
2.3 (1 - 5)	Vocalizes 2 different sounds
4.6 (3 - 8)	Vocalizes attitudes (pleasure, displeasure, etc)
5.8 (4 - 8)	Interest in sound production
7.0 (5 - 12)	Vocalizes 4 different syllables
7.9 (5 - 14)	Says "da-da" or equivalent
12.0 (9 - 18)	Jabbers expressively
14.2 (10 - 23)	Says 2 words
17.8 (13 - 27)	Names 1 object (ball, watch, cup, etc)
18.8 (14 - 27)	Uses words to make wants known
19.3 (14 - 27)	Names 1 picture
20.6 (16 - 30)	Sentence of two words
21.4 (16 - 30)	Names 2 objects
22.1 (17 - 30+)	Names 3 pictures
24.0 (17 - 30+)	Names 3 objects
25.0 (19 - 30+)	Names 5 pictures

Table 2.

BAYLEY SCALES OF INFANT DEVELOPMENT

MENTAL SCALE

Verbal Comprehension Items

Age (range)	Item
1.5 (.5 - 4)	Social smile:E talks and smiles
7.6 (5 - 12)	Cooperates in games (pat-a-cake, peek-a-boo)
7.9 (5 - 14)	Listens selectively to familiar words
9.1 (6 - 14)	Responds to verbal request
9.4 (6 - 13)	Puts cube in cup on command
10.1 (7 - 17)	Inhibits on command
15.3 (11 - 23)	Shows shoes or other clothing, or own toy
17.8 (14 - 26)	Follows directions, doll (chair, cup)
19.1 (15 - 26)	Points to parts of doll (hair, mouth, ears)
19.7 (14 - 30+)	Finds 2 objects
19.9 (16 - 28)	Points to 3 pictures
21.6 (17 - 30+)	Points to 5 pictures
23.4 (16 - 30+)	Discriminates 2: cup, plate, box
24.7 (19 - 30+)	Points to 7 pictures
25.6 (18 - 30+)	Discriminates 3: cup, plate, box
28.2 (22 - 30+)	Understands 2 prepositions
30+ (21 - 30+)	Concept of one
30+ (23 - 30+)	Understands 3 prepositions

The Denver Developmental Screening Scale (Frankenberg & Dodds, 1967) is primarily used as a method for screening children from birth to 6 years for developmental delays. The scale contains four scales: gross motor, language, fine motor-adaptive, and personal-social. Items on the language and motor scales are shown in Tables 5-8. When compared to the Bayley Scales, there was a 68% agreement in both Scales identifying children as abnormal and a 92% agreement in both scales identifying children as normal (Frankenberg, Goldstein & Camp, 1971).

These two Scales are chosen for comparison purposes because each contains a sufficient number of language, fine motor and gross motor skills to permit reasonable comparisons, both include mean age and age range for each item and because the scales differ in how the "skill levels" are assessed. The Bayley Scale relies on behavioural testing in which the tester presents a behavioural task and the child is expected to perform it. The Denver scale permits a higher reliance on mother's report in addition to some behavioural testing. Thus, with the Denver Scale if the child does not perform the skill during the testing period, for whatever reason, mother's report can be used. The Bayley Scale, on the other hand, is strongly performance biased and would be considered a more conservative assessment than the Denver Scale.

Table 3.

BAYLEY SCALES OF INFANT DEVELOPMENT

MENTAL SCALE

Examples of Fine Motor Items

Age	Item
5.4 (4 - 8)	Exploitive string play
5.7 (4 - 8)	Picks up cube deftly and directly
5.7 (4 - 8)	Pulls string: secures ring
5.8 (4 - 11)	Lifts cup with handle
6.5 (5 - 10)	Manipulates bell: interest in detail
7.1 (5 - 10)	Pulls string adaptively: secures ring
8.9 (6 - 12)	Fingers holes in peg board
10.4 (7 - 15)	Attempts to imitate scribble
11.8 (9 - 18)	Puts 3 or more cubes in cup
12.0 (9 - 17)	Uncovers blue box
13.0 (10 - 17)	Places 1 peg repeatedly
13.6 (10 - 20)	Blue board: places 1 round block
16.4 (13 - 20)	Places pegs in 70 seconds
16.7 (13 - 21)	Builds tower of 3 cubes
17.8 (13 - 26)	Imitates crayon stroke
19.3 (14 - 30+)	Blue board: places 2 round, 2 square blocks
20.0 (16 - 29)	Pegs placed in 30 seconds
23.0 (17 - 30+)	Builds tower of 6 cubes
24.4 (19 - 30+)	Imitates strokes: vertical and horizontal
26.1 (19 - 30+)	Train of cubes
30+ (22 - 30+)	Blue board: completes in 60 seconds
30+ (22 - 30+)	Builds tower of 8 cubes

3. RESULTS

The data from the longitudinal sample and the test items were analysed to test the two hypotheses.

Hol: LANGUAGE MATURATION IN INDEPENDENT OF MOTOR-SKELETAL MATURATION

From this hypothesis it can be inferred that performance on a behavioural assessment scale, such as the Bayley Scales of Infant Development or the Denver Developmental Screening Scale, would be such that a child's performance on the language items should not be related to performance on the motor items. The hypothesis can be tested by using the

Table 4.

BAYLEY SCALES OF INFANT DEVELOPMENT

MENTAL SCALE

	Gross Motor Items
2.6 (1 - 5)	Manipulates red ring
2.8 (2 - 5)	Simple play with rattle
3.1 (1 - 5)	Reaches for dangling ring
3.2 (1 - 6)	Fingers hand in play
3.8 (2 - 6)	Closes on dangling ring
4.1 (2 - 6)	Reaches for cube
4.6 (3 - 7)	Picks up cube
4.8 (3 - 7)	Exploitive paper play
5.0 (3 - 8)	Reaches persistently
5.2 (4 - 8)	Lifts inverted cup
5.4 (4 - 8)	Bangs in play
7.8 (5 - 13)	Rings bell purposively
9.7 (8 - 15)	Stirs with spoon in imitation
10.5 (8 - 17)	Unwraps cube
11.3 (9 - 15)	Pushes car alone
12.2 (8 - 19)	Pats whistle doll in imitation
19.9 (15 - 27)	Broken doll: mends marginally

performance of the infants in our longitudinal study of the Bayley Scales. Since the items on the Bayley mental subscale are ordinally scaled according to average age in which each item is passed, it is possible to identify at each testing age (i.e., 6 months, 12 months, 18 months and 24 months) the highest language item passed and the highest motor item passed by each infant. If the hypothesis is correct, there should be a non-significant correlation between language items and motor items at each age.

Table 5.

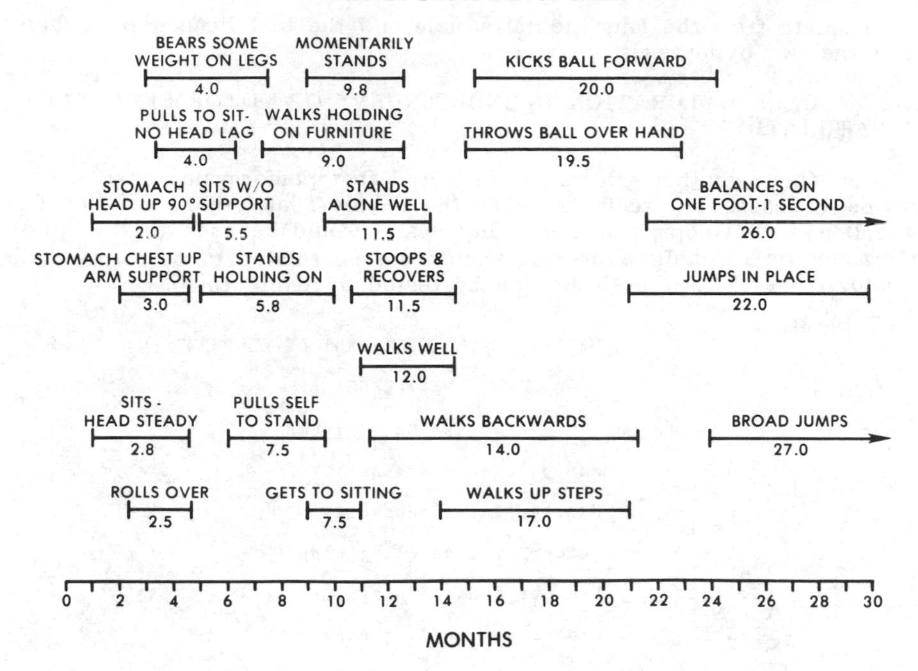

Table 6.

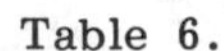

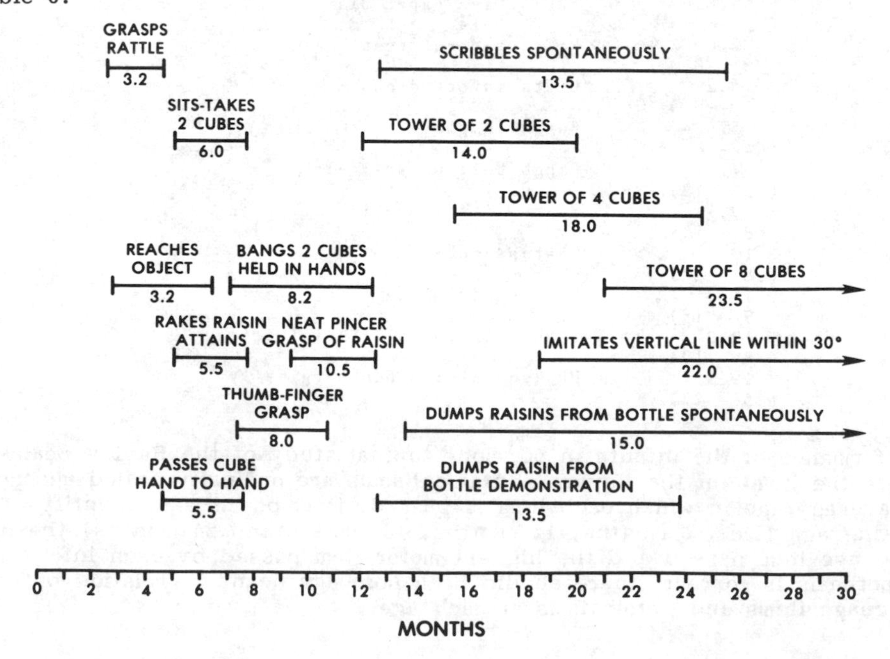

Table 7.

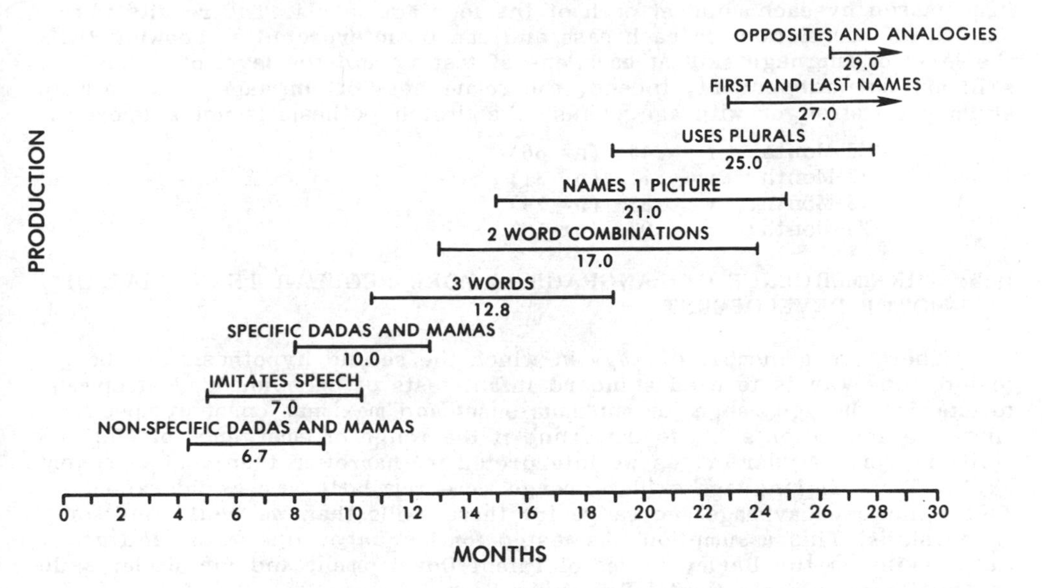

Table 8.

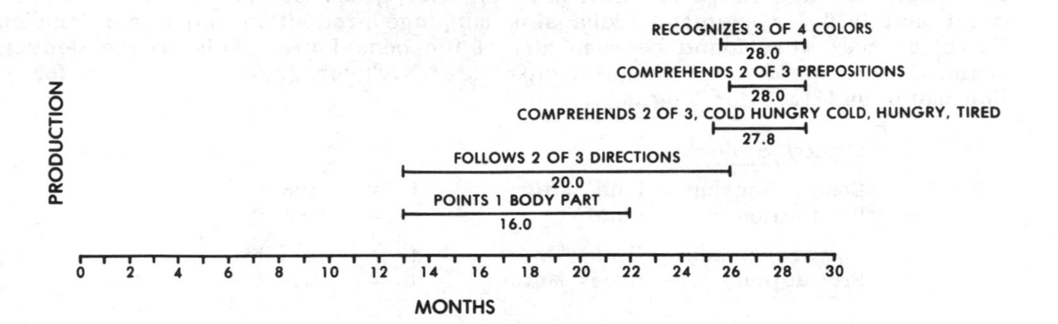

Pearson correlation coefficients were computed on data from our longitudinal data set using the item number corresponding to the last language item passed and the item number corresponding to the last motor item passed by each child at each of the four age levels. The results were significant correlations in each case and can be interpreted as showing that the level of language skill at each age of testing and the level of motor skill are not independent. Indeed, the relatedness of language skills to motor skills grew stronger with age. Thus, the first hypothesis is not supported.

6-Month:	r= .43	(n= 66)
12-Month:	r= .71	(n= 31)
18-Month:	r= .83	(n= 24)
24-Month:	r= .92	(n= 16)

Ho2: THE EMERGENCE OF LANGUAGE IS MORE REGULAR THAN THAT OF MOTOR DEVELOPMENT

There are a number of ways in which the second hypothesis can be tested. One way is to used standard infant tests of behavioural development to examine the age range for minimum onset and maximum onset of specific language and motor skills to determine if the range of emergence of language skills is more regular or, as we interpreted it, narrower than that of motor skills. Thus, if language skills ermerge more regularly, we would expect to find a narrower average age range for these skills than we would find for motor skills. This assumption was tested for language, fine motor and gross motor skills on the Bayley Scales of Infant Development and for similar skills on the Denver Developmental Screening Scale.

We looked at the specific items on the two scales and the range of onset of each item. Using t tests it was possible to compare the range of variation in onset for language skills, fine motor skills and gross motor skills. The results were somewhat different for the two scales. For the Bayley Scales, the language comprehension and language production items were not different in range of onset compared to that found for the fine motor items. However, the range of onset of gross motor items were different from the range of onset of both the language production and the language comprehension items. The means for age range of onset are: 4.98 for gross motor, 9.45 for fine motor and 10.0 for language (collapsing language production and comprehension) No differences were found between any of the behavioural skills on the Denver Scale. The means for age range of onset are: 8.09 for gross motor, 8.56 for fine motor and 12.0 for language.

<u>Bayley Scales:</u>

Comprehension	- Fine Motor	t = ns
Production	- Fine Motor	t = ns
Comprehension	- Gross Motor	t = 4.13**
Production	- Gross Motor	t = 3.04**

<u>Denver Scale:</u>

Language	- Fine Motor	t = ns
Language	- Gross Motor	t = ns

From the data it seems as if the emergence of specific language abilities is not more regular than the emergence of fine motor abilities, although language and gross motor abilities on the Bayley Scales were found to differ.

It must be recognised that for the gross motor items on the Bayley Mental Scales there are many fewer items at each age and at the older ages (after age 19 months) there are no gross motor items, thus, accounting for the low mean age range of onset for gross motor skills. The fewer number of gross motor items is due to the Bayley Scales inclusion of a separate gross motor scale. Thus, the relationship between language emergence and gross motor emergence is not really adequately tested on the Bayley Scales. However, on the Denver Scales, which do contain more of the traditional gross motor items (e.g., sits without support, throws a ball, jumps in place, rides a tricycle), there were no differences between language emergence and either fine or gross motor emergence and the means for the age range of onset of the skills on this scale are more similar. The difference in the items that both scales contain make it hard to come to a conclusion concerning gross motor emergence, but it is interesting to note that different types of gross motor behaviours may emerge differently from language and fine motor behaviours. This may reflect a difference between what we believe is a "cognitively driven system" in the case of language and fine motor abilities and a "physical/structural system" in the case of gross motor behaviour.

4. DISCUSSION

The results of these analyses are interpreted as showing that development of language does not seem to be a special case of cognitive development that "come(s) to maturation...somewhat independent from the other, more general processes", as Lenneberg assumed. Indeed, attainment of specific language abilities was not independent of the attainment of specific motor abilities in a longitudinal sample of infants. Nor is the development of language abilities more regular than the development of motor abilities. These data only include scores up to two years of age, and it is possible that the independence of language and motor abilities might manifest itself later. However, in testing the first hypothesis, the correlations between language and motor skills were growing stronger with age and seem likely to continue to do so.

An explanation of the relationship between motor and language development seems to require an accounting of regularities as well as potential deviations in the onset and development of specific abilities. Such an explanation might make use of a conceptual model of creodes and the epigenetic system introduced by Waddington (1962) and discussed by Piaget (1971), Gibson (1981) and McClearn (1970). Creodes are defined as "necessary routes" or canals through which development of each individual ability passes. The epigenetic system refers to the "sum of creodes, taken as being - to greater or lesser degree - channeled" (Piaget, 1971, p. 19).

In this channeled process, "the genetic system is programmed to interact with the normal successions of environments (both internal and external) in a manner which assures that structures mature in a given sequence and reach a particular end point" (Gibson, 1981, p. 76). If the process deviates too much from the programmed route due to environmental influences, an "interplay of coersive compensations" (Piaget, 1971, p. 19) referred to as "homeorhesis", is brought into force.

The epigenetic system is illustrated in Figure 1 and has been described as a surface containing channels (creodes) and behavioural development is conceptualised as a ball rolling over the surface. Early in infancy, the

Table 9.

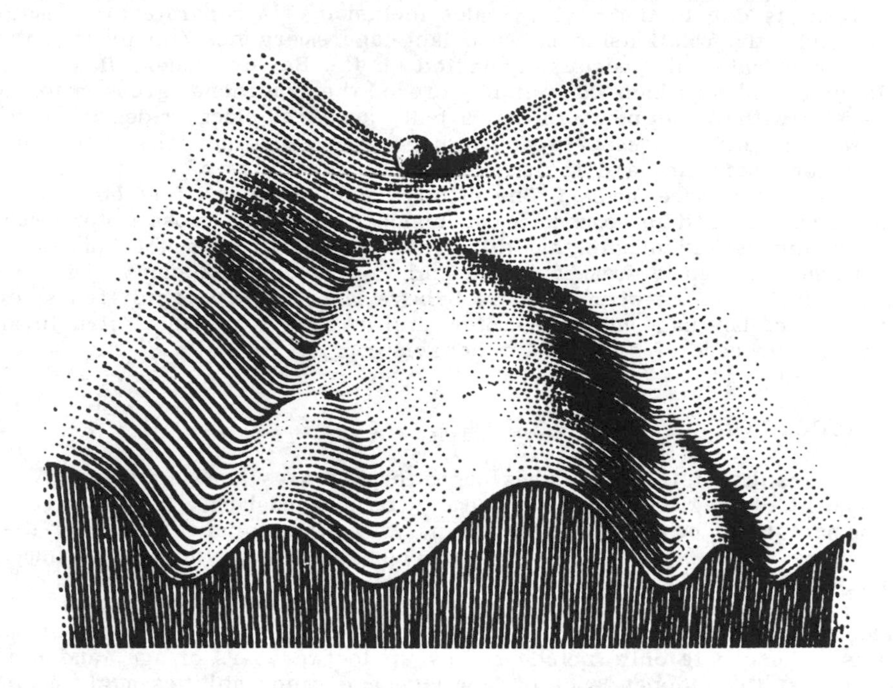

Waddington's "epigenetic landscape."

channels in the surface are deep and the chances of the ball rolling out of (or of deviating from) the channel are not great. However, later in infancy, the channel may broaden or contain alternative routes and greater variations in developments may be seen. Ultimately, however, each ability has a certain end point that is genetically programmed. While the environment can influence to some extent the rate and direction of the development of specific abilities, the epigenetic system does not allow major deviations.

If motor and language development are conceptualised as abilities represented on the ball, and development is conceptualised as occurring as the ball passes along the channel, it might make sense to think that fastest and most regular development would occur the deeper the ball is in the channel. However, as the ball slides from side to side (or wobbles) within the channel, development would occur more slowly and less consistently - much as the speed and progress of bobsled teams are impeded as they deviate from the trough of the run. In the normal course of development, abilities of individuals would generally emerge and develop in a constant and fairly similar fashion but might show temporary deviations as the ball wobbles in the trough. To hypothesise that the emergence and development of one ability is more regular than another, one would have to think of a ball with a differentially weighted surface such that the heavy side would be in the trough more deeply than other sides of the ball and the deep in trough edge would be subject to less deviation than the other points on the ball. Such a differential weighting does not seem to be the case with the development of language and motor abilities, according to the data we have presented. Rather, both Waddington's Epigenetic System model and our data seem to be consistent with a view of parallel development of motor and language abilities.

For the most part, behavioural development across individuals generally shows a normal, regular course. However, there are individual differences that show up as deviations from the normal development model described above. Some of these deviations have been the subjects of antecdotal accounts. For example, one antecdote is about a child who has normal motor skills but does not talk. One day, upon entering the kitchen, the child notices that the toaster is on fire. "Daddy", cries the child, "The toaster is on fire". The father, of course, is astounded. "You have never uttered a word before. Why now?" asks the father. To which the child replies: "Well, up until now everything has pretty much been all right". Individual differences in development such as this might be thought of in the epigenetic model as balls varying in degree of sphere - with some balls less spherical than others ("odd balls"). These balls might run through some differently than the spherical balls (i.e., might run more slowly through some troughs, unable to enter others, etc.). It seems possible that environmental perturbations (such as a toaster on fire) might influence the travel of these balls, possibly influencing both the rate and direction of movement. The influence of environmental perturbations on the flow and course of development has not yet been clearly conceptualised using the model described above primarily because such perturbations are difficult to document without using frequent subject testing and analysing the various environmental events at work on individual subjects. However, it is only through attempts to account for normative as well as individual differences in the development of specific abilities that challenges for existing models of development are raised and new, more inclusive models are developed.

5. SUMMARY

The notion of parallel development of motor and language abilities seems to be supported by two lines of evidence: a) from a longitudinal study of development between 6 months and 3 years of age in which the data showed that correlations between motor ability items and language ability items correlated highly at each age and b) from comparisons of age ranges in onset of specific skills as determined from items on the Bayley Scales of Infant Development and the Denver Developmental Screening Test in which similar ranges in onset of abilities were found for each scale. Lenneberg's views of motor and language development as representing very different developmental processes do not receive support from these lines of evidence.

References

Bayley, N. (1969). *Bayley scales of infant development: Birth to two years.* New York: Psychological Corps.

Frankenburg, W. & Dodds, J. (1967). The Denver Developmental Screening Test. *Pediatrics, 71,* 181-191.

Frankenburg, W., Goldstein, A. & Camp, B. (1971). The revised Denver Developmental Screening Test: Its accuracy as a screening instrument. *Pediatrics, 79,* 988-995.

Gibson, K. (1981). Comparative neuro-ontogeny: Its implications for the development of human intelligence. In G. Butterworth (Ed.), *Infancy and Epistemology: An Evaluation of Piaget's Theory.* Sussex: The Harvester Press Limited.

Lenneberg, E. (1967). *Biological Foundations of Language.* New York: Wiley.

McClearn, G. (1970). Genetic influences on behavior and development. In P. Mussen (Ed.), *Carmichael's Manual of Child Psychology.* New York: Wiley.

Molfese, D. & Molfese, V. (1985a). Electrophysiological indices of auditory discrimination in newborn infants: The bases for predicting later language development? *Infant Behavior and Development, 8,* 197-211.

Molfese, V. & Molfese, D. (1985b). Predicting a child's preschool language performance from perinatal variables. In R. Dillon (Ed.), *Individual Differences in Cognition.* New York: Academic Press.

Piaget, J. (1971). *Biology and Knowledge.* Chicago: University of Chicago Press.

Waddington, C. (1962). *New Patterns in Genetics and Development.* New York: Columbia University Press.

LATERALISATION AND MOTOR DEVELOPMENT

D.L. Molfese and S.E. Linnville

A. INTRODUCTION

Scientists for many years have held the view that the brain is a non differentiated mass from birth until perhaps two years of age (Orton, 1928; Lenneberg, 1967). Proponents of this view have argued that, because of this lack of specialisation in the early years of life, the brain does not display any lateralised biases. Instead, the brain, and the behaviours controlled by it develop initially in a symmetrical fashion. Only later, perhaps between 18 months and 24 months-of-age would positional and processing biases begin to emerge. These biases would be forced in part by the brain's attempt to deal more effectively with related linguistic, cognitive, and motor functions by restricting them to the same hemisphere (usually the left hemisphere in most people). Such restrictions would avoid the longer temporal delays involved in transcollosal communications (via the corpus collosum) and allow the various brain areas which subserve these related functions to communicate more rapidly with each other. Other non-linguistic skills and their related motor patterns would be relegated to the non-language dominant hemisphere, usually the right hemisphere. Lateralisation of these linguistic and non-linguistic functions was thought to continue to develop until puberty, at which time it would have reached an adult level.

This historical position has been used to generate a number of hypotheses, some of which have gained almost the status of scientific law in certain scientific circles. These include the views that: (1) lateralisation is not present at birth but emerges for the first time with the development of language skills (usually between 18 months and 24 months-of-age); (2) the degree of lateralisation increases during development until the onset of puberty; (3) handedness and other motor skills provide a "sign" which indicates which hemisphere of the brain controls language functions; (4) individuals who are "poorly lateralised" (i.e., do not show a clear cut motor asymmetry) are at risk for potential linguistic and cognitive deficits. In the paper that follows, we will review the scientific literature concerned with the development of lateralisation as it relates to motor and cognitive behaviours. Although clear parallels may be seen between the emergence of lateralised motor behaviours and shifts in brain responses, it is of course not clear that one process necessarily directly or indirectly influences the other. Rather, the emergence of lateralised responses in both cases could result from their relationship to some as yet unknown third factor. It is hoped that through this review a clearer understanding of the interaction between laterality and motor development will emerge.

B. LATERALISATION AND ITS AGE OF ONSET

As noted above, Lenneberg (1967) argued quite strongly that lateralisation was not present at birth but emerged later during the last half of the second year of life. Given the higher levels of right hemisphere aphasia in children than adults (30% versus 3%, respectively), Lenneberg believed that language and its associated abilities were not completely restricted to the left hemisphere. However, Woods and Teuber (1978), in an extensive review of the early literature concerned with the incidence of aphasia following childhood brain lesions, concluded that this higher incidence reflected bilateral damage which may have occurred in the absence of antibiotic treatments. Other arguments supporting the absence of early hemisphere differences were based at least in part on the reports of Basser (1962) with hemispherectomised children. However, a number of serious questions have challenged Lenneberg's interpretation based on these data. Basser's criteria for identifying the locus of the lesion was problematic. Apparently, a number of children with bilateral lesions were actually classified by Basser as having right sided lesions. Moreover, his tests for language skills were, to say the least, primitive. Children were identified as having developed language if they could at least say "moma" or "papa" before the onset of the lesion. Clearly, this is a very simplistic view of language and fails to recognise the complexity of a linguistic system beyond that of a single word utterance.

1. Studies with clinical populations suggest early hemisphere asymmetries

More recent research with brain damaged populations of infants and children is clearly at variance with Basser's and Lenneberg's contention regarding early equipotentiality. For example, although Annett (1973) found that children who experienced damage in either hemisphere prior to 13 months of age demonstrated some type of language impairment, left damaged children were more often impaired than those with right hemisphere damage. In a series of studies by Dennis and her colleagues (Dennis, 1977; Dennis & Whitaker, 1978; Dennis & Kohn, 1975; Kohn & Dennis, 1974) employing very sensitive measures of linguistic and cognitive abilities, differential damage to the left hemisphere was found to have a more marked negative effect on long term language development than comparable damage involving the right hemisphere. Dennis (1977) and Dennis and Whitaker (1978) report the results of extensive cognitive and linguistic tests with three children who had undergone hemidecortication in early infancy. The one right hemidecorticate child reportedly developed greater linguistic proficiency while the two left hemidecorticate children became more proficient at visuospatial skills. While generalisations based on results from studies involving such small samples are impossible, these findings seem to be supported by other studies with larger populations (Dennis & Kohn, 1975; Kohn & Dennis, 1974).

Studies involving adults who had undergone hemidecortication during late childhood for injuries sustained in infancy, have reported differential linguistic skills depending on the site of the brain damage. Adults with only an intact left hemisphere were found to perform better and faster on some language tasks as compared to adults with only an intact right hemisphere (Dennis & Kohn, 1975). However, adults with only an intact right hemisphere demonstrate more age-appropriate visuospatial abilities than those with only an intact left hemisphere (Kohn & Dennis, 1974). Taken together, these findings with hemispherectomised populations fail to support Basser's and Lenneberg's contention of early equipotentiality. In fact, it appears that early damage to one hemisphere relative to the other has very specific and long term effects which involve and influence the acquisition of skills which are not yet present at the time of the brain insult.

2. Electrophysiological studies indicate early functional asymmetries: The emergence of a body of research conducted with nomal populations of infants has also indicated that lateralisation of function is in fact present quite early in development. The first study to indicate a functional difference between the two hemispheres early on in development was conducted by Molfese (1972). This work used a procedure called evoked potentials to monitor the electrical responses of the brain to a series of speech and non-speech sounds. The evoked potential is a portion of the ongoing electrical activity of the brain which can be detected by recording electrodes placed on the scalp and which is time-locked to the onset of some stimulus. In this study a group of infants between one week and 12 months of age, 11 children between 4 and 9 years of age, and 10 college aged adults were tested. Analyses which compared the amplitudes of the brain responses which were recorded from the left and right hemispheres revealed that the speech sounds elicited larger brain responses from over the left side of the head than the right side while non-language related sounds evoked larger amplitude responses over the right side. This was the case even in the youngest of the subjects tested, a one-week old infant. Molfese concluded from this that the two hemispheres are not initially equipotential but rather that the two sides of the brain are structured from birth to process the world in different ways. More specifically, the left hemisphere appears to have some advantage over the right hemisphere from birth in the processing of language related materials while the right hemisphere appears to have a number of advantages over the left hemisphere when non language related materials are processed (Molfese, Freeman & Palermo, 1975). Related electrophysiological studies (see also Molfese & Molfese, 1979a; 1979b; 1980; 1985; Molfese & Hess, 1978) since that time have continued to support the view that the two sides of the brain are not identical in the manner in which they process the world. Confirmatory research for this position has come from a number of diverse laboratories. Barnet, de Sotillo and Campos (1974) investigated evoked potential responses of infants to their names and found that the left hemisphere was more sensitive to these stimuli. Davis and Wada (1977) reported that the left hemispheres of 2-10 week old infants were more responsive to click sounds while the right hemispheres were more responsive to light flashes. These results, like those of Molfese, indicated that the two cerebral hemispheres were not equipotential but instead were differentially sensitive to different environmental events. In addition, these patterns of responses found with infants did not differ from those typically found with adults, further support for the view that complex hemisphere differences typical of adults undergo little change from early infancy (for information regarding developmental patterns see Molfese and Molfese, 1979a; 1979b; 1980; 1985; Molfese & Hess, 1978).

3. Early perceptual abilities appear to be lateralised: Other studies using quite different techniques have also reported the presence of functional hemisphere differences early in life. Work by Turkewitz, Birch, Moreau, Levy and Cornwell (1966) suggests that the right ear (which supplies information to the left hemisphere) has a lower auditory threshold than the left ear. Entus (1977) reported such differences in infants between 43 and 100 days of age. She presented either different speech syllables or muisical notes produced on different instruments to infants through earphones placed over the infant's ears while the infant sucked on a blind passifier connected to a pressure transducer and polygraph which in turn recorded the infant's rate and pressure of sucking. After the continuous repetition of one stimulus to

both ears over a period of time, the sucking decreased. Once it reached a predetermined level, the stimulus presented to one ear was changed while the other remained the same. Differences in sucking rates before and after the stimulus change for each ear were determined and analysed. Entus found that the sucking rate increased most markedly following a stimulus change if it involved a change in the speech stimulus presented to the right ear while the recovery was more marked in the left ear relative to the right ear if the changed stimulus was a musical note presented to the left ear. Since sounds processed in the left ear are generally believed to be processed in the right hemisphere while sounds detected by the right ear involve left hemisphere processing, these data were interpreted as support for the position of early hemisphere differences in young infants. It should be noted that one attempt to replicate the Entus findings using a slightly different procedure has not succeeded (Vargha-Khadem & Corballis, 1979). Finally, Glanville, Best & Levenson (1977), using a dichotic listening procedure somewhat like Entus' but in combination with heart-rate measures, did not hemisphere differences in somewhat older infants than tested by either Entus or Vargha-Khadem and Corballis (93 to 130 days of age).

4. Early motor asymmetries suggest the presence of lateralised processes: Infants when placed in a supine position display a right facing bias (Tonic Neck Reflex) from birth until approximately 3 months of age (Coryell & Michael, 1978; Turkewitz, Gordon & Birch, 1965). These infants also show a marked tendency to turn their head to the right after the head was moved to a midline position (Turkewitz & Creighton, 1974). Eye movements also reflect this right turning bias. Wickelgren (1967) noted that newborn infants spent more time looking to the right than to the left. In a related study, Hammer (1977) reported that even infants in the first week of life will more often turn their eyes to the right when listening to speech sounds while they will turn their eyes to the left when attending to musical sounds. Since gross movements of the right side of the body are controlled primarily by the left hemisphere of the brain, such right sided biases are usually interpreted as support for the view that one side of the brain, the left hemisphere, is more active.

Studies of early infant hand reaching activities clearly demonstrate a right hand bias (Young, Bowman, Methot, Finlayson, Quintal & Boissonneault, 1984; von Hofsten, 1980; Mebert, 1984; Goodwin & Michel, 1981; Korczyn, Sage & Karplus, 1978; McDonnell, 1975; White, 1971; Flament, 1963). Typically, in these studies, an object is presented to the infant in the midline of the infant's body and then the observer records the hand which reaches for the object. This pattern of an early right hand preference for reaching seems to be present within days of birth (Korczyn, Sage & Karpluus, 1978). There are a few reports of early left hand preferences at different ages (Gesell & Ames, 1947; Seth, 1973; DiFranco, Muir & Dodwell, 1978; Hawn & Harris, 1984). However, analyses of data from the first three of these studies do not indicate a reliable left hand effect (see Young, Segalowitz Misek, Alp & Boulet, 1984).

While some might argue that the studies outlined above reflect only the involvement of gross muscle groups and consequently do not reflect the types of asymmetries usually measured with children and adults, other studies which specifically assess fine motor skills in young infants also report right sided preferences. Studies of grip strength reflect this right sided bias. While such differences do not seem to be noted at birth (Flament, 1963; Pollack, 1960; Roberts & Smart, 1981; see Halverson, 1937 to this), they do seem to emerge by 3 to 4 weeks of age (Petrie & Peters, 1980; Hawn & Harris, 1984; Halverson, 1937a, b; Caplan & Kinsbourne, 1976; Flament, 1963).

4. Anatomical differences between the two hemispheres: There appears to be some anatomical basis for these early functional hemisphere differences. Wada and his colleagues (Wada, 1969; Wada, Clark & Hamm, 1975), Witelson and Pallie (1973), LeMay and Culebras (1972) and Teszner, Tzavaras, Gruner and Hacaen (1972) have all reported that certain anatomical regions centered around the planum temporale of the left hemisphere are larger than comparable areas in the right hemisphere in preterm, term, and post term infants. These anatomical asymmetries, they note, are very similar to those reported for adults by Geschwind and Levitsky (1968). While there is a well documented concern regarding the generalisation from anatomical to functional relationships, the temptation is certainly there to suggest such a relationship. As Wada et al conclude, "the human brain (may possess) a predetermined morphological and functional capacity for the development of lateralised hemisphere functions for speech and language" (p. 245).

C. CHANGES IN LATERALISATION FOLLOWING BIRTH

1. Electrophysiological studies: In the years since the early evoked potential studies of hemisphere differences, numerous studies have been conducted with preterm and term infants as well as with older infants in attempts to further differentiate the brain mechanisms which appear to be lateralised to the two hemispheres early in life and to chart the development of these processes into adulthood (Molfese & Molfese, 1979a; 1979b; 1980; 1985; Molfese & Hess, 1978). In general, these studies have indicated that while some forms of hemisphere differences are present at or before the end of the normal gestational period (Molfese & Molfese, 1979b; 1980; 1985; Molfese, 1978a; 1985; Molfese & Schmid, 1984), other processes later emerge for the first time as lateralised to either the left or right hemisphere (Molfese, 1978b; 1979a; 1980; Molfese & Hess, 1978). In addition, there is even some data to indicate that other lateralised responses may shift over time from infancy into adulthood while other processes show no pattern of lateralised responses (Molfese & Erwin, 1982).

In the first of these studies, Molfese and Molfese (1979b) noted that the left hemisphere of newborn infants' brains can discriminate between certain types of speech sounds (i.e., place of articulation contrasts) and in this respect is advantaged over the right hemisphere. They reported that during the time in which an infant attends to a speech sound, the brain reacts with two different and apparently independent responses. First, one region of the evoked brain response that is restricted to only the left hemisphere discriminates between sounds such as /b/ and /g/, sounds produced in different parts of the vocal tract and which are characterised by different frequency information. This response is then followed in time by a second shift in the brain response, this time occurring over *both* hemispheres which discriminates between exactly the same sounds. A comparable pattern of responses was found with premature preterm infants (mean age = 35.5 weeks gestational age), thereby suggesting that lateralisation for this process is established long before birth. Intriguingly, this pattern of left hemisphere lateralised followed by bilateral discrimination responses is also found in older infants and adults (Molfese, 1980; 1985; Molfese & Schmidt, 1984), thereby suggesting that there is not much change in the degree of lateralisation for this process after birth.

Other discrimination abilities in infants, however, appear to follow a different pattern of development (Molfese, 1978a; 1980; Molfese & Hess, 1978; Molfese & Molfese, 1979a). A second speech cue, voice onset time (VOT), which reflects a temporal relationship between laryngeal pulsing and consonant release, is used by the language listener to discriminate between speech sounds such as /b/ and /p/. These sounds, unlike /b/ and /g/, are produced in the same place in the vocal tract but are distinguished from each other by a relatively small difference in the delay of vocal fold vibration following production of the sound. Numerous attempts have failed to find evidence for this discrimination in newborn term infants (Molfese & Molfese, 1984). Rather, the discrimination ability seems to emerge for the first time by one to two months of age, at which time it has been verified both behaviourally (Eimas, Sequeland, Jusczyk & Vigorito, 1971) and electrophysiologically (Molfese & Molfese, 1979a). In addition to the difference in appearance of this skill as compared with the perception of place of articulation, there is also a difference in the direction of lateralisation. Molfese and Molfese (1979a) reported a very marked right hemisphere lateralised response which discriminated between consonants with different voicing cues. This pattern of right hemisphere responding did not appear to change further until after four years of age (Molfese & Hess, 1978). The lateralised patterns found in adults, while in the same direction as those noted for infants and young children, were characterised by additional lateralised responses not found in the younger age groups (Molfese, 1978a; 1980). Thus, while the side of lateralisation seems to be relatively constant for a specific skill from some point of infancy to adulthood (much like the results found in behavioural studies investigating possible discrimination abilities across these ages), the electrophysiological studies usually display a much more complex pattern of change. While it is clear from these data that hemisphere differences in fact are well established during infancy, the time of their emergence may differ for different functions. In addition, the patterns of lateralisation may also differ with the left hemisphere assuming additional roles in some cases while the right hemisphere may show some advantages with other processes.

2. Motor asymmetry studies: As in the case of the electrophysiological studies, changes in motor lateral patterns occur after birth. Apparently the head positional biases of infants do change during the early months following birth. This, in part, then suggests that some form of change in lateralisation is occurring during this time. Gardner, Lewkowitz & Turkewitz (1977) reported that 35 week-old gestational age preterm infants displayed a marked right facing bias which increased in extent until by 39 weeks it matched that of full term normal newborn infants. However, when the preterm infants' heads were positioned in the midline it was noted that their tendency to turn their head to the right side from this position was almost totally absent. Consequently, while some forms of postural asymmetries appear present at or before birth, certain motor asymmetries do not emerge until later in development.

As noted earlier, asymmetries of both fine and gross motor activities, while apparently present at or shortly after birth, undergo further changes with development. For example, a lateralised difference in grip strength, while absent at birth, does emerge towards the end of the first month of life (Caplan & Kinsbourne, 1976; Flament, 1963; Hawn & Harris, 1984; Halverson, 1937a, b; Petrie & Peters, 1980). Grosser arm movements as reported by Michel (1981) show little in the way of lateralised biases at birth and during the first few months of life when these movements originate from the midline towards objects placed on either side of the infant. However, the infant will apparently show a strong right side movement bias by the end of the third month following birth. Another relatively gross postural pattern, the asymmetric tonic neck reflex, while rare in newborn infants, appears most pronounced by approximately 2 months after birth (Coryell & Michel, 1978). For motor patterns, then, as well as for linguistically related functions, there does seem to be evidence for continued lateralisation following birth. Even though some behaviours and brain patterns show a marked lateral pattern at birth, other behaviours and brain responses show shifts towards lateralisation well into the first year of life if not later.

Although changes in motor patterns obviously continue to occur during the infancy period and at least parallel in direction (to some extent) asymmetrical patterns found in brain responses and anatomical features, do such changes by themselves provide sufficient evidence to conclude that there is indeed a direct link between the emergence and modification of various postural and motor asymmetries and those asymmetries of the brain usually associated with cognitive and linguistic function? Could such early motor asymmetries bias the organism to develop asymmetries for skills in the cognitive-linguistic domain (Kinsbourne & Lempert, 1979; Michel, 1984)? While this point has been argued a great deal in recent years, the final verdict still seems to be out. Segalowitz has argued on a number of occasions that such diverse behaviours could be as readily argued to develop from a single overlying asymmetrical pattern of development instead of one behaviour necessarily giving rise to other diverse behaviours (Segalowitz & Gruber, 1977). Alternatively, various lateralised patterns (language and motor related) could result from not a single shared lateralising dimension in the organism but rather from several independent processes. In this latter case, lateralisation clearly becomes a multidimensional process; one which allows for different behaviours to be lateralised in different ways and at different times during the development of the organism. Such a view does not stress as much the *fact* that a behaviour is or is not lateralised. Rather, what becomes important is the *structure and nature* of the interaction between these different skills and processes. It is this last view which seems more appropriate at this time, given the range of available data.

References

Annett, M. (1973). Laterality of childhood hemiplegia and the growth of speech and intelligence. *Cortex, 9,* 4-33.

Basser, L.S. (1962). Hemiplegia of early onset and the faculty of speech with special reference to the effects of hemispherectomy. *Brain, 85,* 427-460.

Barnet, A., de Sotillo, M. & Campos, M. (1974). EEG sensory evoked potentials in early infancy malnutrition. Paper presented at the Society for Neurosciences, St. Louis, MO.

Caplan, P. & Kinsbourne, M. (1976). Baby drops the rattle: Asymmetry in duration of grasp by infants. *Child Development, 47,* 532-534.

Coryell & Michel (1978). How supine postural preferences of infants can contribute toward the development of handedness. *Infant Behavior and Development, 1,* 245-257.

Davis, A.E. & Wada, J. (1977). Hemispheric asymmetries in human infants: spectral analysis of flash and click evoked potentials. *Brain and Language, 4,* 23-32.

Dennis, M. (1977). Cerebral dominance in three forms of early brain disorder. In M. Blaw, J. Rapin and M. Kinsbourne (Eds.), *Topics In Child Neurology.* Bloomington, Indiana: Spectrum.

Dennis, M. & Kohn, B. (1975). Comprehension of syntax in infantile hemiplegics after cortical hemidecortication: Left hemisphere superiority. *Brain and Language, 2,* 472-482.

Dennis, M. & Whitaker, H.A. (1978). Language acquisition following hemidecortication: Linguistic superiority of the left over the right hemisphere. *Brain and Language, 3,* 404-433.

DiFranco, D., Muir, D. & Dodwell, P. (1978). Reaching in young infants. *Perception, 7,* 385-392.

Eimas, P.D., Siqueland, E., Juusczyk, P. & Vigorito, J. (1971). Speech perception in infants. *Science, 171,* 303-306.

Entus, A.K. (1977). Hemispheric asymmetry in processing of dichotically presented speech and nonspeech stimuli by infants. In S.J. Segalowitz and F.A. Gruber (Eds.), *Language Development and Neurological Theory.* New York: Academic Press.

Flament, F. (1963). Developpement de la preference manuelle de la naissance a 6 mois. *Enfance, 3,* 241-262.

Gardner, J., Lewkowitz, D. & Turkewitz, G. (1977). Development of postural asymmetry in premature human infants. *Developmental Psychobiology, 10,* 471-480.

Geschwind, N. & Levitsky, W. (1968). Human brain: left-right asymmetries in temporal speech regions. *Science, 161,* 186-187.

Gesell, A. & Ames, L.B. (1947). The development of handedness. *Journal of Genetic Psychology, 70,* 155-175.

Glanville, B., Best, C. & Levinson, R. (1977). A cardiac measure of cerebral asymmetry in infant auditory perception. *Developmental Psychology, 13,* 54-59.

Goodwin, R.S. & Michel, G.F. (1981). Head orientation position during birth and in infant neonatal period, and hand preference at nineteen weeks. *Child Development, 52,* 819-826.

Hammer, M. (1977). *Lateral differences in the newborn infants' response to speech and noise stimuli.* Unpublished doctoral dissertation, New York University.

Halverson, H. (1937a). Studies of the grasping responses of early infancy. I. *Journal of Genetic Psychology, 51,* 371-392.

Halverson, H. (1937b). Studies of the grasping responses of early infancy. II. *Journal of Genetic Psychology, 51,* 393-424.
Hawn, P.R. & Harris, L.J. (1984). Hand differences in grasp duration and reaching in two- and five-month-old infants. In G. Young, S.J. Segalowitz, C.M. Corter and S.E. Trehub (Eds.), *Manual Specialization and The Developing Brain.* New York: Academic Press.
Kinsbourne, M. & Lempert, H. (1979). Does left hemisphere lateralization of speech arise from right-biased orienting to salient percepts? *Human Development, 22,* 270-276.
Kohn, B. & Dennis, M. (1974). Selective impairments of visuo-spatial abilities in infantile hemiplegics after right cerebral hemidecortication. *Neuropsychologia, 12,* 505-512.
Korczyn, A.D., Sage, J.I. & Karplus, M. (1978). Lack of limb motor asymmetry in the neonate. *Journal of Neurobiology, 9,* 483-488.
LeMay, M. & Culebras, A. (1972). Human brain-morphologic differences in the hemispheres demonstrated by carotid anteriography. *New England Journal of Medicine, 287,* 168-170.
Lenneberg, E. (1967). *Biological Foundations of Language.* New York: Wiley.
McDonnell, P. (1975). The development of visually guided reaching. *Perception and Psychophysics, 18,* 181-185.
Mebert, C.J. (1984). Laterality in manipulatory and cognitive-related activity in four- to ten-month-olds. In G. Young, S.J. Segalowitz, C.M. Corter and S.E. Trehub (Eds.), *Manual Specialization and The Developing Brain.* New York: Academic Press.
Michel, G. (1981). Right handedness: A consequence of infant supine head-orientation performance? *Science, 212,* 685-687.
Michel, G. (1984). Development of Hand-use preference during infancy. In G. Young, S.J. Segalowitz, C.M. Corter and S.E. Trehub (Eds.), *Manual Specialization and The Developing Brain.* New York: Academic Press.
Molfese, D.L. (1972). *Cerebral asymmetry in infants, children, and adults: Auditory evoked responses to speech and music stimuli.* Unpublished Doctoral Dissertation, The Pennsylvania State University.
Molfese, D.L. (1978a). Neuroelectrical correlates of categorical speech perception in adults. *Brain and Language, 5,* 25-35.
Molfese, D.L. (1978b). Left and right hemisphere involvement in speech perception. *Perception and Psychophysics, 23,* 237-243.
Molfese, D.L. (1980). Hemispheric specialization for temporal information: Implications for the perception of voicing cues during speech perception. *Brain and Language, 11,* 285-299.
Molfese, D.L. & Erwin, R.J. (1982). Interhemispheric differentiation of vowels: Principal component analysis of auditory evoked responses to computer-synthesized vowel sounds. *Brain and Language, 13,* 333-344.
Molfese, D.L., Freeman, R.B. & Palermo, D.S. (1975). The ontogeny of brain lateralization for speech and nonspeech stimuli. *Brain and Language, 2,* 356-368.
Molfese, D.L. & Hess, T. (1978). Hemispheric specialization for VOT perception in the preschool child. *Journal of Experimental Child Psychology, 26,* 71-84.
Molfese, D.L. & Molfese, V.J. (1979a). VOT distinctions in infants: Learned or innate? In H.A. Whitaker and H. Whitaker (Eds.), *Studies in Neurolinguistic, Vol. 4.* New York: Academic Press.
Molfese, D.L. & Molfese, V.J. (1979b). Hemisphere and stimulua differences as reflected in the cortical responses of newborn infants to speech stimuli. *Developmental Psychology, 15,* 505-511.

Molfese, D.L. & Molfese, V.J. (1980). Cortical responses of preterm infants to phenetic and nonphonetic speech stimuli. *Developmental Psychology, 16,* 574-581.

Molfese, D.L. & Molfese, V.J. (1985). Electrophysiological indices of auditory discrimination in newborn infants: The bases for predicting later language development. *Infant Behavior and Development, 8,* 197-211.

Molfese, D.L. & Schmidt, A. (1984). An auditory evoked potential study of consonant perception in different vowel environments. *Brain and Language, 18,* 57-70.

Orton, S.T. (1928). A physiological theory of reading disability and stuttering in children. *New England Journal of Medicine, 199,* 1046-1052.

Petrie, B.F. & Peters, M. (1980). Handedness: Left/right differences in intensity of grasp response and duration of holding in infants. *Infant Behavior and Development, 3,* 215-221.

Pollack, S.L. (1960). The grasp response in the neonate. *Archives of Neurology, 5,* 108-115.

Roberts, A.M. & Smart, J.L. (1981). An investigation of handedness and headedness in newborn babies. *Behavior and Brain Research, 2,* 275-276.

Segalowitz, S.J. & Gruber, F.A. (1977). What is it that is lateralized? In S.J. Segalowitz and F.A. Gruber (Eds.), *Language Development and Neurological Theory.* New York: Academic Press.

Segalowitz, S.J. & Chapman, J.S. (1980). Cerebral asymmetry for speech in neonates: A behavioral measure. *Brain and Language, 9,* 281-288.

Seth, G. (1973). Eye-hand coordination and "handedness": A developmental study of visuomotor behavior in infancy. *British Journal of Educational Psychology, 43,* 35-49.

Teszner, D., Tzavaras, A., Gruner, J. & Hecaen, H. (1972). L'asymetrie droit-gauche du planum temporale: A propos de l'etude anatomique de 100 cerveaux. *Revue Neurologique, 126,* 444-449.

Turkewitz, G., Birch, H., Moreau, T., Levy, L. & Cornwell, H. (1966). Effect of intensity of auditory stimulation on directional eye movements in the human newborn. *Animal Behavior, 14,* 93-101.

Turkewitz, G. & Creighton, S. (1974). Changes in lateral differentiation of head posture in the human neonate. *Developmental Psychobiology, 8,* 85-89.

Turkewitz, G., Gordon, E.W. & Birch, H.G. (1965). Head turning in the human neonate: Spontaneous patterns. *Journal of Genetic Psychology, 107,* 143-158.

Vargha-Khadem, F. & Corballis, M. (1979). Cerebral asymmetry in infants. *Brain and Language, 8,* 1-9.

von Hofsten, C. (1980). Predictive reaching for moving objects by human infants. *Journal of Experimental Child Psychology, 30,* 369-382.

Wada, J. (1969). Interhemispheric sharing and shift of cerebral speech function. *Excerpta Medica International Congress Series, 193,* 296-297.

Wada, J., Clarke, R. & Hamm, A. (1975). Cerebral hemispheric asymmetry in humans. *Archives of Neurology, 32,* 239-246.

Wada, J. & Davis, A. (1977). Fundamental nature of human infant's brain asymmetry. *Le Journal Canadien des Sciences Neurologiques, 4,* 203-207.

White, B.L. (1971). *Human Infants - Experience and Psychological development.* Englewood Cliffs, New Jersey: Prentice Hall.

Wickelgren, L.W. (1967). The ocular response of human newborns to intermittent visual movement. *Journal of Experimental Child Psychology, 8,* 469-482.

Witelson, S.F. & Pallie, W. (1973). Left hemisphere specialization for language in the newborn: Neuroanatomical evidence of asymmetry. *Brain, 96,* 641-646.

Woods, B.T. & Teuber, H.L. (1978). Changing patterns of childhood aphasia. *Annals of Neurology, 3,* 273-280.

Young, G., Bowman, J.G., Methot, C., Finlayson, M., Quintal, J. & Boissonneault, P. (1984). Hemispheric specialization development: What (inhibition) and how (parents). In G. Young, S.J. Segalowitz, C.M. Corter and S.E. Trehub (Eds.), *Manual specialization and the developing Brain.* New York: Academic Press.

Young, G., Segalowitz, S.J., Misek, P., Alp, I.E. & Boulet, R. (1984). Is early reaching left handed? Review of manual Specialization Research. In G. Young, S.J. Segalowitz, C.M. Corter and S.E. Trehub (Eds.), *Manual Specialization and the Developing Brain.* New York: Academic Press.

AUTHORS INDEX

SUBJECT INDEX